Pandemic Influenza
in Fiction

ALSO BY CHARLES DE PAOLO

The Ethnography of Charles Darwin: A Study of His Writings on Aboriginal Peoples (2010)

Epidemic Disease and Human Understanding: A Historical Analysis of Scientific and Other Writings (2006)

Human Prehistory in Fiction (2003)

Pandemic Influenza in Fiction

A Critical Study

CHARLES DE PAOLO

McFarland & Company, Inc., Publishers
Jefferson, North Carolina

Library of Congress Cataloguing-in-Publication Data

De Paolo, Charles, 1950– author.
Pandemic influenza in fiction : a critical study / Charles De Paolo.
p. cm.
Includes bibliographical references and index.

ISBN 978-0-7864-9589-4 (softcover : acid free paper) ♾
ISBN 978-1-4766-1692-6 (ebook)

1. Plague in literature. 2. Influenza Epidemic, 1918–1919.
3. Fiction—History and criticism. 4. Epidemics in literature.
5. Diseases and literature. I. Title.

PN56.P5D4 2014
809'.933561—dc23 2014022621

British Library cataloguing data are available

On the cover: figurine wearing medical mask © 2014 Anton Stolar/Hemera/Thinkstock; flu virus © 2014 Aloysius Patrimonio/Hemera/Thinkstock

Printed in the United States of America

McFarland & Company, Inc., Publishers
Box 611, Jefferson, North Carolina 28640
www.mcfarlandpub.com

Table of Contents

Acknowledgments

I am grateful to the Faculty Publications Program at Manhattan Community College, The City University of New York, for an award supporting my work on chapter 5, "Terrorism and the Biological-Attack Scenario: 1999." I would also like to thank Patrick Anthony DePaolo for his advice and help in preparing the manuscript.

Introduction

Historiography and the Outbreak Narrative

The influenza pandemic of 1918–1919, the worst widespread outbreak in recorded history, claimed an estimated 100 million lives globally, yet only in recent decades has it captured the attention of historians, scientists, and imaginative writers (N. P. Johnson & J. Mueller).[1] Alfred Crosby, author of the definitive work on the 1918 pandemic, points out that major studies of early twentieth-century U.S. history hardly mention the deadliest pandemic on record (311,314). Even more surprising is that most histories of World War I either ignore the pandemic completely or treat it cursorily.

Of the nearly two dozen U.S. and World War I histories consulted for this study, four cite the pandemic and then only summarily.[2] Edward M. Coffman, for example, identifies the pandemic as a life-altering occurrence: "For the generation which lived through the war, the world-wide influenza epidemic was a common denominator. Whether at home, in the camps, at sea, or in France, all—soldiers, sailors, civilians—remembered the uncertainty and the fear; and some—the loss" (84). Perceiving the close relationship between the war and the pandemic, Martin Gilbert cites startling mortality statistics: the first, announced on 10 October 1918, is that, from September to November 1918, 20,000 American troops died in France, "not in battle, but of influenza and pneumonia" (477); the second, that pneumonia, an influenza complication, had been responsible for the deaths of 62,000 U.S. soldiers, sailors, and Marines, more "than were killed in combat" (540); and the third is that, as the war wound down, and as battlefield casualties diminished, in the presumed safety behind the Allied lines, thousands more would die of influenza on Armistice Day, 11 November 1918 (499). W. P. Willmott mentions four important facts: in the phrase "Spanish Influenza" the adjective "Spanish" is a misnomer; the disease occurred in three waves, originating either on the U.S. mainland or in American army camps in France; that its three concurrent foci were Freetown (Sierra Leone), Brest, and Boston; and that its third wave, in the spring of 1919, ravaged an already-malnourished civilian population, causing millions of deaths (287). Adam Hochschild observes that this "deadly cataclysm" was closely connected with the war; that it originated in a Kansas cantonment and was transmitted to Brest, France, on troop transports; that its victims came from every walk of life; and that Germany lost 400,000 citizens to influenza in 1918 (350–351).

Literature on the pandemic has been accumulating for nearly a century and is an eclectic and multidisciplinary record of humanity's experience with it and its recrudescent forms. This trend is especially evident in the biomedical and fictional corpora and in their interrelationship: since 1890, biomedical investigations in a wealth of articles and books have constituted an important and neglected aspect of the pandemic account; in semi-autobiographical fiction and autobiography of the period, from 1921 to 1946, survivors recreate and come to terms with their terrible ordeals; in historical fiction, imaginative writers, from 2005 to 2007, retell stories involving biomedical, social, and ethical dilemmas unique to the pandemic; and contemporary writers, from 1998 to 2010, have prospectively imagined the consequences of refractory outbreaks and of bioterrorist attacks.

Despite differences in content, methodology, and purpose, both scientific and fictional literature on pandemic influenza belong to a unified, 96-year-old narrative. Priscilla Wald (2008) describes such a unified corpus as an "outbreak narrative" (2). A body of literature on contagious disease, it is a living document containing scientific, journalistic, historical, and fictional writings (Wald, 2). From multiple perspectives, such a narrative records influenza's global effects and the concerted effort to contain its spread. Consistent with Wald's inclusive definition, this study explains how scientists and writers of fiction have tried to understand and to manage pandemic influenza. A cross section of this account is presented in this study.

Overview

In chapter 1, "The Discovery Period: 1892–1940," I survey a central motif of the biomedical literature: the search for the pathogen that caused influenza. By 1912, the virus had been recognized as a parasitic life form, varieties of which had been implicated in nearly 30 plant, animal, and human disorders

(Wolbach, "Filterable Viruses"). Medical scientists, since 1918, have learned about the pathology of influenza, reasoning inductively from fragmentary information to identify its unknown, non-bacterial cause. In the period from 1890 to 1940, through the interactivity between the fields of medical bacteriology, of plant pathology, of veterinary medicine, and of immunology, serology, and vaccinology, the existence of viruses would be confirmed (Taubenberger et al., "Historical Context," 586). The influenza virus itself would be isolated in 1933.

Veterinary medicine, beginning with Dr. J. S. Koen's comparative insight relating human to porcine influenza in 1918, motivated Dr. Richard Shope, from 1928 into the mid–1930s, to isolate swine flu virus, to establish that bacteria were co-infective organisms, and that the presumptive cause of influenza could be pursued through the serial passage of the infectious filtrate. These experiments studied porcine immunological responses, as animals were inoculated with filtrate presumably containing the pathogen. Shope's work paralleled British investigations on the mechanisms of dog distemper, of the common cold, and eventually of the influenza virus. Anglo-American work in the pre–World War II period, notably in the laboratories of Dr. Alphonse Dochez and colleagues at Rockefeller University and of Drs. Smith, Laidlaw, and Andrewes at Mill Hill, in the UK, exemplify the idea that the culture of science is a collaborative, social activity (Campbell, Reece et al., 24; Bresalier, "Uses of a Pandemic"). As medical researchers and historians have pointed out, "efforts to characterize influenza were a driving force behind the development of whole fields of investigation and new research methods" (Taubenberger et al., "Historical Context," 586).

The isolation of the influenza virus led to the development of vaccines. "By 1950, virology had truly come of age," and scientists could now study it with modern technology (Taubenberger et al., "Historical Context," 586). Through genetic engineering medical scientists, from 1995 to 2005, reconstructed the genome of the 1918 virus, the complete complement of its genes and of all nucleic acid sequences (Campbell, Reece et al., "Genome," G-16; Taubenberger et al., "Historical Context").[3] This achievement has allowed for the investigation of its molecular and biochemical characteristics and of new modalities to manage its effects. Over the last decade, experiments with avian viruses in animal models have disclosed the genetic processes behind the emergence of novel viruses. These accomplishments are surveyed here, chronologically through primary texts, and they are analyzed in the fiction.

This study is subdivided into four biomedical/literary periods: Recovery (1892–1946), Recursion (2005–2006), Characterization (1949–2005), and Novelistic (1997–2014). The Recovery comprises biomedical and literary works and two overlapping timelines: the history of early influenza research or Discovery Period (1892–1940) and a survey of the fictional and autobiographical literature (1921–1946). The imaginative writers of this period stand in contrast to renowned contemporaries who had experienced the disease at home or during the war, but who found no place in their writings for influenza. Cultural amnesia, according to Crosby, affected John Dos Passos (1896–1970) (notably in *Nineteen Nineteen* and in *Three Soldiers*), F. Scott Fitzgerald (1896–1940), William Faulkner (1897–1962), and Ernest Hemingway (1899–1961) (315–317). On the other hand, the Recovery writers—Willa Cather (1873–1947), Thomas Wolfe (1900–1938), Katherine Anne Porter (1890–1980), William Maxwell (1908–2000), Wallace Stegner (1909–1993), and John O'Hara (1905–1970)— did take notice and, in a variety of ways, transmuted their influenza experiences into fiction; in addition, Mary McCarthy (1912–1989), who also belongs to this generation, found a place for her childhood remembrances of the outbreak in the context of non-fictional lifewriting. These authors view the disease from a deeply personal rather than scientific perspective, communicating accounts of their sufferings imaginatively (in McCarthy's case, autobiographically). Their writings conform to the original definition of *pathography* or illness narrative.[4] Semi-autobiographical works of this kind are, at once, eyewitness records and memoirs, providing future generations with reliable accounts; and the authors, with a measure of consolation. A dramatic re-enactment of the 1918 pandemic, as witnessed by a contemporary, is both a valuable historical resource and a reminder that pandemic influenza is a perennial concern.

From 1892 to 1946, two intellectual communities, the biomedical (in chapter 1) and the literary (in chapter 2), each operating with distinct methods, responded to a crisis that had engulfed them both. The two cultures were existentially of one mind. Although the Recovery and biomedical writers of the period felt the impact of influenza personally and socially, each understood the cataclysm in different ways, and their writings reflect their thinking. On the one hand, dealing with a dangerous biological phenomenon, scientists urgently struggled to bring its unseen causes to light and to neutralize its effects on humanity. The first-generation fictionists, on the other hand, sought consolation in artistic expression and in the recreations of what they had lived through. Although the cognitive and discursive methods of scientists and novelists are fundamentally distinct from one another, in the greater narrative, as two cultural responses to a common predicament they are complementary. Writers of the Recovery Period chose literary self-portraiture because this modality provided a degree of *emotional* distancing (a correlative to *social distancing*, limiting exposure to disease by avoiding crowds): their suffering, loss, and post-traumatic stress remains in the private domain. Yet, at the same time, survivors such as Katherine Anne Porter and William Maxwell, Jr., restore cultural memory with each reading, for their stories of suffering and loss are archetypes, not artifacts. The stories they tell are universal.

Chapter 3 covers the Recursion Period. Novels by Myla Goldberg, Reina James, Thomas Mullen, and James Rada, Jr., published from 2005 to 2006, revisit the pandemic. The contrast between scientific determination and futility links these four novels. Each novel in the chapter reveals that, in 1918–1919, biomedical investigators and public health institutions, despite their best efforts, were unable to meet the challenge of influenza. The scientific community of the period was theoretically and technologically disadvantaged since they practiced at a time when the concept of the virus as a "filter-passing" agent was not fully understood; hence, medical professionals could do very little, especially since the production of vaccines and medications was mistakenly based on a bacterial hypothesis. At first, the existence of the virus was inferred; not until 1933 was it isolated. Progress had been underway in the period from the late 1890s to 1918: though both invisible and not cultivable, viruses were routinely being isolated through filtration techniques. Other than sequestration and palliation, the public health community in 1918 had no protocol for the treatment of influenza. Recursion novels enter into public health and social areas unique to the crisis, recreating the pandemic through a historiography that brings ideas, predicaments, and human trials to life.

Since virology in the post–World War I period was in a formative stage, it did not influence the Recovery authors to the extent that it would the Recursion writers who live in the age of molecular biology. From a contemporary vantage point, the Recursion writers excavated the lost history of the pandemic and reconstructed the period, inspired, no doubt, by the reconstitution of the H1N1 genome from tissue archives and corpses, a landmark in archaeovirology.[5] Fictionists in this group were sensitive to contemporary influenza history. The 1997 emergence of avian influenza in China, the Characterization research (1995 to 2005) and the development of new vaccines and antiviral medications, inspired them to explore timeless public health issues. In the context of 1918–1919, they bring to light a number of themes and dilemmas: for example, the ethics of human experimentation, the spirit of volunteerism, the necessity of inter-agency and international cooperation in a health crisis, the moral implications of quarantine, and related issues.

The Characterization Period, which extends from 1995 to 2005, is the biomedical context of chapters 4, 5, and 6. In this period, medical scientists reconstructed the genome of H1N1, the virus responsible for the 1918 pandemic, and their story is told in chapter 4 (Taubenberger, "The Origin and

Virulence"). They had successfully retrieved RNA fragments from archived autopsy specimens and from cadavers, buried since 1918 under permafrost. The reconstructed genome has furthered inquiry into the virus' origin, lethality, and transmissibility, among other characteristics. The project and its use of genetic engineering to rebuild the organism, from 1995 to 2005, fascinated another set of authors. Instead of looking back to the social and medical history of 1918–1919, as did the Recursion writers, the Characterization authors imagine a weapon of mass destruction, the product either of the reconstituted microbe or of a virulent hybrid. In this period, biomedical science inspired fiction and, as shown in chapter 8, influenced national defense policy in regard to bioterrorism.

Chapter 5 deals with a fictive subgenre which also developed in the context of modern virology and bioterrorism. Biosecurity writers use scenarios to simulate either man-made or natural outbreaks. Scenarios such as these rehearse the popular and institutional effects of an influenza pandemic (and other contagious diseases). Though synoptic in form, the scenario has a tripartite dramatic structure (i.e., rising action, climax, and falling action). Unlike a novel or a play, however, its motive is utilitarian rather than aesthetic. Participants in this kind of exercise test the authenticity, and estimate the probability, of a natural occurrence or an attack. If the former is extreme and the latter high, they suggest ways of shoring up the public health system; and, with respect to bioterrorism, they devise ways of interdicting aggressors, of strengthening national defense, and of containing a possible outbreak.

Chapter 6 is concerned with the use of the influenza virus as a weapon and with how novelists employ it as ordnance. Their informative novels subsume under current events the history of bio-warfare, of bioterrorism, and of virology. Distilled into plot outlines, these writings resemble attack scenarios. The premise of the 1998 fiction, that the revivified H1N1 virus is suitable ordnance, has been debated over the last decade. In contrast to the 1998 novels of Case and Crane, a third novel Kalla's *Pandemic: A Novel* (2005), more plausibly depicts terrorist cells and rogue nations spreading recombinant influenza strains via suicidal carriers.

The survey of scientific papers on avian influenza in chapter 7 provides the biomedical context of the Novelistic Period, 1997 to the present. In imagining the relentless movement of avian influenza, outbreaks of which originate in the U.S. and in Canada, three writers reveal the potential danger of the pathogen, and they forecast its devastating effects. These novels are important additions to the debate over ongoing research intended to render H5N1 avian flu virus transmissible to, and between, human beings (a natural trait not yet acquired). Some scientists favor experimentation of this kind, arguing that the benefits outweigh the risks: containing a dangerous form of the avian virus in a secure laboratory will facilitate the preemptive development of vaccines and antivirals, anticipating the virus' natural emergence. They remind the public that the scientists who successfully reconstructed H1N1 (1995–2005) did so for the same reason and that their initiative also drew criticism. Opponents were apprehensive about the accidental release of a dangerous virus or about it falling into the hands of criminals or hostile powers. As the research continued, scientists learned about H1N1: an exaggerated immune response, in 1918–1919, was proven to have been the cause of many deaths in the early stage of influenza. Although most recovered from the inciting attack, the greater proportion of fatalities, as medical historians and scientists have recently confirmed, was caused by secondary, bacterial pneumonias. These insights suggest that modern vaccines, antivirals, and antibiotics (to treat secondary infection), had they been available, would have made a significant difference in the outcome of the 1918 pandemic (Taubenberger & Morens, "The Pathology of Influenza Virus Infections"). A similar strategy is at work in the campaign against avian influenza.

In the Novelistic Period (chapters 7 and 8), 1997 to 2014, both medical scientists and fictionists react to the emergence of avian influenza. Imaginative extrapolations, written from 2008 to 2010, envision the disastrous potential of an avian influenza outbreak in under- or unprepared cities, even in industrial societies. Psycho-social themes are also present in these novels. The emphasis in this study, however, is not so much on the pandemic's sociocultural effects as it is on human behavior under stress.

Today's biomedical scientists, equipped with astonishing technology and with the advantage of global networks and immediate communication links, have not underestimated avian viruses, which are unstable, ubiquitous, and an evolutionary step ahead of institutionalized medicine. The writers reviewed in chapter 8 advertise these ideas: even in the industrialized world, the morbidity rate will far exceed the capabilities of public health and care, that is, at the outset of the pandemic (Craig DiLouie); the emergence of a novel Type A influenza virus is neither fantastic nor statistically improbable; nor is its immediate detection guaranteed (D. W. Hardin); and Western society, however rich and resilient, is fragile if unprepared in time of pestilence (Steven Konkoly).

Recent Scholarship, 2012–2013

This study complements two important books that appeared in 2012. Nancy K. Bristow and Jane Fisher analyze the literature of the pandemic milieu from an interdisciplinary perspective and with a common sociocultural emphasis. Bristow's contributions to the field are significant. The idea that the pandemic was slipping away from cultural memory informs her important articles (2003, 2010) and book (2012). She emphasizes the need to reconstruct fragmentary sources, "to hear voices previously unheard and [to] elucidate the range of ways Americans experienced the pandemic" (*American Pandemic*, 6), and she agrees with Alfred Crosby that, "for millions of Americans, both those who suffered from influenza and those who lost loved ones to the disease, the 1918 pandemic lived on in vivid memories and in lives indelibly marked by those experiences" (*American Pandemic*, 6–7). Bristow also points out that cultural trends and the national ethos shaped influenza narratives. Enumerating two interesting reactions to the catastrophe, one literary and the other nationalistic, she shows how both modalities obscured the historical record to some degree. One is the "preferred narrative," a mode of writing conforming to "a culture's beliefs about itself and about its past, present, and future." Preferred narratives, reinforcements of the status quo during and after the pandemic, helped to induce public amnesia and tended to interpret the causes and effects of the pandemic in terms of social identity, gender, race, and class (*American Pandemic*, 8–9). Remembering the pandemic's ravages was not in the country's interest, especially at the war's end. For Americans to recall the pandemic as a public health debacle was, in Bristow's view, to admit to "vulnerability and weakness that contradicted their fundamental understandings of themselves and their country's history" (*American Pandemic*, 11). In contrast to preferred historiography were more realistic writings "on the experiences of Americans as they endured the influenza pandemic and on the public and private narratives they created and give meaning to those experiences" (*American Pandemic*, 11).

Jane Fisher's interests, in *Envisioning Disease, Gender, and War* (2012), are the political and social effects of the war and the pandemic on contemporary (Cather, Porter, and Woolf) and later women writers (Alice Munro, the poet Ellen Bryant Voigt, and the Nigerian novelist Buchi Emechita). Fisher's analysis of the literary and mass media representations of the milieu, including posters, music, poetry, and photographs, demonstrates how women endured the dual trials of war and disease and how literature had a restorative effect. The trauma of war and disease ultimately allowed women to reprise traditional gender roles in post–World War I culture, as they acquired suffrage rights (26 August 1920) and new social opportunities.

Like Wald, Bristow, and Fisher, I believe that the literature of pandemic influenza, while generically diverse, is nevertheless a unified narrative. The primary emphasis of the present study is to demonstrate that pandemic fiction and biomedical history have been intimately connected for nearly a century. The imaginative literature, situated in its scientific matrix, has proven to be a therapeutic medium for survivors, a valuable historical resource, and a discussion forum for ethical, sociopolitical, theological, national defense, and public health issues.

Part One

The Recovery (1892–1946) and Recursion (2005–2006) Periods

1

The Discovery Period: 1892–1940

The Bacterial Hypothesis

The search for the cause of influenza began in the wake of the 1889–1890 pandemic in the laboratory of the German physician and bacteriologist Robert Koch (1843–1910). Ironically, the misapplication of his method, in 1892, was the opening chapter in the history of modern influenza research.

Koch had developed an experimental methodology to determine disease causation and employed it in his work on anthrax, on tuberculosis, and on cholera. In 1884, he described a sequence of steps in the hope of proving that *B. anthracis* caused anthrax ("Etiology" [1884], 116–118). Using blood samples extracted from an animal dying of the disease, he searched for the preponderant organism. Under the microscope, he observed in anthrax-infected blood samples a rod-shaped microbe arising from spores belonging to "the class of lower plants." These spores and rod-shaped microbes, if inoculated into a healthy animal, induced the very same disease; and, if the inoculated animal also died of anthrax, its blood would be expected to contain the rods and spores.

Even if blood-borne rods and spores were present in the secondary animal, Koch realized that this did not constitute definitive proof that these organisms caused anthrax. The possibility remained that something in the blood other than the bacillus was the cause of the disease. To move further in the direction of proof, one had then to cultivate the host animal's blood, isolating the organism: the rod-shaped bacillus was expected to be the only living organism in the *in vitro* culture. Culturing a pure colony of the anthrax bacillus required placing samples of infected blood on solid nutrient media (either gelatin or potato), in order to permit the organism to proliferate, from culture to culture, and eventually to be harvested in progressively purer form. By the second or third day of the experiment, the bacilli reproduced as expected, forming a white covering on the potato.

Because the cultured specimen retained its virulence and infectivity when inoculated into a healthy animal, Koch concluded that laboratory-grown germs, anthrax-laden blood from a dead animal, and spores in the wild each had the capacity to induce fatal disease. The laboratory method outlined above strongly suggested that in both domestic animals and man this bacillus was the causal agent of anthrax. The question facing bacteriologists during and immediately after the 1889–1890 influenza pandemic was whether Koch's postulates could be used to isolate the agent responsible for influenza.

While Koch's students at the Berlin Institute of Infectious Disease, Drs. Richard F. J. Pfeiffer (1858–1945) (the former's protégé and son-in-law) and Shibasaburo Kitasato (1853–1931), both of whom were distinguished researchers, applied their mentor's procedure to influenza, hoping to identify the cause of the 1889–1890 pandemic. In a 16 January 1892 paper, Pfeiffer declared that *B. influenzae*, a bacillus isolated from human secretions and dubbed Pfeiffer's bacillus, was the inciting cause of influenza, and the scientific community would accept this as a valid conclusion for nearly two decades. Embracing the claim that this bacillus caused influenza, the medical community had done so precipitously. I would like to review the steps in this momentous experiment and its ironic outcome.

The Pfeiffer-Kitasato experiments, guided by Koch's method, drew purulent bronchial secretions from thirty-one cases of influenza (including six autopsies) during the 1889–1890 pandemic (Pfeiffer, "Influenza Bacillus"; Kitasato, "Mode of Cultivating It"). These samples, Pfeiffer suspected, would contain the causative micro-organism. He presumed it was bacterial. Transferring the organism using his father-in-law's method, he tried to make a pure culture, one calculated to induce influenza if inoculated into laboratory animals; using control experiments, he claimed that these particular bacilli were found *exclusively* in flu cases, not in patients with other pulmonary diseases. With the suspected bacilli in culture, Pfeiffer transferred the organism from one animal to another, inoculating apes, rabbits, guinea pigs, rats, pigeons, and mice, but obtaining positive results with apes and rabbits alone. It is not clear from the published work whether or not Pfeiffer or Kitasato tried to complete the cycle by re-introducing the cultured bacillus into healthy apes and rabbits to see if these animals would develop influenza. In all likelihood, had they done so, their results with respect to influenza would have proven inconclusive, as later experiments would soon demonstrate.

The root of the problem, of course, was Pfeiffer's erroneous *assumption* that *B. influenzae* was the inciting entity.[1] He could not have known that an invisible, submicroscopic organism, later identified as a virus, was the pathogen. Viruses are described, not as organisms, but as "infectious units" or "obligate intracellular parasites" lacking functional ribosomes, cellular organelles, or energy-producting enzymes; though replicable in a host cell, they do not increase in size (Mahy 492). With no other starting point, they had proceeded with the idea that the cause was a form of bacteria and used incomplete laboratory evidence to support their assumption. Their hypothesis, however, would not stand the test of accumulating data, leading up to the 1918 pandemic and thereafter. Pfeiffer and Kitasato would have profited from Koch's 1890 caveat that proof depended on exhaustive experimentation using the appropriate methodology:

> We know nothing about the disease agents of influenza, whooping cough, trachoma, yellow fever, Rinderpest, Lungensuche, and many other undoubtedly infectious diseases. All existing technology has been skillfully and carefully used in the examination of these diseases. The negative results of the efforts of numerous researchers can only mean that the methods of investigation, which until now have proved themselves in so many cases, no longer suffice. I suspect that these diseases involve organized disease agents that are not bacteria but rather belong *to completely different groups of microorganisms* ["Research," 184; italics added].

Virology was in its earliest stages when Pfeiffer and Kitasato committed themselves to an exclusively bacterial route of investigation (Taubenberger et al., "Historical Context," 584). Apparently, neither scientist had considered the possibility that the 1889–1890 pandemic had a nonbacterial cause. Neither did they take Koch's 1890 advice nor seem to be aware of current biological developments in virology. Before the 1889–1890 pandemic, the idea of the virus and its disease-causing properties was not a matter of crypto-biology. Pasteur, in 1881, had been making breakthroughs with fowl cholera (actually a viral disease) and with rabies vaccines ("On a Vaccine" 131–132). Although he did not know what caused rabies, he was still able to isolate the pathogen in animal tissue, to make filtrates containing the agent, and to use this material in animal experiments to create a vaccine ("Prevention of Rabies," 379–387). The distinction between bacteria and the unknown organism tentatively called a *virus* was unclear. The semantics of the term illustrate this fact: in correspondence of 3 and 5 October 1882, pertaining to vaccinology experiments, for example, Pasteur uses the word *virus* interchangeably to describe both anthrax (a visible bacillus) and rabies (an invisible virus) (Pasteur and Thuillier, 197, 201).

The discovery of the virus depended on technology, especially on the development, in 1884, of the Pasteur-Chamberland (Charles Chamberland,

1851–1908) porcelain filter and, in 1891, of the earthenware Berkefeld filter (Wilhelm Berkefeld, 1836–1897), devices that trap bacteria but allow viral filtrate to pass through and be utilized in experimentation ("Chamberland"; "Berkefeld Filter"; Waterson & Wilkinson, 15–17). It is important to remember that these filtration systems also had varying levels of permeability; for this reason, a filter-passing organism was not necessarily a virus; nor was every impassable organism a bacterium. Three examples illustrate this fact: Celli and De Blasi, in 1904, filtered *Mycoplasma agalactia*, an infectious bacterial disease of goats and ewes, through a Berkefeld filter, and consequently misidentified it as a virus; similarly, the microbe Petrie and O'Brien filtered in 1910, presumed to have been the virus responsible for Guinea-pig epizootics, was actually a tiny, filter-permeating bacillus; and, on the grounds of permeability, what Bertrelli and Cecchetto in 1908 thought was the viral cause of trachoma, an infectious disease of the conjunctiva, was later to be reclassified as a bacterium, *Chlamydia trachomatis* (Wolbach, "Filterable Viruses," 8–11).

Despite these exceptions, early versions of filtration systems allowed plant virologists to make important contributions. Iwanowski (1892) and Beijerinck (1898) had successfully transferred Tobacco Mosaic Virus from one plant to another ("On the Mosaic Disease," 124–126). Beijerinck went a step further, identifying viral properties and speculating that the unseen pathogen was "a soluble living germ" or *contagium vivum fluidum*, an agent that incorporated itself into cells "in order to reproduce" ("*Contagium Vivum Fluidum*," 156). The first proof that viruses could attack animals came in 1899 when Loeffler and Frosch identified an infected filtrate from calves afflicted with foot-and-mouth disease ("Report," 149–153). They determined that Beijerinck's soluble agent was a submicroscopic particle, not a fluid: "the activity of the filtrate is not due to the presence in it of a soluble substance, but due to the presence of a causal agent capable of reproducing. This agent must then be obviously so small that the pores of a filter which will hold back the smallest bacterium presently known will still allow it to pass. The smallest bacterium presently known is the influenza bacillus of Pfeiffer" ("Report," 152). Walter Reed, following Carlos Finlay's research, proved through trial-and-error and the process of elimination that viruses could attack human beings: mosquitoes, as vectors, could carry yellow fever from person to person ("Yellow Fever," 479–484). Bacteria-destroying viruses or bacteriophages were indirectly manifested, in 1896 and in 1915, through the lysis of bacterial cultures. In 1917, Felix d'Herelle discovered that these ultra- or submicroscopic organisms were active in bacterial cultures ("Invisible Microbe," 157–159).

All of these breakthroughs, the products of logical and patient experimentation, were made without ever seeing a virus or knowing its makeup. Even though the technology leading to the invention of the electron microscope was decades away, scientists at the turn of the twentieth century were able to infer, extrapolate, and imagine reasonable possibilities. Clearly, at the time of Pfeiffer's experiments on influenza, the scientific community already suspected that an infectious agent existed beyond the visualizing capacity of the light microscope. The science of virology was founded on intuition and indirect evidence. Koch's 1890 advice about jumping to conclusions from incomplete evidence was sound.

The Co-Pathogen Theory[2]

Pfeiffer's single-pathogen assumption stood fast for decades because the experimental technology needed to invalidate it was unavailable. But gradually medical science challenged this claim. The etiology of influenza (its origin and cause) was as-yet nebulous; however, between 1890 and 1904, medical scientists were recording important observations regarding its epidemiology (i.e., its incidence, distribution, and control) and its associated pathology. Medical literature, such as Franklin Parson's 1891 report on the sanitary districts in England and Wales, Otto Lichtenstern's 1896 study of influenza in Hermann Northnagel's pathology handbook, and the medical textbooks of the American physicians Frederick Lord and William Osler, were important resources for the understanding of influenza during the inter-pandemic period (Eyler, "The State of Science," 28, 30–32).

Osler, for one, looked at the disease from epidemiological and pathological viewpoints. In *The Principles and Practices of Medicine,* for example, he describes influenza as an irregularly-occurring pandemic disease that spreads rapidly, indiscriminately attacking a "large proportion of the inhabitants [of a region]." From 1890 to 1904, outbreaks recurring in different regions had been difficult to diagnose. Although known to attack "the respiratory mucous membranes," its clinical manifestations were considered "protean" or variable (*Principles and Practices*, 95). The mortality rates for pandemics before 1889–1890 had been relatively low; however, the 1889–1890 outbreak suggested that influenza had *"sequels and complications"* (96; italics added).

As early as 1904, Osler suspected that influenza involved a sequence of infections. While taking for granted the claim that Pfeiffer's bacillus was the cause of the disease, he also entertained the possibility that secondary infection could be a factor in influenza. Conceiving of influenza as a complex, dual-stage disease, and following Lichtenstern, Osler proposed a threefold nosology or disease classification: epidemic influenza *vera* (genuine or true influenza), presumably caused by Pfeiffer's microbe; endemic-epidemic influenza *vera*, also attributed to Pfeiffer's microbe, emerging seasonally or cyclically during inter-pandemic periods; and endemic influenza *nostras* [*sic*], "a special disease, still of unknown etiology" (Osler, 96; Eyler, "The State of Science," 28). The Latinate phrases suggest that Pfeiffer's bacillus *and* an unidentified "special disease," in Osler's view either were coextensively or sequentially active in some cases. Osler learned from autopsies that pandemic influenza had an affinity for the respiratory system and had three levels of severity: a "simple" form inducing fever, achiness, inflammation, prostration, and debilitation; a complicated form typified by worsening respiratory symptoms, continuing fever, and developing bronchitis; and a serious form causing purulent sputum, bronchial tube dilation, cyanosis, and asphyxiation. In this paradigm, Osler again uses the word "sequel"; thus, he was mindful of the possibility that the serious condition of "influenza pneumonia" was distinct from the "simple" form and that its pathogen might be opportunistic (96).

Osler's exposition of the influenza concept, in 1904, is an index of what the medical community knew about the disease: it had identifiable phases (the "simple" and the "complicated"); it could arise solitarily, coextensively, or sequentially; bacteria (he thought wrongly) were responsible for the simpler form, but some unknown agent acted in the complicated form. Medical scientists, in the inter-pandemic period, realized that "their knowledge of the cause of epidemic influenza was still quite limited" (Bristow, *American Pandemic*, 31).

Doubts about Pfeiffer's hypothesis mounted during the inter-pandemic period (Eyler, "The State of Science," 30). As early as 1915–1916, scientists found little evidence of the germ during the influenza epidemic of that period (Bristow, *American Pandemic*, 31). In the winter of 1915–1916, when a respiratory infection had broken out resembling the 1889–1890 flu, Dr. George Mathers and colleagues in Chicago were able to test Pfeiffer's assertions directly. They studied 61 cases using bacteriological methods. In only one case was Pfeiffer's microbe found (86). Clinical and postmortem data indicated that hemolytic streptococci were dominant; and in no autopsy was *B. influenzae* (Pfeiffer's bacillus) found (87). Mathers circumspectly concluded that streptococcus seemed to be "*an important factor*" in the etiology of influenza (87; italics added).[3]

Referring to the 1889–1890 pandemic, Mathers points out, in 1917, that "no observer has satisfactorily prove[n] that one species of bacteria is of primary importance in the causation of the disease" (85). Investigators had found that patients were infected by several forms of bacteria, considered to be "secondary invaders" (85). Although Pfeiffer was able to isolate *B. influenzae* from the sputum and bronchi of patients, Mathers reports neither finding them in the bloodstream nor being able to reproduce the disease in animals. Furthermore, recent investigations had failed to corroborate the claim that these Gram-negative, hemolytic bacilli caused true influenza, which was evidenced by "a local inflammation of the respiratory tract" (85). Nor did Pfeiffer's bacillus appear to be specific to influenza (85). In fact, this ubiquitous organism was also found in patients with tuberculosis and chronic bronchitis; therefore, with respect to influenza, it was considered unimportant. Mathers' review of the evidence led him to state flatly that, since 1890, "this organism [had] not been found with any regularity associated with the epidemics of acute respiratory infections" (85–86).

Military physicians at work during the 1918 pandemic learned firsthand how contagious the disease was in crowded environs. Dr. Roy Grist, in a 29 September 1918, letter from Camp Devens, in Ayers, Massachusetts (west of Boston), gives us a sense of how conditions in this cantonment had quickly deteriorated. In a letter to a colleague describing the crisis, Grist relates what was happening at the base hospital for the Division of the Northeast, where fifty thousand men were housed. The epidemic broke out at the beginning of September (early in the second wave), exploding so rapidly that all military plans were put on hold, and the camp was rapidly "demoralized." Orders proscribed gatherings to control contagion; but, in an overcrowded installation, this was impossible.

Grist's observation that the sickness had two clinical phases links up with Osler's and Mathers' notions of a mixed infection. At the outset the medical staff at Devens was certain it was influenza because of the symptoms of fever, pain, and prostration; but once the patient was brought into the hospital, Grist was impressed by "the most viscous type of pneumonia that has ever been seen." It was typical for a patient's skin to take on a mahogany discoloration, with cyanosis "extending from their ears and spreading to their face." In a matter of a few hours, soldiers in this condition perished. Grist watched them die without being able to do anything: "it is simply a struggle for air until they suffocate." Even an experienced physician had difficulty dealing with the scene. For Grist, the impact of these events was worsened by the sheer numbers of patients: "One could stand to see one, two, or twenty men die, but to see these poor devils dropping like flies sort of gets on your nerves." One hundred men, on average, died each day, and no relief was in sight. At this point in the letter, Grist offers an acute clinical interpretation, one that the medical community would echo for another decade: "There is no doubt in my mind that there is a new mixed infection here, but what I don't know." These difficult conditions permitted Grist to learn about the disease, the clinical manifestations of which were symptomatically consistent with influenza; but, at the same time, what struck Camp Devens was unprecedented in virulence and involved a mixture of infections.[4]

While investigations into a nonbacterial cause of the disease were in the early stages, two *JAMA* editorials of 5 and 12 October 1918, respectively, anticipate modern understandings of influenza epidemiology: (1) the disease "never spreads faster than human travel"; (2) it appears suddenly, "in the course of evolutionary processes"; (3) "the infectious agent" is a new form, to which large numbers of people have little or no resistance; (4) "it is transmitted readily from person to person under the most diverse hygienic and geographic circumstances"; and (5) the outcome of the etiologic investigation is incomplete. A 12 October 1918 *JAMA* editorial loudly proclaimed in upper-case type:

> THE PRECISE CAUSE OF THE PRIMARY ACUTE RESPIRATORY INFECTION IS NOT KNOWN—IT MAY BE THE INFLUENZA BACILLUS; AS YET DEFINITE PROOF IS WANTING—BUT THE MOMENTOUS PERIL SO FAR IS THE DEVELOPMENT OF PNEUMONIA, AND THIS APPEARS TO BE ASSOCIATED WITH AND IN ALL LIKELIHOOD CAUSED BY DIFFERENT BACTERIA, OF WHICH THE INFLUENZA BACILLUS, HEMOLYTIC STREPTOCOCCI, AND PNEUMOCOCCI ARE THE MOST IMPORTANT ["Quarantine and Isolation," 1220].

These editorial statements are indices of where medical research stood as the second wave intensified. If we collate the editorial staff's cautionary observations of 5 and 12 October 1918, one finds that the cause of influenza, as yet unknown, had suddenly appeared through some evolutionary process; that people had no immunity to it; that it was highly and indiscriminately contagious; that human travel spread the disease efficiently; and that two kinds of pathology were involved, the sequel, a very dangerous pneumonia, being attributed to bacteria. Although influenza was "veiled in mystery," the lifting of that veil had begun as the crisis worsened.

Research on the filterable-virus theory continued in earnest. On 14 December 1918, Gibson, Bowman, and Connor published a landmark paper experimentally corroborating the recent results of the French researchers, Lebailly and Nicolle, who had been trying to find the virus as well. After inoculating monkeys with sputum from human influenza patients, they found upon dissection, "haemorrhagic exudate affecting especially the lower lobes of both lungs." They were able to differentiate between lesions associated with the nonbacterial filtrate, on the one hand, and those attributed to secondary bacterial infection, on the other; moreover, the initial infection "was ... in many respects comparable to that noted in certain human cases of influenza in which a fatal issue had supervened before the occurrence of marked secondary infection" (646). An unknown agent, in some influenza cases, killed the patient before a secondary pneumonia set in, and the pathology it caused was, again, distinct from that associated with bacteria. A breakthrough, therefore, had come at the end of the second wave: a submicroscopic entity, in a monkey model, had been associated with the inciting, nonbacterial cause of influenza pneumonia. It was only a matter of time for the proof to crystallize.

On the basis of lab results, prominent medical researchers continued to raise doubts over Pfeiffer's single-pathogen theory. A variant of the mixed-infection idea was that influenza could involve sequential bacteria other than Pfeiffer's microbe (Osler's notion in 1904). Ernest W. Goodpasture, renowned for his work in the 1920s on the herpes viruses and in the late 1930s on viral culturing in chicken eggs, was convinced that influenza was a dual-stage disease. Though he used the word "virus" in its indiscriminate sense, the infectious agents in both stages of influenza, in his view, were bacterial ([1919]: 724–25; Waterson & Wilkinson, 190). Corroborating Mathers' 1916 findings, post-mortems during the second wave, at the Chelsea Naval Station near Boston, indicated that Pfeiffer's bacillus was not the primary cause of infection: pneumococci predominated in pulmonary cultures of six cadavers, examined in autumn 1918; in December and January, streptococci were found most often in lung cultures, taken from sixteen cadavers. Of these sixteen, only two exhibited Pfeiffer's bacillus; and those two, only in December (Crosby, 219). This was further evidence that bacteria played a prominent role in influenza but that Pfeiffer's microbe, though harmful, was of minor importance.

If influenza had two infectious stages, further evidence was needed to explain how bacterial infections could succeed one another, and which flora initiated the disease. As expert opinion became stronger, Pfeiffer's claim weakened proportionally. Drs. Sheldon F. Dudley (Surgeon-Commander of the Royal Navy), Edwin O. Jordan, and S. W. Patterson were three such experts. Dudley reported, on 9 March 1919, that influenza "renders its victims more prone to invasion by other pathogenic bacteria" (37). In July 1919, on the basis of daily microbiological examinations of influenza secretions, Jordan, like Goodpasture, found no evidence of a predominating organism "in the upper respiratory tract of influenza patients" ([1919], 147–48; [1927], 251, 271). The clinical and laboratory work of S. W. Patterson, whose March 1920 paper is summarized here, is an index of the early study of influenza etiology as it gradually disengaged from Pfeiffer's claim.

Patterson's findings represent an intermediate phase in the theoretical revision of Pfeiffer's hypothesis. As director of the Walter and Eliza Hall Institute of Research in Pathology and Medicine, Melbourne, Australia, Patterson recounted his first-wave experiences at the army hospital in Rouen, France,

April 1918 (207–210). The infection sent patients to their cots, was unbelievably contagious, and induced a 3-to-5-day fever. Patterson accepted Pfeiffer's hypothesis at the outset, but lab results and pathology reports forced him to revise his thinking. First of all, blood cultures revealed the presence of Pfeiffer's microbe, but over a 12-to-17 day period, *and though the patient was still ill,* bacilli gradually disappeared. Patterson observed something else: pulmonary edema that later investigators identified as not resulting from bacterial infection. He, therefore, correctly assumed that the inflamed and engorged lung disease of the first stage had "paved the way for secondary infections, the results of which dominated the whole field in the later stages." Areas of hemorrhagic edema in the lungs preceding the secondary infection had amounted to "an excellent culture medium for the activities of the bacteria of the respiratory system, of which *B. influenza* [Pfeiffer's bacillus] is probably the first and most important invader, followed in the more prolonged cases by streptococci and pneumococci" (italics added). For Patterson, then, the initiator of the disease was an unknown pathogen which caused tissue damage, permitting secondary bacterial infections to set in; Pfeiffer's bacillus, though harmful, had been reduced to a complication.

The idea of an unknown nonbacterial, primary cause of influenza had become the target of investigation. The pathological changes observed in the initial stage of influenza strongly suggested that something other than bacteria was at work. Drs. Peter K. Olitsky and Frederick L. Gates, for example, arrived at this conclusion through their study of influenza pathology in rabbits they had inoculated with human secretions over consecutive time periods (in 1918–1919, in late autumn 1919, and in winter 1921). They reconfirmed that bacteria were responsible for a secondary effect in influenza but stressed that the "essential effects" of influenza "were produced *by a substance wholly unrelated to bacteria*" (1499; italics added). Thus, influenzal etiology had, by the early 1920s, reached a crisis point. If the co-pathogen hypothesis was valid, the most important step was to identify the prequel unequivocally.

At this point in time, researchers were still very much in the dark about the existence of infectious viruses. Without the appropriate technology, they could only approach the unknown pathogen indirectly. Here are the basic facts: (1) the suspected agent, labeled a filterable virus, was small enough to pass through the least porous filter; (2) it was invisible under the light microscope; (3) it could not be grown in artificial media (Waterson & Wilkinson, 78); (4) the lesions attributed to this agent, as pathologists frequently observed, were different from those caused by bacteria; and (5) the mysterious agent was considered responsible for predisposing the lungs to secondary invasion.

From 1900 to 1914, medical researchers had been unsuccessful in their attempts to isolate the suspected cause. For want of a better method, they had tried to cultivate them, not *in vivo* through animal experiments, but on artificial media in glass (Waterson & Wilkinson [1978], 35). John Rose Bradford and colleagues, in 1919, thought they had made a breakthrough (127–128). Tiny by bacterial standards, the organism they found seemed to be a hybrid. On the one hand, it had bacterial characteristics: it was visible under a light microscope, was Gram-positive, had a circumferential range from 0.15 to 0.50 micrometers, could be cultivated from blood, sputum, and pleural specimens, and was isolable from lymphatic tissue during postmortems. In several respects, this organism also resembled the elusive agent: it, too, could pass through the least penetrable of filters; if injected into animal models, it sickened guinea pigs and monkeys; and, when dissected, these animals were found to have pulmonary lesions and bleeding suggestive of influenza.

Using Koch's method, they isolated an unusual organism, but its visibility through a light microscope meant it had more in common with bacteria. Bradford and coworkers then passed the infectious agent on from slightly ill to healthy animals by injecting them with infectious bodily fluids. As a result, healthy animals became sicker than the original donor, and the former group suffered fatalities. The inoculated animals, at postmortem, had the germ in their bloodstreams, and the organism, as expected, was successfully cultured from their tissue; thus, they had followed through with Koch's cycle. They thought they had found the elusive cause; but, as we now know, they had found something else.

In the early 1920s, investigators had neither the laboratory methods nor the hardware to isolate a virus. Methods for cultivating invisible viruses, however, were being developed slowly and would be in use within the decade. Woodruff and Goodpasture, in 1931, would introduce the technique of growing influenza virus in developing eggs, and F. M. Burnet would perfect the technique in 1936 (Waterson & Wilkinson, 138; Woodruff and Goodpasture, 209–22; Burnet, 282–293). With the development of electron microscopy, the presence of viruses would no longer be suspected through indirect evidence. The evolution of electron microscopy belongs to the history of physics (Palucka [2001]). In 1939, Kausche, Ruska, and Pfankuch published the first micrographs of Tobacco Mosaic Virus; and, in 1940, of bacteriophage (Kausche et al., 292–299; Pfankuch et al., 46).

The organism that Bradford's group had isolated at Étaples, France, in early 1919, was likely *Mycoplasma pneumoniae*, a bacterium, not a virus. In several respects, this organism could be mistaken for the cause of influenza since it was responsible for a disease similar to seasonal influenza. Morphologically, it was an unusual bacterium. Devoid of a cell wall, it was eventually classified as "the smallest known free-living microorganism" (Bono, "*Mycoplasma and Pneumonia*"). The organism Bradford's group found had a circumferential range from 0.15 and 0.50 micrometers, comparable to *Mycoplasma*'s range of 0.15 to 0.30 micrometers (Bono). Thus, in contrast to a virus, however, *Mycoplasma* is gigantic. Since most bacteria range in size from 1.0 to 10.0 micrometers, Bradford's microbe was actually a tiny bacterium. Electron microscopy would determine that viruses fall in the range of 60 to 100 *nanometers* (1 nanometer = 0.001 micrometers); apparently, the Bradford organism, while much larger than a virus, was at the lower end of the bacterial size scale.

Because this little bacterium acted like a virus, it intrigued the Bradford group. Having "a selective affinity for respiratory epithelial cells," as do Type A/influenza viruses, it has been implicated in the activation of "inflammatory mediators, including cytokines" (Bono); thus, it is understandable why Bradford's group thought they had solved the influenza mystery. *Mycoplasma*'s rightful place in the prokaryotic domain would eventually be confirmed.

The Bradford investigation, however, was not groundbreaking. In 1898, pathologists at the Pasteur Institute had identified the *Mycoplasma* through a light microscope, found it cultivable in "collodion sacs implanted in the peritoneum of live guinea pigs," and able to multiply by binary fission. Thinking, then, that a filterable virus had been found, pathologists tried to grow it and other filter-passers and make them visible through staining or through resolution upgrades in light microscopes (Waterson & Wilkinson, 32–33). In 1938, R. A. Reimann, investigating human cases of *M. pneumoniae*, confirmed that it caused "primary atypical pneumonia" (2377–2384). The Bradford group, it seems, was unfamiliar with the 1898 research.

Drs. Goodpasture, Walker, McCallum, and Opie, as early as 1919, had begun to study influenza etiology using interdisciplinary methods. Coupled with technological advancements, this approach proved to be revolutionary. Pathology, histology, microbiology and other branches of medical science, therefore, were drawn into the search for the pathogen, to find out how it attacked the respiratory system (Taubenberger & Morens, "The Pathology").[5]

Reports continued to favor the idea that influenza was a dual-stage syndrome in which an unknown, virulent pathogen incited the infection, leaving the respiratory system vulnerable to the colonization of harmful bacteria. Through pathology, scientists could further differentiate the effects of the unknown agent from those of harmful bacteria. Winternitz, Mac Namara, and Mason asserted, in 1920, that the massive edema of the respiratory system in influenza decedents, upon microscopic study, was unmistakably the result of "the inflammatory process in the early stage of the disease" (*Pathology*, 20). This process, especially evident in the aveoli, was the typical and "dominating expression ... in the early stage" (*Pathology*, 20). They drew an analogy between influenza and the effects of poison gas, both of which caused edema and ruptured aveoli ("Symptomology," 321–325; "Pathology," 201). When aveoli rupture, air escapes into the interstitial tissue, creating a form of emphysema of the lung that spreads throughout the neck and thorax, and this phenomenon, which is well known, occurs more frequently and extensively in influenza "than in any other disease" (*Pathology*, 22). Once the initial process of inflammation, edema, and tissue damage subsided, pneumonia could result, "varying in extent from peribronchial to lobar," and this pneumonia most often develops in a necrotic lung, where abscesses and gangrene can be found (*Pathology*, 26). Even though the initiating pathogen was unknown, the authors had firm evidence that, as the sequel, "bacteria ... find their way into the damaged lung," producing various, undifferentiated complications (*Pathology*, 43).

Wolbach and Frothingham, in 1923, studied the dissected lungs of 26 influenza decedents at Camp Devens and from the Boston area who presented with both gross and microscopic lesions. These investigators recognized that, in many fatal cases, pulmonary disease included both nonbacterial and bacterial lesions (1–30). The problem, as Winternitz et al. had noted, was that discrete organisms—filter-passer and bacteria—produced typical pathology; but, when coextended, their respective effects were not easily differentiated from each other. The confusion arose because a variety of complicating organisms were involved, and because "manifold gross pathologic appearances" were evident (Wolbach & Frothingham, 14). To demonstrate the differences between areas of diseased tissue, the authors provided photographs of lung surfaces damaged (they believed) only by viral infection. The lung tissue was hard, exhibiting acute alveolar emphysema, hemorrhagic exudate, a "dusky red" and mottled pleura, the formation of a hyaline membrane in the aveoli, and blood tinged or bloody serous liquid in the lungs (Patterson had described similar findings in 1920). By 1923, the consensus was that the lung lesions appearing at the onset of influenza were *unlike* those associated with typical lobar and bronchopneumonia and, therefore, probably not caused by bacteria (Wolbach & Frothingham, 15; italics added).

Although the pulmonary characteristics of influenza were obvious to trained eyes, when bacteria colonized the inflamed tissues, even for specialists like Wolbach and Frothingham, it became difficult to tell one lesion from another: "This gross appearance of the lungs, which was considered to be due to the virus of the disease, was quickly complicated by the lesions of *different bacteria*, and in the gross more than microscopically in some instances the characteristic features of the virus lesions were obscured by the superimposed reactions" (17; italics added). In one instance, these investigators point to a photomicrograph of lung tissue showing an unusual double lesion in an area of "pneumococcus lobar pneumonia": a bacterial lesion was superimposed over a healing viral lesion, while in another area of the lung "a fresh virus lesion was found with all the usual histologic findings." Though influenza made for "a complicated pathologic picture," the authors conclude that an acute inflammatory reaction was typical and that its effects remained in the bronchi even after lesions had healed (26, 29). Although the inciting cause had not yet been isolated, it most likely was not bacterial.

Although viral and bacterial lesions were, at times, indistinguishable from each other, this was not the case when attempting to identify specific *bacterial* lesions. The authors knew, for example, that disease caused by colonizing bacteria varied from species to species and that lesions were distinctive. Pneumococcus lesions appeared in lobular, lobar, or patchy distributions; staphylococcus caused multiple abscesses; and the influenza bacillus (Pfeiffer's germ), though it did not mask viral lesions entirely, was nonetheless implicated in serious bronchial disease, "after the initial virus lesion had subsided" (Wolbach & Frothingham, 17). Although Pfeiffer's bacillus predominated (in 22 of 26 cases) in several mortality cases occurring within two weeks (7 to 10 days from the start of the epidemic; in Camp Devens, 7–14 September 1917), this bacillus *could not be found* at postmortem (italics added). They inferred from these cases that Pfeiffer's bacillus was, indeed, among the secondary invaders; thus, for want of a better term, patients dying before the bacterial invasion had succumbed to a *virus* (19–20).

For Wolbach and Frothingham, the virus concept was apprehended in two ways: empirically, in terms of tissue damage, observed and ascribed to the unknown pathogen; and comparatively, in terms of how the tissue damage differed from that which was known to result from bacterial pathogens. In all but one case (the 27th and sole survivor), viral pathology was present: "It was felt ... that this lesion was not produced by any of the bacteria present since the lesion was found in one early case in which the only bacterium present was an unidentified *coccus* found in the stained sections in the bronchial exudate" (Wolbach & Frothingham, 20). Additional negative evidence weakening the candidacy of Pfeiffer's bacillus came to the fore: three decedents presented with the viral lesion and no influenza bacilli. Nor was any other organism detected in the majority of cases (20). By 1923, as the Wolbach-Frothingham study illustrates, medical scientists had learned to differentiate between the sequential processes affecting the respiratory system, based on visual examination of damaged tissue. Through the process of elimination, they inferred what the effects of the non-bacterial pathogen were.

These authors admit that, despite steady progress on the etiological front, the cause of the influenza epidemic was not definitively known. However, they reiterate Patterson's observation: Pfeiffer's bacillus, rather than being the prequel, was "one of the secondary invaders." The Wolbach-Frothingham study points out that the invisible virus, the newly presumptive cause of influenza, had distinct pathological and symptomatic effects of its own: a febrile reaction, severe inflammation, edema, toxicity, and characteristic lesions in the lungs (i.e., alveolar emphysema, hemorrhagic exudate, hyaline membrane, and hardened lung).

It is amazing to learn that influenza, in 1918–1919, was usually "mild and self-limited": "For most affected populations, the case-fatality incidence was [less than] 2 percent [;] and the overall mortality rate was [less than] 0.5 percent" (Brundage & Shanks, "Bacterial Pneumonia"). Shanks and Brundage learned from the study of contemporaneous records that the "immuno-pathologic" reactions in 1918–1919 influenza patients (the so-called "cytokine storm") accounted for the high mortality rate among young adults ("Pathogenic Responses"). They attribute the severity and high mortality figures, in 1918–1919, to the synergistic effect of three processes: "infection with the virus, aberrant immune responses to the virus, and secondary opportunistic bacterial pneumonias [which] were severe and often fatal" ("Bacterial Pneumonia"). Viral infection induced toxic shock-like symptoms as the immune system overreaction caused bleeding capillaries, edema, and organ failure (Harrison, 330–331; Webster & Walker, 124–125).

By 1927, the sequential infection and co-pathogen hypothesis had all but discredited Pfeiffer's claim (Jordan, *Epidemic Influenza*, 251, 271). Morens and colleagues conclude that "the majority of individuals who died during the 1918 pandemic succumbed to secondary bacterial pneumonia, caused by *Streptococcus pneumonia*, *Streptococcus pyogenes*, *H. influenzae*, *Staphylococcus pyogenes*, and other organisms," whereas a subset died within five days from the effects of the viral infection which produced acute pulmonary hemorrhages, pulmonary edema, and the effects of cytokine overproduction (Morens et al., "Predominant Role of Bacterial Pneumonia"; Sheng et al., "Autopsy Series"). The pursuit of the causative agent in the pandemic, begun in 1918, indirectly and inferentially, gained momentum after 1931, as veterinary and medical science joined in a common enterprise. Pigs and ferrets led the way.

Swine Influenza Hypotheses

Swine influenza was first recognized at the Cedar Rapids (Iowa) Swine Show, which was held 30 September to 5 October 1918 (Shope, "Neutralizing Antibodies" [1936]; "History," 171–172; Appendix). Local veterinarians discovered that many hogs at the exhibition had become ill and died as the result of a mysterious disease. Fatalities occurred in only two or three days. After the show ended, and after the hogs had been returned to their farms, swine influenza broke out, spreading throughout the Midwest, the epizootic lasting until January 1919. The disease became endemic thereafter, reappearing annually and at varying levels of intensities, from 1919 to 1936.

Dr. J. S. Koen had been the first veterinarian to point out the uniqueness of the disease. An inspector in the Division of Hog Cholera Control of the U.S. Bureau of Animal Industry, he was especially struck by the similarity between the swine disease and the contemporaneous human pandemic, and he is credited with having coined the phrase "swine flu" (Shope, "History," 172). He noted that the swine disease had not existed prior to 1918 and that its appearance coincided with the onset of the deadly second wave of the human pandemic. This coincidence inspired him and other veterinarians to find out if the human and porcine diseases were in any way related to each other (Shope, "History," 172).

Koen outlined the etiology of hog flu in terms similar to those describing the disease in human beings (469). Hog flu had a "sudden and severe onslaught." The animals became very distressed, had labored breathing, a heavy, painful cough, were sore, nervous, excitable, and exhibited watery discharges from eyes and nostrils. The temperature elevated as high as 108 degrees Fahrenheit, and an animal could lose as much as five pounds per day. Despite the extreme physical weakness, an entire herd could quickly recover after four or five days. At the crisis point, animals either would rapidly recuperate or quickly die. The parallel between the human and porcine diseases was striking:

> Last fall and winter [1918] we were confronted with a new condition, if not a new disease. I believe I have as much to support this diagnosis in pigs as the physicians have to support a similar diagnosis in man. The similarity of the epidemic among people and the epizootic among pigs was so close, the reports too frequent, that an outbreak in the family would be followed immediately by an outbreak among the hogs, and vice versa, as to present a most striking coincidence if not suggesting a close relation between the two conditions. It looked like "flu," it presented the identical symptoms of "flu," it terminated like "flu," and until proved it was not "flu," I shall stand by that diagnosis [Koen, 475].

The swine outbreak, to Koen, appeared to be influenza of some type, but definitive diagnosis was not yet possible.

In the same issue of *The American Journal of Veterinary Medicine*, Koen mentions that the swine outbreak was unlike any other illness he had ever seen or studied. He thought it to be a new condition, and he called it "flu," simply because "it resembled that condition among people." It could be compared to human influenza in another respect: swine morbidity was high but mortality was low, analogous to the ongoing human pandemic. Confronting a critic, Koen simply restated his viewpoint: "I do not say that this diagnosis is right. It has not been proved what it was" (476).

Dr. Richard E. Shope (1901–1966), who would become a professor of animal pathology at the Rockefeller Institute for Medical Research, in the 1930s contributed significantly to the understanding of swine influenza and to the etiology of virus diseases. Finding Koen's article, he "began to play with the hunch that the pursuit of the cause of swine influenza might lead to the cause of human influenza" (Crosby, 298). He and his colleagues began to test swine influenza in the autumn of 1928, putting Koen's comparative insights to the test (Shope, "History," 165–169).

Shope recalled that, in 1931, after passing the swine flu infection on from hog to hog, through the nasal instillation of mucous or by close pen contact, he was able to isolate eight strains of swine flu, active during three epizootics and all producing similar disease in pigs. The organism's presence was confirmed through clinical manifestations in animals and not through laboratory or microscopic tests ("Swine Influenza. I" [1931], 349–359).

Shope and Dr. Paul A. Lewis (1879–1929), in a second experiment, cultured specimens taken from the respiratory tracts of swine, experimentally infected with swine flu, and also from several animals in the field ("Swine Influenza. II" [1931], 361–371). Specimens yielded a hemophilic bacillus which could be seen under a light microscope and cultured through conventional methods. They describe the morphological and cultural characteristics of the microbe, naming it *Hemophilus influenzae* (variety *suis*); however, 11 out of 13 tries at inducing swine flu symptoms in uninfected animals with intra-nasal pure cultures of the *suis* microbe were negative. The porcine analogue of Pfeiffer's bacillus, it seemed, was not the inciting cause of influenza in pigs.

The bacillus, when introduced into healthy pigs, did not bring on influenza. Continuing to hunt for the presumed cause, Shope made headway. In a third experiment, using Berkefeld filtrates from infected swine, he reported having isolated a "virus" ("Swine Influenza. III" [1931], 375–385). When administered intra-nasally to susceptible swine, the filtrate induced mild disease. Although the respiratory effects of the inoculation were mild, they still resembled those found in naturally-occurring swine influenza cases. The bacillus alone caused no disease, whereas the filtrate brought on mild influenza-like symptoms. Shope then decided to mix pure cultures of *H. influenzae suis* with the viral filtrate and to instill the mixture into healthy swine. The result was a disease clinically and pathologically *identical* to swine influenza.

What conclusions did Shope draw from this experiment? One, based on the 1931 experiments, was that the filterable virus and the bacillus "act in concert to produce swine influenza and that neither alone is capable of inducing the disease." In this variant of the co-pathogen hypothesis, the virus and the bacillus were thought to be synergistic: that is, in combination, they presumably generated swine flu, enhancing each other's virulence. By the same token, if swine flu affected pigs like influenza affected human beings, it might be reasonable to suggest that a pig, debilitated by the viral infection, could also be susceptible to secondary bacteria. Since Shope could not replicate his theory in humans, and since his detractors rejected the idea of synergy, his hypothesis was "shelved"; but it was not forgotten (Crosby, 219). Research in 2013 discovered "a strong but short-lived interaction [between influenza virus and bacteria], with influenza infection increasing susceptibility to pneumococcal pneumonia [approximately] 100-fold" (Sherestha, et al.). Shope may have been on to something after all.

Shope's work with filterable virus in connection to influenza was important but not unprecedented. It aligns him with the 1918 French researchers, Lebailly and Nicolle, whose investigations of filterable viruses were corroborated by Gibson, Bowman, and Connor. All of them suspected that influenza was a viral disease. Furthermore, Shope's porcine immunology investigations align him with Pasteur's vaccine experiments which led to a rabies vaccine in 1885. In 1911, having isolated an agent in tumor filtrate that induced the same neoplastic growth, Dr. Peyton Rous (1879–1970) hypothesized the presence of a "self-perpetuating agent active in this sarcoma of the fowl as a minute parasitic organism." Although Rous draws an analogy between the activity of this "agent" and "several infectious diseases of man and the lower animals, caused by ultramicroscopic organisms," he recognizes that, without definitive proof, "an agency of another sort is not out of the question" (that is, "an agent separable from the tumor cells" [409]). In 1914, Rous and Murphy replicated the 1911 findings, isolating a "causative agent" from three different chicken tumors. Each agent was a "distinct entity," capable of causing the very same tumor from which it was derived. The "agent" or "entity" was obtained from dry or glycerinated tumor, filtered through Berkefeld filters. They go as far as to suggest that the three invisible entities are "of the same natural class" and possibly a new group of entities altogether ("On the Causation of Filterable Agents"). Rous had found a virus.

Shope's multidisciplinary approach to swine flu in the 1930s involved microbiology, pathology, immunology, and, of course, veterinary medicine. He suspected, in 1932, that porcine influenza involved co-morbidity. Of the two pathogenic microbes involved in swine influenza, he found that only the filterable virus stimulated immunity. "*H. influenza suis*" (the porcine bacillus), on the other hand, "while essential to the production of the disease, played only a subsidiary role and, alone, conferred no immunity." He confirmed his findings serologically: blood serum from swine recovering from the filtrate-induced disease neutralized what he called "the swine influenza etiological complex or organism and virus"—a bulky phrase reflecting the uncertainty over how the two pathogens interacted with one another. He suggested that the swine virus had a predilection for the respiratory tract (Shope, "Immunity" [1932], 575–585).

In conjunction with Shope's experiments on swine flu, Alphonse Raymond Dochez (1882–1964) and colleagues, in 1933, attempted to isolate influenza pathogens using human nasal and throat washings. They cultivated the disease-causing organism after serial transmission in chicken embryo cultures, an innovative laboratory method ("Etiology" [1930], 1017–1022). For Dochez and co-workers, a virus and bacteria could be sequentially involved in influenza disease: "agents belonging to the group of filterable viruses" are "primarily infectious," and "the resulting etiology may be complicated by one or more of the well-known bacteria." Pfieffer's unitary theory of infection and the dual-bacteria variant were fast becoming obsolete. Positive results of viral transmissibility were obtained in Dochez's laboratory, not with influenza specimens, but with common cold secretions. Through transmission experiments, coupled with "negative controls with material derived from normal individuals," Dochez's group showed that a filterable virus was present in the upper-respiratory tract in cases of acute colds ([1933], 1442). They also saw the therapeutic importance of recognizing co-pathogenicity and the need to treat both disease processes independently. Thus, if it were known that two or more organisms could be involved in influenza etiology, Dochez et al. advise that, "more rational methods of control may be undertaken" ([1933], 1444).

The experiments of Dochez et al. paralleled those of Shope, with the difference that Dochez's team used human cold secretions. Both labs suspected, nevertheless, that the active agent of influenza was likely a filterable virus, having a role in "the complex nature of infections of the upper respiratory tract." Furthermore, in conjunction with Shope, Dochez and colleagues examined the interactivity of "filterable viruses and visible bacteria" and experimented on the transmissibility of influenza and cold viruses during seasonal outbreaks ([1933], 1443; "Studies in Influenza," 581–598). Dochez and co-workers eventually discovered that the cold virus was *transmissible*; pathogenic bacteria in the upper-respiratory tract of the inoculated volunteers *did not* appear to affect the course or the nature of the experimental infections; and, after prolonged cultivation using chick embryos, a virus became attenuated to the point of being non-infectious.

A British group, at The National Institute for Medical Research Farm Laboratories, at Mill Hill, England, in collaboration with Dochez et al. at Rockefeller University, made further progress towards isolating the influenza virus (Taubenberger et al., "Historical Context,"). Drs. Wilson Smith, P. P. Laidlaw, and C. H. Andrewes, in "A Virus Obtained from Influenza Patients," describe having taken throat-washings from human influenza cases during a 1933 outbreak, having extracted the filtrate, and then having instilled it intranasally into ferrets, animals with the closest affinity to man with respect to influenza susceptibility ([1933], 66–69). The original idea that human beings and ferrets were vulnerable to the same strains of influenza was illustrated, serendipitously, when a sick ferret is said to have sneezed in Dr. Wilson's face, communicating the flu to the researcher; the 1933 strain of influenza central to the study was appropriately labeled *W.S.*, for *Wilson Smith*.

The Mill Hill ferrets became ill with human influenza, and the induced infection was propagated serially from ferret to ferret, either through intranasal instillation or through close contact. The virus-laden solution was then found solely in the nasal passages of sick ferrets. Of eight throat-washing specimens taken from influenza patients in the early stages of the disease, only five produced disease in ferrets. Of greater significance was that throat-washings, either from convalescent *or* healthy persons, had no adverse effect on ferrets.

For Smith, Laidlaw, and Andrewes, experimental results were significant but not definitive. Their experiments showed that, 60 percent of the time, human virus in filtrate infected ferrets via inoculation, and that the disease could be communicated serially from animal to animal. Cross-immunity between man and ferret was proven when human antibodies to the virus, present in blood serum, immunized ferrets against human influenza filtrates.

At this critical point, they introduced a third species into the loop. Andrewes' group took Shope's swine influenza virus that had been isolated in bacillus-free filtrate and instilled it into ferrets. The ferrets came down with an illness *indistinguishable from that which the human virus caused.* This demonstrated that the porcine and human viruses had a close antigenic affinity (the antigen being the protein inducing the immune response), since both viruses affected ferrets in similar ways. The ferret model, as an experimental bridge between human and swine influenza research, demonstrated that the viruses were related to one another (Shope, "History," 172–173).

The 8 July 1933, Smith-Laidlaw-Andrewes paper proposed that: (1) with some degree of certainty, there was "a virus element in epidemic influenza"—a supposition of great import to understanding the etiology of the disease; and Shope's 1931 discoveries had furnished indirect support for their conclusions in 1933; (2) porcine virus rather than the bacillus was "the essential factor in swine influenza," the bacillus being a concomitant factor in the illness; (3) Shope's synergistic hypothesis, of an enhanced viral-bacterial interaction in swine flu, was left in abeyance.

Smith, Laidlaw, and Andrewes subscribed to the co-pathogen variant of "two separate agents": the virus alone causing mild disease; and the bacillus alone, none at all. Furthermore, their ferret experiments went a long way in confirming Shope's suspicion that influenza was caused "primarily" by a virus. The researchers at Mill Hill state what is now known to be true: "in certain cases this infection facilitates the invasion of the body by visible bacteria giving rise to various complications." Thus, the human and porcine bacilli associated with influenza disease in each species—Pfeiffer's bacillus and *H. bacillus suis*, respectively—were opportunistic organisms. Wilson and his colleagues based this finding on their experience with dog distemper in which bacterial could follow viral infection. They were fully aware that the only way to prove this theory was to perform human experimentation during an epidemic. The remarkable research contribution of the Mill Hill group was made possible, at that time, because a human influenza virus was circulating in the population during a seasonal epidemic. In 1935, Laidlaw, in "Epidemic Influenza: a Virus Disease," asserted that the virus of swine influenza was, in fact, *derived from the virus of the 1918–1919 pandemic*: it had adapted to the pig and persisted endemically in that species (1118–1124; italics added).

After recovering a virus from eight cases of human influenza during the epidemic of early 1935, Andrewes, Laidlaw, and Smith learned that these filtrates caused disease in ferrets ("Human Sera," 566–582). Of the eight samples, six were serologically identical to the 1933 *W.S.* virus. The results of animal tests, however, were inconsistent. Most of the human sera examined had neutralizing antibodies to *W.S.* influenza virus, probably because of exposure to the 1918–1919 pandemic sixteen years earlier. Fourteen children under ten, however, had no neutralizing antibodies to swine influenza virus, which likely meant that persons born after 1919—those who had not been exposed to H1N1 (the influenza viral strain of 1918)—would not have antibodies either. This deduction corresponded to what Shope had learned through porcine immunity studies. Additionally, because two volunteers had neutralizing antibodies in their sera *before testing*, they resisted influenza virus that had been passed serially through ferrets.

Both human and swine flu, it became clear, were closely related to one another in terms of contagiousness. Shope conjectured on the basis of these insights that the second wave of the 1918 pandemic had been caused by a virus serologically related to the one that caused swine influenza. The porcine virus was also closely related to the Type A human influenza viruses that, at least since 1933, had been appearing seasonally (Shope, "History," 173). Furthermore, Shope posited that, in the autumn of 1918, swine had likely acquired the disease from man and that, in pigs, the two distinct pathogens—a Type A human influenza virus and the bacillus *H. influenzae*—coexisted with one another (173).

2

Literature of the Recovery Period: 1921–1946

The Recovery or post-pandemic corpus consists of one novella, one author's childhood reminiscences, and chapters from novels. In the fiction of 1921 to 1946, factors related to contagion and the determination of health care professionals during the crisis are prominent themes. These authors share a common experience in the pandemic and uniquely portray human behavior under duress. Their fiction was concurrent with the emergence of the co-pathogen and the sequential-infection hypotheses; with the discovery of the influenza virus; with the development of egg-culturing procedures, essential to immunological experimentation; and, in 1939, with the invention of the electron microscope. The Recovery corpus emphasizes not the cause or cure of influenza but, rather, its morbid and mortal effects. As pathographers, these authors were also seeking emotional resolutions.

Contagion

Invisible and ubiquitous, influenza afflicted multitudes, was unpredictable and impervious to medical remedies. During the 1918–1919 pandemic, public activities ground to a halt and health-care systems were overburdened. The idea that influenza could be spread through aerosolized secretions was well established before the pandemic. That is why, at the time, sneezing, spitting, and coughing in public were outlawed, and why masks (of arguable value) were recommended for public use. The Latin word *contagium*, correlating to the verbs "to pollute" and "to come in contact with," meant that physical proximity to carriers, breathing in their air space, or even touching contaminated surfaces, could be life-threatening (*Pocket Oxford Latin Dictionary*, 282).

The idea of the human carrier has anti-social implications. During an influenza pandemic, introversion and reclusiveness were preferred, medically-justified lifestyles. Respiratory droplet contagion weirdly inverted reality: breathing could cause death. Because human beings carried and spread whatever caused this pestilence, people themselves were seen as sources of infection and as vectors; they were that, indeed. How many of us, today, hold our breaths as long as possible in a crowded elevator or train if someone has the nerve not to muffle a sneeze? Public precautions, in 1918–1919, included avoiding group activity, being wary of strangers, avoiding conversation and community worship, not commuting in public transportation, and so on. If a neighbor called for help, then one bolted the door. In 1918–1919, ignoring these precautions could be perilous. The most robust and the youngest, ironically, were the most susceptible. Like the bubonic plague or leprosy, influenza disfigured, turning patients blue or black, asphyxiating some, and driving others mad. The conditions were set for panic, for irrationality, for the persecution of scapegoated minorities, for quackery, and for every imaginable form of anti-social behavior.

Influenza was a mystery. A wave of disease could recede, and life could gradually become routine, only to be disrupted as a succeeding wave commenced. It seemed to be malicious, striking again when people celebrated its apparent cessation. This occurred twice: in the late summer of 1918 and in the winter of 1918–1919. Scientists understood that they were dealing with the worst set of circumstances: a rapidly-spreading, lethal infection, the pathophysiology of which, although evident clinically and at postmortem, was protean (a word frequently used in the contemporaneous medical literature). From previous outbreaks, medical scientists were familiar with the wave phenomenon in influenza, and they had other information as well (Taubenberger et al., "Historical Context," 583). However, what caused influenza could neither be isolated with certainty, nor could the infection be treated with existing regimens.

Although, in 1918, the incubation period of influenza was a mystery and its pathogen uncertain, medical scientists speculated about how it was contracted, but did so crudely and improvisationally. Two period documents describe field experiments on contagion. British physicians, Peter MacDonald and J. C. Lyth, for example, tried to ascertain approximately how long it took for one to develop symptoms after exposure (488). The obvious difficulty was how to pinpoint the time when one came in contact with a carrier of the germ. Traveling by rail (commutation being a motif central to the writings of McCarthy and Maxwell), McDonald and Lyth left King's Cross, at 5:30 a.m., on Thursday, 3 October 1918, and were bound for York at 9:30. At York, the doctors recollect that during the trip they had shared a carriage with a flying officer who had been coughing and sneezing. The officer told the doctors that he had had "influenza" for several days prior to the journey. On Saturday, 5 October, both doctors became symptomatic, coming down with laryngitis and severe coughs, and the onset for both of them was some time between 2:00 and 2:30 p.m. on Monday, 7 October. One doctor had a mild case, his fever rising no higher than 101 degrees Fahrenheit, while the other, who had more severe respiratory symptoms, had a fever of 104.5. The family of one doctor was infected.

Both MacDonald and Lyth were convinced that they had picked up the infection from the traveling companion on the York-bound train. Estimating the time of initial exposure to be 9:30 a.m., the doctors approximated the period of incubation for both of them to have been a minimum of 41 hours, with a maximum margin of error of four hours. One entire family became symptomatic 48 hours after coming in contact with him. Full-blown influenza, the doctor surmised, would occur about two hours beyond the appearance of symptoms. Though their findings were not scientific, they believed that the family's incubation period and that of their own (41–48 hours) was more than coincidental and could prove to be a valuable starting point for more accurate investigations. A step in that direction, though futile in hindsight, was taken on 10 October when throat cultures taken from one of the doctors showed Pfeiffer's bacillus, the organism incorrectly assumed to be the primary agent in the pandemic.

As the second wave rose to a critical level, doctors continued to speculate about the mode of transmission and about incubation periods. With no scientific means of approaching these problems, many conjectured anecdotally; and some, like MacDonald and Lyth, used common sense methods to consider ways of limiting exposure. Captain George T. Palmer, of the United States Sanitary Corps, illustrated how the germ could be picked up in public. Assuming that the pathogen could be passed from person to person through simple contact, he asked the question: "How many chances would the average man have to acquire infection in the course of a single day [?]" (Collier, 139–140). Routine morning activities in the barracks uncovered seven distinct contact risks, such as the bathroom doorknob and the toilet flush-handle. Commuting to the Officers' Club brought even more hazards, especially in the cramped confinement of a trolley car. At breakfast, Palmer cited 22 hand-to-mouth contacts, aside from the more obvious instances of hand-shaking, blowing one's nose, or using the toilet. Nine more contacts are recorded at lunchtime which included visits to the post office and bank. Palmer's unbelievable total was 119—119 ways to pick up the flu-causing germ, whatever it was (Collier

140). We are made aware of viral communicability today when we see disinfectant soap stations at every entrance of a public or private institution, and in the vestibules of hospitals, colleges, and businesses. What Richard Collier rightly called "the era of the mask" had begun in mid–October 1918. Whether or not the wearing of gauze face-masks prevented infection was strongly debated. An industry of mask producers sprung up, nevertheless, and the practice became widespread, especially in San Francisco (Collier 193).

Willa Cather, One of Ours *(1922)*

A transatlantic troop ship, packed to the superstructure with passengers, is the worst place to be in an epidemic. Willa Sibert Cather (1876–1947) claims to have anticipated the problem while planning the novel, *One of Ours* (1922). She lived through two influenza pandemics, that of 1889–1890 (when she was 13) and that of 1918–1919 (when she was 31). She recorded experiences with influenza in the aftermath of the 1918 pandemic, at a time when the disease had become seasonal and less virulent than the 1918–1919 strain. Her Pulitzer Prize–winning novel is a historical, rather than a pathographic, addition to the fictional corpus. Her fictional hero, Claude Wheeler, enlists and is killed in combat while in France. Wheeler's fate mirrors that of Cather's cousin, Grosvenor Cather, who died while serving in the First Infantry Division at the Battle of Cantigny on 28 May 1918 (Harris "Getting Claude," 248).

In correspondence of 1922, 1923, 1933, and 1936, Cather mentions having had bouts with influenza, having been hospitalized, and having been sent to a sanatorium to recover (Stout, ed., 88–89, 101; O'Brien, 146–158).[1] If indeed she had genuine influenza on each occasion, and not common respiratory infections or a combination of somatic and of psychosomatic ailments, then, from 1922 to 1936, she had endured seasonal strains of the flu at least five times. This is not to imply that recurrent bouts were innocuous, far from it. She was debilitated by them and even had influenza while writing *One of Ours*. There is no doubt that influenza inspired her writing, in part. Her recurrent bouts and reliance on first-person accounts lend authenticity to her fictional account of a transatlantic outbreak, and it is a valuable addition to the canon.

The transport outbreak in her novel is consistent with historical records. Cather's sources were direct accounts of the naval experience during the pandemic. As Joshua Doležal points out, *One of Ours* (1922) is considered to be a rare contemporary "recounting [of] the ravages of influenza on American soldiers ... bound for France" (82–83). She adapted her story from at least two eyewitness documents, one unpublished and the other published; and, undoubtedly, her narrative is informed, to some degree, by seasonal flu episodes. Dr. Frederick Sweeney's World War I unpublished diary is one major source ("Diary"). Dr. Sweeney had treated Cather for influenza in the spring of 1922, when she had been working on the novel while recuperating in Jaffrey, New Hampshire (Doležal, 90; Letter 588 [26 April 1922], Stout, ed., 89–89). During World War I, Sweeney had treated patients onboard his ship, survived the flu himself, and recorded the experience in the diary, which Cather read, and which influenced the chapters on the voyage in *One of Ours* (Doležal, 90–91). Cather was also influenced by Joseph Husband's *A Year in the Navy* (1919) (Doležal, 87; Harris "Getting Claude," 246–256).

Even though Sweeney's diary was never published, it is still possible, from actual accounts, to ascertain some sense of what servicemen endured on infected transports and in overcrowded barracks, as well. Once again, the connection between contagion, transportation, and crowding is evident. The realism of Cather's fictional transport outbreak is evident, once we contrast her text to a documentary of a U.S. naval operation during the pandemic.

The medical literature reported the problem at the beginning of the first wave. A *JAMA* article of 28 September 1918 states that, from 28 August to 11 September 1918, a severe and rapidly spreading epidemic of influenza had arisen in the northeastern First Naval District. Within two weeks, doctors had recorded more than 2,000 cases and that the disease was spreading relentlessly. The authors are reasonably certain that this was the very same disease first heard of in Spain that year, and for that reason misleadingly labeled "Spanish Influenza." During the spring of 1918, it had made its way through Germany, Italy, France, England, and Ireland, striking 30–40 percent of the overall population. Like its predecessor of 1889–1890, this disease had moved inexorably from east to west, and it did so "along the lines of travel" (Keegan [1918], 1051).

Documents related to actual conditions onboard transports voyaging from the American East Coast to Brest, France, provide contrasting perspectives. One such document is Rear Admiral William B. Caperton's personal account of the influenza outbreak in October 1918, on the armored cruiser USS *Pittsburgh*, en route to Rio de Janeiro, Brazil ("Personal Account"). With startling suddenness, the disease erupted in the ship. Admiral Caperton explains that they knew about the disease that had swept through Europe and also had been forewarned that it had arrived in Brazil, Bahia, and Pernambuco, most likely via transatlantic shipping. Another ship, the SS *Dannemara*, bound from Lisbon and Dakar, Africa, had preceded the *Pittsburgh*. When it had arrived at Rio de Janeiro, the captain reported that four had already died and that there were several other cases. At that crucial moment, the local health authorities in Rio failed to isolate the Portuguese ship and its passengers. The consequences were predictable: the disease was carried onshore.

Judging from Caperton's narrative, it appears that the *Dannemara* had brought its fatal cargo to Rio on or about 4 October. HMS *New Castle,* arriving in Rio on 6 October, had come from Bahia. Onboard were 60 cases of a "benign" form of influenza. One can infer from this remark that the *New Castle* had picked up the disease in Bahia. Whether a "benign" form (the milder first wave infection in the summer?) was on that ship is difficult to determine. By 7 October, however, the terrible effects of the autumn disease were being felt as hundreds became incapacitated, forcing the shipping company to close the port entirely.

By 7 October, several cases of flu had been reported on the *Pittsburgh*. The morbidity rate began increasing exponentially. The record of 8 October shows that 33 cases had been diagnosed on the American cruiser, while cases on shore were multiplying at an even more alarming rate. On 9 October, *Pittsburgh*'s sick bay, with 92 patients, was nearing or had reached capacity. By this time, "hundreds ashore were dying without medical attention." It became obvious to the admiral and to his officers that the safer place to be, at least for the moment, was shipboard rather than on shore or inland. Word came to the *Pittsburgh* that a disease was raging on the coast. Hospitals were overcrowded, and so many people died in the space of one week that the city had run out of coffins.

Early on 10 October, the *Pittsburgh* entered the floating dry dock for needed repairs because they were slated to embark on patrols. Despite the widespread disease in the nearby village of Candelaria, putting politics above good sense, Caperton and his officers left the relative safety of the *Pittsburgh* to attend memorial services for more than one hundred Brazilian sailors, victims of influenza while at sea. Efforts to refit the *Pittsburgh* for a forthcoming West Indian mission were severely hampered by the medical conditions of crewmen. The sick roll, by 10 October, had risen to 418 men. Caperton urgently wired Washington, D.C. that the *Pittsburgh* had to be delayed. Work on the ship centered wholly on caring for the sick, the level of which had risen over four days to 644, with 350 others symptomatic but ambulatory. The first death on the *Pittsburgh* occurred on 13 October. Three more perished on 15 October and at that point even the commanding officer, the department heads, and members of the admiral's staff were confined to their bunks.

Caperton made it absolutely clear to the Department of the Navy that the *Pittsburgh* had no choice but to remain in Rio. As people died "like flies" on shore, more than one-half of the *Pittsburgh*'s hospital corps became incapacitated. By 18 October, 12 cases of pneumonia onboard ended fatally. The urgent necessity arose, at that time, to inter these men in Rio, but caskets were at a premium. After six more American servicemen died on 20 October, the Brazilian Minister of Marine, Admiral Alexandrino de Alençar, requisitioned fifty hospital cots for American use. But when the *Pittsburgh*'s cortege arrived, they found that no graves had been prepared. The crew of the *Pittsburgh* dug the graves of their shipmates themselves.

Cemetery conditions were indescribable. Eight hundred decomposing bodies were strewn about the grounds awaiting burial, while vultures circled overhead. The City of Rio was without medicine, food, or wood for coffins. Hundreds of naked bodies had to be piled in the public hospital. Thanks to the intervention of an American businessman in Rio, proper transportation and other necessities were procured, allowing 40 patients to be taken from the ship and transported inland to an army hospital; presumably, resources on the *Pittsburgh* had been stretched too thin. Food, clothing, and clean bedding were running out. Meanwhile, on the cruiser, morbidity had risen to 654, 102 or 6.4 percent of these men having pneumonia; but of this group, the case mortality rate was very high (46 of 102 died).

Under these deteriorating conditions, the crew reversed its sequestration policy and began to transfer its sick to the onshore U.S. Army hospitals, while an American company, Rio Power and Light, furnished naval personnel at the hospitals with much-needed kitchen equipment, glassware, and ranges. Although 58 more men were to die, the disease appeared to have reached its peak. Health gradually returned to many, and men began to return to work. Contrary to the trend in the army hospitals in Rio and on the *Pittsburgh*, more than one thousand Brazilians in Rio continued to die each day, sometimes unexpectedly and with grotesque suddenness.

The work of a selfless medical staff, of the soldiers, sailors, and Marines on the cruiser, and the kindness of people in Rio whose ordeal was more dreadful, helped the *Pittsburgh* weather the ordeal, which lasted from 4 October to 5 November. "The most thoroughly savaged of all the major fighting vessels," Alfred Crosby writes, "was the USS *Pittsburgh*" (122). Caperton's narrative, though not intended as an epidemiological report, records 126 deaths in one month. On the *Pittsburgh,* the mortality rate derived from the admiral's figures amounts to 14 percent, nearly six times the norm for the pandemic; and 45 percent of pneumonia patients died, which also exceeds the statistical norm. It is probable that conditions on the vessel and in the port contributed to the high morbidity and mortality statistics. It also reveals that, although contagion was explosive, most of those who were stricken survived. The account in mind, we can now move to Cather's imaginative depiction of the HMS *Anchises.*

Cather's maritime story begins in the spring of 1918, as recruits from the

Kansas regiment ship out on the transport, HMS *Anchises*, from Hoboken, New Jersey. The ship is bound for the coast of France and its troops for deployment on the Western Front. On the third day of the voyage, Claude Wheeler, along with two other soldiers, learns that one of the men, Corporal Fritz Tannhauser, had experienced a violent nosebleed during the night. Gradually, after a prolonged morning medical examination, the doctor guardedly remarks that, "There seemed to be an outbreak of sickness onboard." Two other men, who come to Wheeler's attention, are also showing symptoms of some illness. One is Albert Usher, a Marine who, prior to embarkation, had been in sick bay at the naval hospital in Brooklyn. Usher was destined for France to join his regiment. The only clue we have as to his health prior to embarkation is that he looked "rather pale from the recent illness" (Cather, 168). Usher could have been the index case and a carrier. The other patient is Lieutenant Bird. Both Usher and Bird are examined by Dr. Trueman who directs them into the hold below.

One prescription for influenza was to rely on natural immunity. Though Dr. Trueman may not have known that for a fact, he sensibly prescribes isolation, hot tea, bed-rest, and sweating, a modern therapy for colds and flu. The *Anchises*, like the *Pittsburgh*, was ill-equipped to weather the flu: medical care was insufficient; the staff was shorthanded; the American physician onboard was sick; and the ship's doctor, employed by a British company, refused to care for American passengers. In addition, the *Anchises*, a British liner converted to troop transport duty, was well over its 2,500-passenger capacity.

Wheeler questions Dr. Trueman about the possibility of an epidemic on the ship, but the doctor equivocates. Suspecting further infection, the doctor recruits Wheeler to look after the stricken men down below (Cather, 171). During the night of the third day, Tannhauser's condition worsenes. His nosebleed becomes severe, and he is carried to the infirmary in the morning. By this time, Dr. Trueman's worst fears are confirmed: "a scourge of influenza had broken out on board, of a peculiarly bloody and malignant type." At this point in the text, Cather placed an asterisk and note stating: "The actual outbreak of influenza on transports carrying United States troops is here anticipated by several months" (Cather, 175), ostensibly in the summer of 1918. If this is true, then Cather would have foreseen the first of many troop ship outbreaks, reports of which were first publicized in September (Crosby, 121). The transatlantic medical crisis at the beginning of the second wave, as Crosby explains, was exacerbated by "the proximity of all crew members to one another ... [making] it quite likely that a high proportion will come down with a virulent breath-borne disease all at once, leaving the operation of the ship in the hands of people tormented by high fevers and suffering from extreme prostration." The mortality statistic for the naval transports throughout the pandemic was 4,136 influenza pneumonia deaths of officers and men, from autumn to early winter of 1918 (Crosby, 122).

Cather describes the soldiers' mixed reactions to the news of the outbreak. Some officers immediately sequester themselves in smoking rooms, to drink whiskey all day to fend off infection (Cather, 175), the self-quarantining (not necessarily the booze), in hindsight being a beneficial decision. But the medical reports are dire. Lieutenant Bird, nicknamed the Virginian, dies in the afternoon of the fourth day and, on the morning of the fifth, is buried at sea.

By the morning of the fifth day, the epidemic had worsened considerably. Relying on every ambulatory man, Trueman requests that Wheeler help at sick call, for the number of febrile men had escalated. The doctor treats 70 men in line even though he, too, is symptomatic (suggesting Dr. Sweeney's experience). The morbidity statistic over a five-day span exceeds Caperton's figures by 16 percent (Cather, 177). When visiting Lieutenant Fanning below, Wheeler is shocked to learn that he had been suffering all night, coughing and gasping for breath. A brief examination reveals double pneumonia, a serious diagnosis. All that can be done is to keep Fanning comfortable in the states room. Wheeler is instructed to give him alcohol baths for fever and to feed him raw eggs beaten up in orange juice every two hours, night and day, to keep up his strength, as his immune system had to put up the fight (Cather, 178–79).

Cather represents the facts accurately. Medical care on the *Anchises*, as it was on the *Pittsburgh*, was severely limited. One doctor had to care for nearly two hundred patients, which is reminiscent of Dr. Grist's letter from Camp Devens. Trueman expends all of his medicines and exhausts the ship's ineffective supplies (Cather 178). Since no trained medical staff was onboard, the Kansas military band has to work as stretcher-bearers and orderlies on night and day shifts (Cather 179).

When Wheeler visits Tannhauser, he finds him both febrile and delirious. On his rounds, he must descend from the hospital into the damp, musty, and poorly-ventilated hold where one-half dozen men from his company were lying ill, probably the worst place on the ship to house persons in pulmonary distress. In the fetid air, the band boys help the stewards, while Wheeler feeds Fanning at two-hour intervals, as instructed (Cather, 179). At eleven o'clock, Tannhauser's fever breaks; but, despite the hopeful sign, the ordeal continues. Wheeler hears "the frightful sounds that came from his throat, sounds like violent vomiting, or the choking rattle of a man in strangulation—and, indeed, he was being strangled." The "struggle" lasts until 3 a.m. when Tannhauser dies. At sunrise, he and four others were buried at sea (Cather, 181).

Typical of the pandemic was the high mortality rate among the strongest young men. One theory, formulated decades later and mentioned in the previous chapter, was that robust victims suffered from what would be called the "cytokine storm," the edematous and inflammatory overreaction to the virulent germ that initially invaded the lungs. John M. Barry describes the physiological effects of the condition, called *hypercytokinemia*. Cytokine proteins, released by white blood cells, drive up the temperature and bind to receptors in the hypothalamus, ultimately inhibiting viral growth. Paradoxically, the body's efforts to protect itself cause pulmonary damage, patients succumbing "who were not very sick." As Barry describes it, since the flu virus had a proclivity for the epithelial tissue of the lungs, it penetrates the aveoli, causing viral pneumonia: capillaries then leak profusely, flooding the lung. Inflammation leads to tissue necrosis. The immunological response, so robust in the young, leads to fluid build-up until oxygen exchange is impossible, and the patient suffocates (*Influenza*, 249–250). Crosby explains that edema is another paradoxical effect of the body's effort to protect itself: antibodies, protein inhibitors or destroyers of virus, can only reach the site of infection after an inflammatory process has "engorged the infected area with fluids"; the antibodies can then move via these fluids "from their interior posts to the real site of battle," the lining of the respiratory tract where the influenza virus has seated itself (Crosby, 220). The body's biological reaction to the invader—in cells, proteins, and secretions—causes irreversible damage, setting the stage for secondary, bacterial infection. Cather's depiction of the floating hospital is true to the facts: "Vigorous, clean-blooded young fellows of nineteen and twenty turned over and died because they had lost their courage, because other people were dying,—because death was in the air" (Cather, 186).

The omniscient narrator, more existential in outlook than Wheeler, considers those who succumbed on the *Anchises* to be "merely waste in a great enterprise, thrown overboard like rotten ropes" (Cather, 191). Wheeler gradually comes to this view as well. He reflects on the shipboard death, broadening the definition of war casualty to include disease, accident, friendly-fire events, homicide, and suicide. He is momentarily ambivalent about the meaning of the *Anchises'* voyage. The comfort that he finds in patriotism does not stand up to the morbid atmosphere, as the *Anchises* has become "an emblem of mortality." The senseless deaths undercut Wheeler's idealism. He is happy to disembark but is conflicted about what the outbreak has taught him about the natural world and about human conflict. He seems to waver between patriotism and idea of the just war and skepticism over the cost in lives and treasure; a third outlook, perhaps belonging to the narrator, is that arrogant pride, rather than the mindless virion, is the real nemesis of all soldiers. Arriving at Brest,

Wheeler exults in the cliffs of the French coast, a symbolic affirmation of the Allied cause; but he pauses to reflect on the relative insignificance and frailty of the individual soldier. The sublimity of the scene, unfortunately, is the more illusory and enchanting of the two views. The sheer cliffs at Brest re-confirm his musings on the idea of human history, not in its ecological context, but as an ineffable drama. For Wheeler, arrival on the French coast revives his euphoria about the Great War (Cather, 273).

The ideals that captivate Wheeler, in the reader's view, are meaningless in light of the mortality statistics of the war and the pandemic: from 1914 to 1919: 675,000 Americans died of influenza (summer 1918–winter 1919), and 117,465 died in the war (Clodfelter, ed., 481). Soldiers dying of flu and on the battlefield were thought of as casualties of war, and this could have accounted in part for the national amnesia over the pandemic. Crosby suggests the government mixed the mortality figures of disease and combat intentionally: the influenza obituaries of young servicemen may have become "one general blur with casualty lists, and there is no doubt that the demographic effect of the pandemic intended to be concealed within that of war." For some who acknowledged the flu, it was "simply a subdivision of the war" (Crosby, 320). Cather realized this.

William Maxwell, They Came Like Swallows *(1937)*

In a 1999 interview, William Keepers Maxwell (1908–2000) recollected his childhood experiences in the autumn of 1918, as the second wave was about to strike ("Interview," cited in Burkhardt, 19–22). Maxwell recalls that his father had been reading *The Chicago Times* about an infectious disease that had been spreading in the military camps. Maxwell's parents were worried about the epidemic as it approached their region. His mother, Blossom, who was civic-minded, joined the women of Lincoln, Illinois, in the sewing of masks, thought at the time to protect against contagion. The pandemic apparently reached the city by rail. Once again, inter- and intrastate commuting played an important role in the spread of influenza from its East Coast foci. The main railroad, which figures prominently in the novel, connected St. Louis to Chicago and Lincoln. The 12,000 inhabitants of Lincoln were in the path of commuters who carried the infection westward. When 30 new cases of influenza were reported in Lincoln, the government, on 17 October 1918, finally prohibited public gatherings. Contagion was on everyone's minds.

Maxwell recalls that, on the day of the Armistice (11 November 1918), caution was abandoned, as William Sr. and Blossom drove through Lincoln in a victory parade while Blossom was pregnant with her third child (Maxwell, "Interview"). They were optimistic about the future. She could not restrain her happiness since her husband would not be drafted; she was expecting a child; and influenza's second wave was receding. Lincoln had lifted its second ban on public gatherings on 20 December and, by the 23rd, only two flu cases had been reported. As schools were preparing to re-open, William Sr. and Blossom boarded a train for Bloomington, Illinois, a community 30 miles to the north. Blossom was in the last term of the pregnancy, so the couple took the precaution to stay with Blossom's sister, Edith. Since her husband was an anesthetist at Brokaw Hospital, it seemed like a prudent move for the expectant couple. Meanwhile, William Jr. and older brother Hap were left in good hands with their aunt Mabel, William Sr.'s sister. Every precaution had been taken; every contingency, thought through.

On Christmas Day 1918, as the temperature fell to 10 degrees Fahrenheit, both boys developed influenza. The timing could not have been worse since they got sick the day after their parents had left for Bloomington (Maxwell, "Interview"). On 26 December, even though the second wave had diminished and virtually disappeared from the population, Blossom suddenly became acutely ill with influenza, developed double pneumonia, and, in just eight days, died in childbirth, giving birth to her third son, Robert Blinn Maxwell, on 3 January 1919. William Sr. was also down with influenza but recovered. Mabel heard the bad news from William Sr. on 4 January 1919, as he was about to accompany his wife's body back to Lincoln.

These unexpected events defined William Maxwell, Jr.'s life and shaped his fiction. Caroline Havanec believes that a "dark undercurrent of contagion" flows beneath the appearance of a close family, "though ultimately the novel attempts to recuperate the family structure and its promises of communion, sympathy, and consanguinity" (172). To extend Hovanec's metaphor, this undercurrent erupted seismically for the Maxwells on Christmas Day when the third wave commenced.

Compounding the grief and anxiety that the Maxwell boys must have felt when their family was struck by influenza is the insufferable series of ironies that must have caught everyone off guard. First, precautions had been taken to protect Blossom's health in the trip to Bloomington, Illinois, where adequate medical care was assured; however, the trip itself, ironically, caused both of them to contract influenza since they used public transportation, not an imprudent decision since the second wave had petered out and life seemed to be returning to pre-pandemic normalcy. They responsibly left their children in the capable hands of their aunt Edith, but both boys developed influenza anyway, even though the second wave had dissipated. Though the second wave had indeed gone, unknown to all a third wave was just beginning, bringing all who entertained a false sense of security back to prostrating reality. Few could have anticipated a relatively mild resurgence, but the effects were still severe.

William Maxwell memorializes these events in, *They Came Like Swallows* (1937) (Crosby, 311). In the story, the Morrisons'/Maxwells' home is relocated to Logan, Illinois. The influenza scene begins in November 1918, and the similarities to actual events are obvious and intended as such. Ten-year-old Peter "Bunny" Morrison (William Maxwell, Jr.) hears his father read about the epidemic in the Sunday papers. The article provides important background information for the reader. It describes the infection as "a very contagious kind of 'cold' accompanied by fever, pain in the head, eyes, back, or other parts of the body, and a feeling of severe sickness" (Maxwell, 14–15). Fortunately, the symptoms pass in 3–4 days for most; however, some patients will develop pneumonia, ear infection, meningitis, among other complications, and many will die. The article mentions that it is not known whether the so-called "Spanish influenza" is identical to an outbreak that occurred twenty-nine years earlier, presumably the reference is to the influenza pandemic of 1889–1890 (which has been attributed to an H3, not to an H1, viral Subtype [Taubenberger et al., "Historical Context," 583]). To Bunny, the word "epidemic," which he has been hearing regularly on the news and in the conversations of adults, is meaningless (Maxwell, 15). More information is forthcoming, as James/William Sr. continues to read the article aloud. He relates, for example, that the "epithet Spanish" has no truth to it. The belief in learned circles, as reported in the papers, is that it had originated as early as the fall of 1917, along the Eastern Front. Bunny sensed that his father had more than a casual interest in the epidemic, just as he had in other current events, such as the war, floods in China, and family history. The newspaper reading, a true representation of Maxwell's reckoning, is an effective device that gives the reader important background information.

At this point in the narrative, the disease is nothing more than an abstract and distant concept. Yet, as James Sr. reads further, more ominous facts emerge that will catch Bunny's attention. The entire family learns that, unlike ordinary coughs and colds, influenza epidemics can occur in any season. In 1918, the epidemic raged in Europe in May, June, and July (the first and mildest of three waves). Furthermore, influenza's symptoms are significantly worse than the common cold, during which fever, pain, and depression are mild. As for the Spanish influenza, its symptoms are not described in the narrative. Therefore, much is left to the imagination.

As Bunny continues listening to his father's reading, he is distracted by his mother's effort to stifle a sneeze. At this inopportune point, James Sr. resumes his recitation, stating that influenza has a sudden onset, and, unlike the common cold, spreads rapidly through a community. The more James reads the greater is Bunny's alarm: his mother's sneeze suggests to him that she was coming down with influenza (Maxwell, 17). James Sr. reads that influenza is highly contagious and that "a person who has only a mild attack of the disease may give a very severe attack to others" (Maxwell, 17). Elizabeth then sneezes loudly, just as James utters the words: "When death occurs it is usually the result of complications" (Maxwell, 17). The public health synopsis of the disease, though intended to inform the average adult, has made Bunny anxious. The ten-year-old boy is made aware of an incipient danger, although we cannot speculate how much of this awareness the twenty-nine-year-old author had attributed to his ten-year-old self.

The balance of the newspaper article is concerned with local precautions in Logan. Schools are to be closed until further notice (the Lincoln school district, however, did not take this precaution) (Maxwell, 17). This news impresses Bunny's thirteen-year-old brother, Robert, who, though vague on the details of the impending emergency, realizes that the health office's and school board's decision is serious. He realizes that, "there was more in the notice than that"; but they intuit a deeper and more unsettling implication: "It meant that something was happening in town, all around him" (Maxwell, 83). The kind of public anxiety that had gradually arisen was quite unlike the jubilation that had taken place on 11 November 1918, the day the Armistice was signed. That was a day of public celebration and relief. But the influenza notice had made the atmosphere heavy. An insidious threat had arrived: "a quiet thing that he [Robert] couldn't see or hear; that was in Bunny's room, and on Tenth Street where Arthur Cook lived, and more places than that." Robert, pleased that school is closed, forgets about the indistinct danger. He neither understands that closure is intended to limit contagion nor appreciates the reason for this decision. The Illinois Committee on Public Safety, in an effort to limit contagion, advises citizens neither to gather in public places in large numbers nor to ride public transportation. None of this advice has any relevancy to the day-dreaming Robert. The advisories, however, have serious ramifications: they will halt commerce, education, cultural events, and travel (Maxwell, 83).

In Maxwell's novel, at the onset of the third wave in the town of Logan, James, Sr., Bunny, and Robert are sickened, but, like Mary McCarthy and her siblings (as we shall see), they all survive. Tragically, their mother, Elizabeth succumbs to the disease, leaving James Sr. a widower with two adolescent boys and a surviving infant (Maxwell, 134, 153). James who is distraught, goes through a period of self-incrimination: was it his fault for exposing Elizabeth to the public on an interurban bus ride? Robert also blames himself for his mother's death because he had failed to prevent her from entering Bunny's sickroom.

The narrator makes it clear that Robert could not have been responsible for Elizabeth's having contracted the flu since Bunny was no longer contagious when his mother had entered the room. On the other hand, James agonizes that he is responsible for exposing his family to the infection, as will become clear below. At this point in the narrative, he articulates an unconvincingly fatalistic view of the epidemic and of his wife's death. All human beings, he reflects, live and function the same way. His personal tragedy is not unique, and other human beings will suffer from pneumonia and respiratory collapse (Maxwell, 172).

Through the persona of Irene, Elizabeth's sister and a mourner, Maxwell is able to interject a credible message of consolation for Robert. She counsels that his gnawing guilt is unfounded, since the incubation period for infection after exposure is three days, and weeks had passed since Elizabeth had cared for Bunny. James Sr. accepts her reasoning and will talk to Robert more openly, so his son will not blame himself.

James, however, cannot rely on the incubation period for self-exoneration, for he knows something that Irene does not. On the spur of the moment, contrary to public health advisories, he had thoughtlessly boarded a crowded train with his family, rather than a relatively empty, and presumably safer, interurban on the parallel track. He had, in effect, exposed himself to the jostling crowd in a closed environment. Drs. MacDonald and Lyth, along with Mary McCarthy, reveal the medical perils of crowded commuting during flu season. James Sr.'s frenetic decision is likely to have brought the flu infection to his household (Maxwell, 138). He tries unsuccessfully to rationalize his guilt away. But the probability, however low, still existed that someone on the interurban was a carrier: "With so much sickness, with the epidemic everywhere, it stood to reason that someone with influenza might have been on that interurban, too. They [his family] might have been exposed to the flu there, just as they were on the crowded train. And what point was there in torturing himself like this? What good did it do?" (Maxwell, 153). Furthermore, Elizabeth was in the third trimester of her pregnancy, and it was generally known that pregnant women were especially susceptible to the infection. Dr. Fernando Calderon, an obstetrician, noted in a 27 September 1919, article, that "influenza exerted a pernicious influence on pregnancy," the effects of lobar pneumonia, otherwise a treatable condition, being worse in this segment of the population (Calderon, 982–983; Barry, 239–240).

Through James' predicament, Maxwell expresses a philosophical problem that Camus, one decade later, would explore in *The Plague* (1949). Despite advances, the limitations of medical science are acutely demonstrated as bubonic and pneumonic forms of *Yersinia pestis* sweep through Oran, and the disease persists, despite all that public health authorities and front-line clinicians can do to stop it. As Dr. Rieux treats the dying Tarrou through the night, his task is to watch his friend's struggle, despite the medicines with which he injects him and the abscesses that he lances. "The only way he might help," Camus writes, "was to provide opportunities for the beneficence of chance, which too often stays dormant unless roused to action. Luck was an ally he could not dispense with" (Camus, 256). Rieux's regimen against the plague, though inadequate, had to be applied because his efforts could conceivably afford the patient an opportunity to resist the infection and to rally. Thus, his strategy was to stay the course and to apply current knowledge and practices to the problem, keeping in mind that each patient is unique. As for James Maxwell, Sr., given the epidemiological circumstances, one can say that he was thoughtless, even reckless. By the same token, one can argue that he was lulled into a false sense of security in the hiatus between the two waves.

Mary McCarthy, Memories of a Catholic Girlhood *(1946)*

Contagion is the central motif of Mary McCarthy's (1912–1989) autobiographical account of the pandemic in *Memories of a Catholic Girlhood* (1946). McCarthy who was six in 1918, recalls a fateful train journey from Seattle to Minneapolis taken 28 years earlier that claimed the lives of both of her parents (McCarthy, 12). She distinctly remembers coming down suddenly with chills (McCarthy, 12). The entire family was stricken with flu while in sight of the Rocky Mountains. When they reached Minneapolis and entered a hotel, "they brought the flu with them" (McCarthy, 16). Only one week had passed since the family had boarded the train in Seattle, on Wednesday, 30 October 1918, and McCarthy's mother's death on 6 September; and her father's, on the next day. The grandmother accommodated the sick family in her home because no hospital beds were available. McCarthy remembers vividly that people either "went about with masks or stayed shut up in their houses" (McCarthy, 35).

What McCarthy aptly calls "the awful fear of contagion" had paralyzed all services and created social chaos, making each person "an enemy of his neighbor." Having eagerly boarded at Puget Sound, and with great expectations of a new life in Minneapolis, one week later the family was carried off, "one person at a time" (McCarthy, 35). McCarthy makes it clear that when they started out, no one had the slightest idea that they carried within them an incubating parasite. Irrespective of whether they knew so or not, the McCarthy family "had carried the flu with [them] into their drawing room in the train, and one by one they were struck down as the train moved eastward. Stretchers, wheelchairs, and distraught officials awaited them. Several weeks later, the children understood that they were ill and gradually, from the behavior of the adults around them, they had become orphans" (36). McCarthy's tone, Nancy Bristow writes, effectively conveys "the sense of abandonment and helplessness she suffered as an unwanted child" (*American Pandemic*, 187).

The pandemic remained with Mary McCarthy over the decades—an emotional wound that never completely healed. In her autobiography, she pieced an illness narrative together. Childhood recollections of their deceased parents formed a bond between McCarthy, her brothers, and their grandmother, who filled in the memory gaps during the aftermath of the influenza attacks in early November. McCarthy and her brothers had been "kept in quarantine, like carriers of social contagion, among the rhubarb plants of our neglected yard." The memories their grandmother doled out, even the unpleasant ones, "became [their] secret treasures" (McCarthy, 45).

The chapter, "Ask Me No Questions," is devoted to reminiscences of her deceased grandmother. In ca. 1945, McCarthy recalls the events of November 1918. Before her parents' death, when they were leaving Seattle for Minneapolis to take that fateful train ride (some time just before 30 October, when the second wave was rising to crescendo), she remembers seeing her grandmother wearing "a funny white mask," recalls hearing the word "epidemic and her grandmother cautioning her parents that the children should be masked, too" (McCarthy, 201). Amidst the bits and pieces of memory, McCarthy has an acute flashback: "We were very sick on the train" (201). A blurred transition finds McCarthy recuperating at her grandmother's home, where she lay "on an iron bed." Her other grandparents (the Prestons of Seattle, her mother Tess' parents) visited her while she was semi-lucid. She recounts the six-year-old's confusion and the threads of memory are finally interwoven: "No one enlightened me; I heard the word 'flu,' but it was months before it dawned on me that the occasion had been my parents' funeral. Yet when I surmised, finally, that Mama and Daddy were not coming back, I felt a certain measure of relief. One mystery, at least, was cleared up; the strange lady had come and cried on my bed because her daughter was dead" (McCarthy 201–202). These recollections may have provided comfort. This is clear from her search for these traces of memories pertaining to her life after her parents' death and while in the care of her grandparents.

Thomas Wolfe, Look Homeward, Angel *(1929)*

Recovery authors did not study the disease with the analytical impassiveness of medical scientists; rather, as in Thomas Wolfe's and Katherine Anne Porter's cases, most experienced its physical effects personally: the former, through the death of his brother; and the latter, in her own illness. In *Look Homeward, Angel; A Story of the Buried Life* (1929), Thomas Wolfe dramatizes his direct experiences with the pandemic in a fictionalized outbreak narrative. It is an example of pathographic fiction, biographically accurate and resonant with irrepressible emotions. Wolfe had been a student at the University of North Carolina, when he learned that his brother, Benjamin Harrison Wolfe (to whom he would dedicate the book) had been stricken with influenza. Returning home in late September 1918, Thomas Wolfe witnessed his brother's death, on 19 October 1918, and he returned to UNC grief-stricken (Nowell, 42–44; Donald, 47–48). In communicating Ben's story, Thomas seems to have distanced himself from the event through time and mode of discourse, while perhaps restoring some wholeness to his life.

Wolfe's clinical description compares to the content of the medical reports of the pandemic years, but there are obvious differences in purpose and effect between the two. Whereas Dr. Patterson, whose experiences are recounted in chapter 1, describes influenza pathology in physiological detail, especially in the dissection of corpses, Eugene Gant and family unnervingly witness the effects of the disease while at the bedside of a dying family member. The autopsied soldiers in the military hospitals and Thomas Wolfe's brother, in the persona of Ben Gant, are united by a common experience. Whereas doctors depended on the de-personalizing anonymity of the autopsy report to learn about human disease and, with this knowledge, to care for the living, the depiction of Ben Wolfe's private suffering permits the author to face his loss and to communicate a profound encounter with the pandemic.

Twenty-six-year-old Ben Gant was not a robust person. In fact, he had a pulmonary condition (probably tuberculosis) that pre-disposed him to pneumonic complications. Ben had been repeatedly rejected for military service because of his physical condition (Donald, 48). Lamenting over his failures, he tells his brother that his lungs "are going: they won't even give the Germans a chance to shoot at me" (Wolfe, 444).

The rest of the pandemic story is transparently autobiographical. Eugene Gant/Thomas Wolfe receives a letter from his father, early in October when the second wave of the pandemic was under way. His father writes that the family is besieged by flu: "Everyone has it, and you never know who's going to be next" (Wolfe, 447). It seems, to his father, that "the big strong ones" come down with it first. Men like the young Methodist minister, Mr. Hanby, who died from pneumonia which had "set in" during the course of the infection, were typical. So virulent was his case that no prognosis was given: "The doctors said he was gone from the start" (Wolfe, 447). Unknown to the family, Ben, who was showing early symptoms, was moping around and complaining of having no appetite. Several weeks would pass when Eugene received a telegram from his mother, summoning him home because Ben had pneumonia (Wolfe, 448).

When Eugene arrives home, he learns that Ben is very ill, presumably having caught influenza from one of the sick children, and had been dragging himself around while sick and feverish without getting bed-rest (Wolfe, 449). When he finally got to bed, he improved over a span of two days, which was customary. At this deceptive point, he was most at risk. The doctor recommended that the patient remain in seclusion and to be monitored, in order to prevent a relapse or the development of a secondary, bacterial infection which was more difficult to manage (Wolfe, 449). The idea that flu involved co-morbidity, as surveyed in the previous chapter, was being hotly debated in 1918 and into the mid–1920s. Ben, however, did not heed the medical advice. One day later, after Ben had gone about in his usual "cursing rage," he was struck down with a high fever, having "developed pneumonia in both lungs" (Wolfe, 449). The news "silenced them for a moment with its inexorable sense of tragedy" (Wolfe, 449). Ben's condition was critical (Wolfe, 451).

The reader is brought into the sickroom to witness the effects of viral and/or bacterial pneumonia, a secondary infection. Wolfe's graphic narrative gives us some sense of what doctors had been witnessing each day for months. Wolfe describes his brother's gaunt outline, twisted beneath the bed sheets "in an attitude of struggle and torture." Throughout the ordeal, Eugene senses that Ben's body "seemed not to belong to him," appearing "distorted and detached as if it belonged to a beheaded criminal." The imagery suggests the cleavage of selfhood from body, a divergence of Ben's spiritual self from a body that can longer sustain it. Ben's cirrhotic complexion had turned ashen; his beard, a "stiff black furze," reminiscent of the posthumous growth of hair seen on "a rotting corpse." His thin lips lifted in a fixed "grimace of torture and strangulation." Double pneumonia prevents him from gasping nothing more than "a thread of air into his lungs" (Wolfe, 452).

Eugene's vigil at Ben's bedside reveals a contrast between the latter's physical deterioration and his ineradicable dignity. Gradually, Ben becomes calm "in all his fierce gray lonely beauty" (Wolfe, 461). Despite his deathly pallor and faintly beating heart, he is perceived by all present as having been transformed. The family ceases their bickering as they suddenly perceive Ben's eyes brightening, and all become aware of "the strange wonder, the dark rich miracle of his life." To describe how his wretched body is transfigured in the minds of those present, Wolfe uses figurative and abstract language: the miracle of his life is an "enormous loveliness," a palpable beauty that "surges" over those present. It is a moment of epiphany: the family is brought silently together, "in a superb communion of love and valiance," transcending the horror, confusion, and anxiety of the moment (Wolfe, 461). As he dies, Eugene senses that Ben is finally "detached from the terrible chemistry of the flesh" (Wolfe, 462)—literally, the destruction of delicate lung tissue and the interruption of oxygen transmission to the blood.

Katherine Anne Porter, Pale Horse, Pale Rider *(1936)*

Katherine Anne Porter (1890–1980), while a reporter for *The Rocky Mountain News* in Denver, Colorado, contracted the flu in the fall of 1918 at the age of 28. She recovered, after suffering through the illness and after enduring complications from a subsequent fall. By the spring of 1919, she had physically recovered, but her fiancé died of the disease (Crosby, 317–318). Her experience is memorialized in the novella, *Pale Horse, Pale Rider* (1936), the title of which was adapted from an African American spiritual, the lyrics of which had been derived, in turn, from Revelation 6:8. St. John of Patmos beholds, "a pale green horse! Its rider's name was Death, and Hades followed with him; they were given authority over a fourth of the earth, to kill with sword, famine, and pestilence, and by the wild animals of the earth" ("The Revelation to John," 6:8; 429).

An aspect of the story, which has stimulated commentary, is the nightmare experience of the central character, Miranda. Contemporary medical observers believed that influenza "could alter mental processes," and delirium brought on by high fever was a common and very distressing symptom (Barry, 378). *The American Diagnostic and Statistical Manual of Mental Disorders* defines delirium as an "acute, transient, global, organic disorder(s) of higher nervous system function involving impaired consciousness and attention" (Taylor & Lewis, 742). Diagnostic criteria for delirium are eightfold: (1) the reduced ability to maintain attention to external stimuli; (2) disorganized thinking with rambling, irrelevant or incoherent speech; (3) reduced level of consciousness; (4) perceptual disturbances; (5) sleep-wake cycle disturbances; (6) increased or decreased psychomotor activity; (7) time, place, or personal disorientation; (8) and memory impairment. Delirium is associated with an etiological disorder (743)—in this case, with influenza.

Among the symptoms of delirium, as the Mayo Clinic points out, is difficulty staying focused on an idea or changing topics randomly ("Delirium: Symptoms"). A person in that condition does not respond to questions or carry on conversations well and is easily distracted. The patient, usually with a fever of 105 degrees Fahrenheit or more, can be withdrawn and unresponsive to the environment. Cognitively impaired, this patient has short-term memory loss, is disoriented about location, identity, and time; speaking is difficult, words are hard to find, speech is not understood, and reading or writing is impaired. The person's behavior is affected dramatically: hallucinations, restlessness, agitation, irritability, combative behavior, disturbed sleeping habits, and extreme emotional states (fear, anxiety, anger, and depression) are common. Often overlooked, delirium is a horrific effect of the fevered state. Porter experienced it, and she devotes a significant part of the narrative to describing the condition in an amalgam of recollections, of literary allusions, and of formulaic references.

Porter turned, in part, to Virginia Woolf for a description of the delirium state and was also influenced by Woolf's 1925 essay, "On Being Ill" (Belling, 64–65). Woolf refers to delirious states brought on by seasonal influenza and other disorders, conditions that disclose to mind and spirit, "undiscovered countries." The power of illness to disrupt one's mind and physical condition should be "among the prime themes of literature." Ironically, she quips: "Novels, one would have thought, would have been devoted to influenza" ("On Being Ill," 193).

The nightmare episode in *Pale Horse, Pale Rider* owes a considerable debt to Porter's reading of Woolf's first novel. Catherine Belling astutely observes that "Porter's account is informed as much by Woolf's description of fever as it is by Porter's memory of her own," specifically to the latter's first novel, *The Voyage Out* (1915) (67). The persona of Miranda may have been influenced, specifically, by the character of Rachel Vinace who dies a febrile and delirious death in *The Voyage Out* (Belling, 68–69). Let us look at Rachel Vinace's symptoms using the *Diagnostic Manual* and the Mayo Clinic report as guides.

As Rachel Vinace becomes febrile, she exhibits cognitive impairment consistent with the Mayo Clinic description. Stricken by an infectious disease causing high fever, most likely by influenza, an endemic outbreak of which happened in 1915, Rachel complains of severe headache and becomes prostrate. Unable to keep "her attention fixed" during Terence's recitation of Milton's verse (Woolf, 326–327), she drifts off "upon curious trains of thought suggested by [random] words ... which brought unpleasant sights before her eyes, independently of meaning" (Woolf, 327); thus, she is cognitively impaired. In addition to her inability to understand spoken words, she experiences visual disjunctions between images and their meaning. The garden begins to look strange, and her spatial perception becomes distorted: "the trees were either too near or too far, and her head almost certainly ached" (Woolf, 327). Rachel, achy and febrile, goes to bed and begins to experience "a transparent kind of sleep," as her consciousness is altered. Sensitivity to light and the impression that flat surfaces are curved as in migraine headache are aspects of her visual disturbance. Hallucinations follow: the movement of the blind and the drawing of the cord across the floor suggest animal movements which frighten her. With high fever, chills, and severe headache, she tries but fails to leave her bed (Woolf, 328).

In the afternoon of the second day, when again she attempts to walk, she finds that the fever and discomfort have "put a gulf between her world and the ordinary world which she could not bridge" (Woolf, 329). Though she understands what the doctor is saying to her, she becomes withdrawn: "drowsy and intolerably hot"; and she barely answers the doctor's questions. During the second day of her illness, Rachel's existential space shrinks to the rectangular parameters of her bed; and the outside world, "when she tried to think of it, appeared distinctly further off" (Woolf, 329). Gradually, all "landmarks were obliterated," which includes diurnal periods and points of reference, and the outer world dilates to a point beyond her consciousness. Her short-term memory loss becomes acute: "The recollection of what she felt, or of what she had been doing and thinking three days before, had entirely faded" (Woolf, 330). She had to make an effort "to remember certain facts from the world that was so many millions of miles away" (Woolf, 332). Paralysis ensues, as she "was completely cut off, and unable to communicate with the rest of the world, isolated alone with her body" (Woolf, 330). The preposition "with" instead of "in" signifies that her mind is receding from her physical self. The sense of duration and of time units dissipates: night and day, hours and minutes become meaningless. Night is not a twelve hour period; it had become "interminable." Her nurse becomes a shadowy, sinister figure (Woolf, 330–331). Bad dreams erupt when she shuts her eyes (Woolf, 331).

Rachel deteriorates to the point that her lips are drawn, cheeks sunken and flushed, but colorless. Her eyes are half shut (Woolf, 339). Oblivious to the world outside, she struggles to focus on those around her: Helen, Terence, the nurse, and the doctor. But she cannot concentrate and must begin again. An awful aspect of delirium is the sense of submergence; however, the body is not immersed in an external body of water; instead, the fluid build-up is internal. Thus, she perceives herself "at the bottom of the sea. There she lay, sometimes seeing darkness, sometimes light, while every now and then someone turned her over at the bottom of the sea" (Woolf, 341). Her descent into darkness continues. Conscious of what was around her, she is brought to the surface of awareness on a wave only to re-descend, her perception being translucent, "very pale and semi-transparent" (Woolf, 346–347). She dies peacefully (Woolf, 353).

Porter's Miranda experiences symptoms very similar to Rachel's. To the landlady's query about her being in a dressing gown, Miranda responds, acutely aware of her imminent trial, "influenza, I think." (Porter, 181). The delirious state gradually engulfs Miranda as her temperature spikes. As she experiences chills, indicating the body's reaction to cool itself down, hallucinations occur. She perceives the Rocky Mountains rising around her, "chilling her to the bone" (Porter, 182); in need of warmth, she is instantly plunged into a tropical hallucination, one from her past, but the scene is dense jungle, stifling, dappled with dark shadows, and vultures hover above. The bedroom walls suddenly disappear, and a strange maritime scene develops at the foot of her bed: a ship moored to a pier is shrouded in darkness. A second jungle scene emerges, a mélange of all that she has ever seen or known about such an environment. This tropical hallucination, unlike the idyllic earlier ones, is disturbingly vivid. Porter's imagery is also chimeric: writhing serpents, "rainbow-colored birds with malign eyes," humanized leopards, screaming primates, and tangled, decomposing flora. She envisions herself exiting her body and boarding a slender ship which flies into the jungle. The imagery strangely fuses the hellish triptychs of Hieronymus Bosch (1450?-1516), such as in the *Last Judgment* (1506), the disturbing incubi of Henry Fuseli (1741–1825), as in the *Nightmare* (1782), and cartoonish animals in the tropical paintings of Henri Rousseau (1844–1910), such as *The Jungle* or *The Sleeping Gypsy*. There are auditory hallucinations as well, a cacophony of screams, bellows, and cries of "danger" and "war."(Porter, 182–183).

From this tumult of sensuous imagery, she ascends to semi-consciousness as she sees and hears Adam Barclay arguing with the landlady about Miranda's condition as the ambulance arrives; the landlady, Miss Hobbe, is justifiably agitated that Miranda poses a contagious threat to her and the other tenants: "'I tell you, they must come for her now, or I'll put her on the sidewalk ... I tell you, this is a plague, a plague, my God, and I've got a houseful of people to think about!'" (Porter, 183). Both Miranda and Adam are acutely aware of the pestilence and of the threat of contagion. Adam's leave was extended because men in his camp were "dying like flies," succumbing to "This funny new disease" (Porter, 185). When Miranda is sick, Adam describes how extensive the pandemic had become: "It's as bad as anything can be ... all the theaters and nearly all the shops and restaurants are closed, and the streets have been full of funerals all day and ambulances all night" (Porter, 184). Even though

Miranda is glad to see Adam, she warns him that he is "running a risk" (Porter, 184).

Porter permits the reader to trace Miranda's worsening condition back to the moment of contagion in October, when she had volunteered for the Red Cross and was exposed to mixed convalescent soldiers in barracks (Porter, 150–51); complained of feeling "rotten" (Porter, 159); felt a cold coming on (Porter, 161); and became disorientated and anxious: "This is the beginning of the end of something. Something terrible is going to happen to me" (Porter, 170). She experiences aches and anxiety: "I have pains in my chest and my head and my heart and they're real. I am in pain all over, and you are in such danger as I can't bear to think about, and why can we not save each other?" (Porter, 178). Prostrate and incoherent, she is diagnosed as having influenza (Porter, 180–181).

After her initial hallucinations, Miranda experiences an interlude of fevered semi-consciousness, during which she speaks with Adam about mundane and religious matters. Throughout the dialogue, she clings desperately to waking consciousness, so as not to sink into the abysmal disorder and dissociated thought-patterns of delirium. When she offers to sing a hymn to the Greek god Apollo, Adam thinks she is trying to be funny when, in fact, she is using all her strength to stay awake: "I'm trying to keep from going to sleep. I'm afraid to go to sleep. I may not wake up. Don't let me go to sleep" (Porter, 188). Despite the caffeine intake, she slips momentarily out of conscious awareness, and her head is claustrophobically submerged in darkness, at which point her mind suddenly clears, and she bolts upright, "in panic, throwing off the covers and breaking into a sweat. Adam leaped up with an alarmed face, and almost at once was holding a cup of hot coffee to her mouth" (Porter, 189).

The third nightmarish sequence begins when Miranda, who by this time is completely exhausted, sinks into a delirious fugue in which she, like Rachel Vinace, suddenly has no sense of time and space. Fixed in the present moment, she no longer is aware of Adam's physical presence in the room (Porter, 190). She has now entered a state of consciousness that Porter attempts to differentiate from an ordinary dream, although formulaic imagery might have been included here for literary effect or because it is difficult to retrieve disordered and fleeting recollections; for example, Miranda finds herself in a foreboding world: she is in a forest, and a din of "concealed voices [are] singing sharply." Adam appears and is struck repeatedly by arrows, a classical symbol of plague infection and an obvious literary allusion (*The Iliad*, I, 383–384).

Emerging from this episode, Miranda then perceives Adam deceased and then resurrected. Miranda is immediately running through the forest in terror, at which point she jolts back to ordinary time and out of this "odd sort of dream." At this juncture, the fugue state ends: the dream of running through the forest, in reality, was her jumping out of the bed, running across the room, and into Adam's arms, an act akin to sleepwalking, of which she had no conscious recollection (Porter, 191). Miranda tries to recount her nightmare, which is a lucid and deliberate intention, but she cannot articulate her thoughts, indicating psychomotor dysfunction or what one may experience when awakening from anesthesia.

When an ambulance arrives to transport Miranda to a hospital, she says goodbye to Adam twice, thinking that she was awake; actually, as the narrator explains, she only thought she had said goodbye (Porter, 192). As an intern examines her, she experiences another classic symptom of delirium: a disconnection between intention and action in the neuromotor processes of speech. Believing herself to be awake, she exclaims, "I know what I want to say," but she is shocked to hear babbling. Complaints and chatter are the means through which she maintains a tenuous connection to the external world: "anything, anything at all to keep her small hold on the life of human beings, a clean line of communication, no matter what, between her and the receding world" (Porter, 194). When she tries to read a letter from Adam, she sees the page but simply cannot understand the script. Not visually but cognitively impaired, she sees nothing more "than a page full of hasty scratches in black ink" (Porter, 194). Even as the nurse patiently reads the text, Miranda cannot join two thoughts together coherently; thus, "hearing the words one by one, [she] forgot them one by one" (Porter, 195).

As Miranda is wheeled on a gurney through the hospital corridor, hallucinations encroach upon her from all sides. The walls become white cliffs; the ceiling lights, moons. Opaque against the curtain while preparing a dead body for removal, hospital personnel are perceived as dancing a macabre waltz. As the corpse is bound and wheeled away, the image persists. A delirium terror commences as a white fog rises in Miranda's runaway thoughts. The fog conceals abstract emotions, "all terror and all weariness." Behind the fog is incarnate human suffering, not an abstract symbol but an organic, writhing mass of "wrung faces and twisted backs and broken and abused, outraged living things, all the shapes of their confused pain and their estranged hearts" (Porter, 196).

The fog parts and the hospital scene replays. The staff is transformed in Miranda's mind into executioners who push along an old Lazarus-like man who, for some reason, is slated for execution, even though he pleads that he is innocent of any crime (Porter, 196). She imagines the German-American physician who is caring for her, Dr. Hildesheim in a familiar and graphic propaganda poster: Hildesheim as a German soldier with a baby impaled on his bayonet (Porter, 197). As "her mind tottered and slithered," Miranda hears the doctor comment that she is a shouter rather than a runner, referring to the tendency of the delirious patient to bolt away. Suddenly, an even more terrible phase of the psychological disorder begins.

As Miranda's consciousness, once again, recedes from normal awareness, she experiences a cognitive phenomenon in which "her mind splits in two [and] acknowledged and denied what she saw in one instant." According to the omniscient narrator, Miranda is undergoing a kind of psychic fragmentation in which she no longer distinguishes between waking consciousness and nightmare, and this bifurcation is evident to her from a self-reflective distance, removed from the cascade of disordered perceptions. The cogitations of a divided mind are in full view of "her reasoning coherent self [which] watched the strange frenzy of the other coldly, reluctant to admit the truth of its visions, its tenacious remorse and despairs" (Porter, 198). The bifurcation, in addition, releases irrational thoughts, vividly perceived but understood as being unreal. She knows, for example, that Miss Tanner's hands are her hands, but to Miranda they appear to be white tarantulas (Porter, 198). The nurse, who thinks the hallucination is visual rather than neurological, tells Miranda to shut her eyes. Shutting her eyes, however, makes things worse: it removes her from exterior stimuli. Thus, she replies: "On no ... for I see worse things." But the illness pulls her away, nonetheless, and, as the omniscient narrator remarks, "her internal torment closed about her" (Porter, 198).

Without warning, Miranda descends to an insensate level of consciousness. She imagines a descent or harrowing that is indescribable. Her descent into darkness approaches the "farthest bottom of life." Her senses become inoperative: she knows herself "to be blind, deaf, speechless, no longer aware of the members of her own body" (Porter, 199); and she is separated from all human contact. Although family ties "fell away from her," she is not consumed in the depths; rather, the irreducible core of her being is revealed to, and as, herself. In a state of "serene rapture" and spatiotemporal displacement, she winds up on a rock ledge and then proceeds to run into a meadow and towards the sun. On a beach, she sees all the human beings she had ever known. Each is transfigured in beauty, their features enhanced, and their bodies "cast no shadows." Porter's vision is of living souls, "pure identities," whose presence she apprehends intuitively. Mingling with them, she gazes seaward, beholding an eternal and "overwhelming deep sky" (Porter, 200). The scene evokes a passage in Revelation of the white-robed redeemed souls "who have come out of the great ordeal," and who stand "before the throne of God" (7:13–15, 431).

From this vision, Miranda is instantaneously transported onto a stony path of slippery snow and realizes that she must return. Directionless and confused, she feels a burning pain, which signals her gradual ascent to her senses. The stabbing pain is actually the effect of an inoculation. She smells the odor of her own illness, the fetor typical of the disease, and she awakes to see Miss Tanner, the nurse, and Dr. Hildesheim administering an injection. Miranda awakens from her "dreamless sleep" precisely on 11 November 1918, the day the Armistice was signed. Her battle for life is won on that day of peace.

Has the near-death experience and interior journey affected Porter's persona in any significant way? Miranda states that her physical self is not what constitutes her true self. In fact, she loathes and distrusts her corporeal self, calling her body "a curious monster, no place to live in," and an alien habitation in which her spiritual being is immured ("how could anyone feel at home there?"; and is it possible "I can ever accustom myself to this place?") (Porter, 203). Her post-visionary experience is not a spiritual resolution in the orthodox sense; she has not emerged from her harrowing radically changed by the experience. Instead, she views her surroundings with "the covertly hostile eyes of an alien who does not like the country in which he finds himself" (Porter, 203). Emerging from her great ordeal, Miranda seems to have brought back no profound insight into the mystery of life, other than having being plunged into the organic pit of mortality.

Miranda learns from a one-month old letter, that Adam Barclay, like tens of thousands of other servicemen, had succumbed to influenza in a camp, and it is at this point that her recovery begins (Porter, 206). She must grieve for Adam and for her pre-influenzal self, both now gone. A denizen of a gray area, she stands astride two ontologies, "one foot in either world" (Porter, 207). She yearns to meet others of her kind, not to convey a spiritual message regarding the afterlife, but to commiserate with fellow survivors whose better fortune is attributed, not to providence, but to chance: she, therefore, "shall visit the escaped ones and help them dress and tell them how lucky they are, and how lucky I am still to have them" (Porter 208). Her philosophical resolution is incongruent with the providential vision of Revelation.

Miranda's frame of mind mirrors that of Porter's in the aftermath of the pandemic. Porter recalls how the illness had "divided" her life, altering it in "some strange way." After the disease and subsequent health problems resolved, she needed psychological healing. She had great difficulty going out into the world because she felt "alienated," since she had "participated in death" (*Conversations*, 85). Indeed, Porter had direct knowledge of the modernist conceptualization "of the human subject as a fragmented, hybrid, and self-contradictory being" (Hovanec, 165). Why then did Porter return to the fevered and near-death experience in her fiction? There is no triumph of the human spirit exhorted at its end. The story ends rather anti-climactically and perhaps too realistically. Miranda survives but the character seems to construe her survival as a random event. The delirium state, however, is interesting as a clinical exemplum. Porter seems to be re-exploring the neuropsychiatric effects of influenza, presenting herself as a case study.

John O'Hara, "The Doctor's Son" *(1935)*

John O'Hara's "The Doctor's Son" is a semi-autobiographical story set in northeastern Pennsylvania, in the region of Montgomery, Berks, and Schuylkill counties, where mining is a major industry. There, Dr. Michael Malloy, one of the protagonists, will find himself working excessive hours to treat influenza cases among the impoverished ethnic minorities. O'Hara's fiction has an important epidemiological message: it dramatizes how the pandemic affected urban and rural areas in different ways. If regional populations differed from each other in terms of ethnicity and livelihood, these factors had to be considered in order to assess the incidence, distribution, and control of disease. The problem was complex: the urban poor and the rural poor both had substandard living conditions and inadequate medical care, but the population densities and environments they each inhabited were radically different from one another. These factors were directly involved in determining how quickly the virus spread. A historian (Crosby), a young medical student (Dr. Starr), and an autobiographer/fictionist (O'Hara) help us to understand how people in Pennsylvania faced influenza. So many medical professionals and citizens during the catastrophic second wave acted selflessly and resolutely, and these behavioral characteristics underlies the pandemic fiction of O'Hara and Stegner. Although O'Hara's fiction is set in rural Pennsylvania, I would like to preface the discussion with two authoritative accounts of how the pandemic impacted Philadelphia.

Alfred Crosby's depiction of the pandemic in Philadelphia, an index of the urban experience nationwide, is characterized by three elements: public health unpreparedness, frustration and helplessness on the part of the populous and medical community, and determined volunteerism (70–90). He describes the anticipation and readiness of the first-rate, though understaffed, public health system in the summer of 1918, just before the second wave struck. As the disease became entrenched, three factors weakened the city's ability to withstand the surge: a false sense of security fostered by the unfounded claim that a bacillus was the initiating pathogen; the downplaying of the crisis in the news and in medical literature; and poorly- informed health officials.

When the flu manifested itself on 1 October 1918, the city was unprepared, staggered under the blow, but then tried to right itself by closing amusement venues and schools, and by cancelling public gatherings, but all with little effect. Statistics speak for themselves, and the author uses them to stress how the public health system was inundated in a matter of weeks. Essential services were short-circuited, mortuaries overwhelmed, and the slums—where people routinely struggled with chronic illnesses, poor sanitation, and bad nutrition—had few medical personnel and social workers to help them. Crosby cites the crisis point in Philadelphia as the week of 12–19 October, when a reported 4,597 people died of influenza and of complicating pneumonia. Although the mortality rate was low with respect to the total population, the immigrant slums suffered the worst.

To reinstitute order, the city set up a kind of 9–1–1 service. Non-medical personnel, whom the newly-created Bureau of Information had peremptorily trained, were dispatched to make house calls. The city was subdivided into seven geographical districts to optimize medical care, but these measures, too, fell short. Food centers, shelters, and a medley of transportation alternatives were improvised to sustain those who were not sick and to aid those who were. Many secular and religious organizations pitched in, and volunteers were plentiful, even though risking contact with the disease. The dissemination of a vaccine of arguable worth revived the false sense of security, a kind of placebo effect on a social scale. As the second wave began to recede slightly in late October, schools, theaters, and houses of worship were re-opened—prematurely, they would soon learn. Crosby's research on the Philadelphia experience is built solidly from the brick and mortar of public health, government, and medical reports. These are worked into a chronological matrix, with two dozen newspaper articles, largely from the *Philadelphia Inquirer*, reflecting the public's thinking throughout the crisis.

Crosby was aware that, because of physician shortages, medical school students had been reassigned "from the lecture hall and laboratory directly to the sick rooms and wards and the abrupt assumption of the responsibilities of mature physicians" (81). To see the Philadelphia crisis through the eyes of medical personnel, engaged in feverish and often frustrating duties, imparts a vicarious sense of the catastrophe, Nancy K. Bristow pointing to this genre's capacity to restore the American memory of the pandemic (*American Pandemic*, 8).

Isaac Starr, M.D.'s memoir, "Influenza in 1918: Recollections of the Epidemic in Philadelphia," complements Crosby's historiography. In the summer of 1918, during the hiatus (late August-early September 1918) between the first and second waves, the author was about to enter his third year of medical school at the University of Pennsylvania. Although he and his friends had enlisted for military service, they had not yet been called up. Late in August, as the second wave was about to hit forcefully, Starr heard a news report of an epidemic in Spain. Returning to Philadelphia from a vacation in Massachusetts, he learned that a British freighter with influenza cases was nearing Philadelphia. The British consul arranged for the university hospital to prepare suitable accommodations to receive the sick men. Twenty-five Indian seamen were to be hospitalized when the vessel docked, and it was determined that they suffered from an unfamiliar and severe pneumonia.

After the medical school opened, Starr recalls a mid–September conference and an impromptu lecture on influenza, in which a senior physician described putative forms of the disease but cautioned that no treatment had been effective during the pandemic of 1889–1890. Three days later, Starr and his peers learned that an epidemic was developing and, since medical practitioners were away in the army, the students' services were urgently needed to care for the sick. For third- and fourth-year students, the medical school was closed. An emergency hospital was set up containing 75 beds. When the 25 seamen arrived, fourth-year students acted as interns, while third-year students acted as nurses. One trained nurse was on staff, and all medical personnel, who were attired in gowns, were given infectious disease precautions.

At the outset, the patient population on Starr's floor included Philadelphia residents, none of whom was very ill, except for slight fevers. But the level of concern rose drastically, as patients began to present with acute pulmonary distress, pneumonia, cyanosis, delirium, incontinence, and bloody expectorations. Many patients died without ever receiving medical care. Starr recalled learning techniques and remedies from a cadre of retired physicians; no remedy had any appreciable effect on conditions. As people died, Starr innovated, using atropine and camphor; neither helped. Too tired to experiment and to record evidence, he reflects on how their interventions were useless. Many died after a day or two of agony.

Starr soon learned that a triage system was in place, as the most seriously ill were concentrated on his floor. Hospital deaths reached 25 percent per night during the peak of the pandemic. Bodies were thrown from the cellar into trucks for disposal. Volunteers, both secular and clerical, turned up to help. Any place of public assembly was temporarily closed. Starr and other medical students would drive into the slums and be mobbed by citizens imploring them for help. As reinforcements arrived, conditions improved. After two weeks, presumably by the end of October, deaths declined in number and, by the beginning of November, the worst had ended. A mild febrile condition which Starr contracted appeared infrequently thereafter. Thus, "as mysteriously as it had come, the killer departed." Medical school resumed after this five-week interruption ("Recollections").

Starr's account, published in 1976 (coincidentally, with the first edition of Crosby's study, originally titled *Epidemic and Peace: 1918*) was prompted by the 1976 alarm over the possibility of another influenza outbreak, and his story gained currency in 1977–1978 when it was learned that human H1N1 viruses (descendants of the 1918 killer virus) had re-entered the human population via a foreign laboratory containment breach, the details of which are obscure (Taubenberger & Morens, "1918 Influenza," 15).

Starr intuited that the 1918 disaster could help with future preparedness. As if in answer to Starr, Drs. Taubenberger and Morens explain that, "Despite an explosion of data on the 1918 virus in the past decade [mid–1990s], we are not much closer to understanding pandemic emergence in 2006 than we were in understanding the risk of H1N1 'swine flu' emergence in 1976" ("1918 Influenza," 21). Starr's Philadelphia experience was not unique, as the survey in chapter 1 shows; in fact, as he points out, the flu's pathophysiology clearly had two stages: a prequel, for most a moderate febrile disease that came and went in one week. However, for a "distressing number of patients," the mild illness gave way to pulmonary complications. The cyanosis that resulted suggested that the "black death" had returned. Each night, about one fifth of the patients died.

A future pandemic, Dr. Starr stated in 1976, could be handled better than that of 1918–1919. Central to the possibility of improvement, he remarks, is the theory that "the initial mild illness was of viral origin and the pulmonary complications of bacterial origin," as some conjectured in 1918. Starr rightly deduces that, if antibiotics had been available in 1918–1919 to have prevented bacterial pneumonia, the mortality rate would have been greatly diminished; thus, in 1976, he attributed most of the fatalities to the pneumonic sequel. Pathologists have recently corroborated Starr's speculations.

John O'Hara's "The Doctor's Son" (1935) was written 17 years after the pandemic. The author who was 13 years old in 1918 had routinely observed his father, Dr. Patrick O'Hara, while at work during the outbreak. Dr. O'Hara received his medical degree at the University of Pennsylvania, in Philadelphia (MacShane, 4–5, 10). According to Frank Macshane's incisive biography, Dr. O'Hara was a gifted surgeon. Moving to Schuylkill Haven, Pennsylvania, he was appointed surgeon at the county hospital and superintendent of the local insane asylum. In 1896, the doctor moved to Pottsville, approximately 70 miles northwest of Philadelphia. There he became a resident surgeon. Establishing a private practice in Pottsville, he regularly treated Irish miners and other European migrants who lived in impoverished villages near coal mines. As noted above, Dr. O'Hara did not lose contact with modern medicine. He travelled weekly to Philadelphia to observe medical procedures at Lackenaw Hospital where he conferred with his mentor, Dr. John Deaver. Accompanied by Dr. Swaving, Doctor O'Hara also went to Europe, at this time, to study modern surgery in Italy. His visits to Rome and Turin allowed him to learn conversational Italian which he would use when treating Italian immigrant patients who lived in Palo Alto, Pennsylvania, on the outskirts of Pottsville. On a weekly basis, he would also visit Philadelphia and his alma mater, the University of Pennsylvania. With his professional career established, Dr. O'Hara married Katharine Delaney of Lykens, a town 30 miles southwest of Pottsville. The couple settled in Pottsville. John, born on 31 January 1905, was the first of eight children.

John, who was 13 in 1918, along with his brothers would accompany their father on house calls. The caseload would increase dramatically with the outbreak. Before the pandemic broke, Dr. O'Hara had established himself as a dedicated and well-respected physician who allowed nothing to impede his work. On call 24/7, he responded to rural locations with the help of his sons. John had acquired some knowledge of medicine in the field when the second wave of the pandemic struck the area and, in 1935, fictionalized the story.

Philadelphia had a population of two million in 1918, and its densely populated ethnic ghettos, according to one historian, were susceptible to rapidly spreading diseases. Because of the war, medical resources were at a reduced level: more than 26 percent of its physicians were overseas, along with 75 percent of hospital-based doctors (Armstrong, "Philadelphia"). As Crosby points out, the flu had arrived in Europe in July; it reached Boston in the third week of September, but Philadelphia did not publicize these facts, nor did it issue a warning. A false sense of security came when Dr. Paul A. Lewis, director of the Phipps Institute of Philadelphia, announced having isolated the inciting pathogen (he would die of yellow fever in 1929) (Crosby 71, 298–299). A high death rate ensued because of these factors and the city's unpreparedness. By early October, all public venues were temporarily and belatedly closed, and the law mandated the wearing of face masks.

Dr. O'Hara was in the midst of the pandemic, his practice having extended from Philadelphia, which he continued to visit, to the mining and farming communities in and around Pottsville. The events described in "The Doctor's Son" are, therefore, both transparently autobiographical and an authentic representation of the pandemic in eastern Pennsylvania. The story, published in 1935, coincided with fantastic strides in the areas of influenza virology and immunology. John O'Hara, though only 13 at the time of the disaster, remembered the period through his father's labors and directly as he assisted him. While much of the scholarship is understandably concerned with characterization and social commentary in the stories, our focus is on the doctor rather than the son, on his microbial antagonist, and on the difficult social barriers with which he, his son, colleagues, and neighbors had to contend.

The accounts by Drs. Grist, Vaughan, Starr, and others convey how overwhelming the pandemic was and how frustrating it was to treat. O'Hara's fiction reproduces these refractory conditions. James Malloy/John O'Hara is acutely aware of his father's labors during the crisis. In the opening paragraph, James describes, in first-person narration, how his father had been making house calls for three days, getting only two hours' sleep per day. Arriving home on the fourth consecutive morning, Dr. Malloy was so exhausted that he forgot to shut the car off, its engine running through the night, but then slept for two days straight through. Because of the non-stop calls for house visits and care, the doctor could only sleep peacefully if sequestered. Thus, he would sleep on an operating table in back of his darkened office. He would have a loaded revolver at his side to protect himself against irate and desperate patients, though this self-defensiveness did not affect his dedication, nor did it cloud his sympathy, especially for immigrants who were dying in great numbers (O'Hara, 5). This kind of dedication was typical of so many overworked doctors. B. Franklin Royer, M.D., in a letter to the editors of *JAMA* complains that large numbers of Pennsylvania's physicians are contracting influenza, "because they are indifferent to danger and careless about protecting themselves from the spray of moisture from the mouth of the patient" (1431). Because physicians had to see so many patients, they were unconcerned about their own health during examinations, not wearing gauze masks and not insisting that the patient cover the cough or sneeze in a handkerchief. "The sick rate among physicians and the death rate are appalling," he writes, but this trend was reversible if physicians observed the kind of precautions used when examining tuberculosis patients (Royer, 1431).

Dr. Malloy's practice during the pandemic had also grown unwieldy. No longer did he see his usual complement of 40 patients per day. When the epidemic worsened, in early October, he simply lost count. Under normal circumstances, if he had become ill, a young physician would have covered him. With the war ongoing, however, that coverage was no longer available: "now every young doctor was as busy as the older men." For young general practitioners who had been trying to acquire patients, the load was becoming unmanageable. The community was hard hit. Mines closed down "with the first whiff of influenza." Anyone with a chronic lung condition, such as the occupational hazard called black-lung disease, never had a chance against "the mysterious new disease" (6); "even the younger men were keeling over," probably due to the unregulated immune response, of which little was known for certain in the period from 1918 to 1935. The Commonwealth of Pennsylvania finally ordered all schools, churches, and public congregating to stop. Simple pleasures were given ominous overtones: ice cream sodas were now served in cardboard containers rather than in fountain glasses. For young James Malloy, the implications of the outbreak are unrealized. He reflects how he and his friends were happy that the schools in Gibbsville had been closed; but, more somberly, they acknowledged that influenza struck mining communities hard.

Just as Dr. Starr had related in his letter, because of the physician shortage, the state had no choice but to deploy fourth-year medical students from a Philadelphia school to unmanned practices, which was how Dr. Myers came to Gibbsville to take over Dr. Malloy's practice while the latter got his strength back. Both Myers (a fourth-year student like Starr) and Dr. Malloy had studied at the University of Pennsylvania and were proud of their institution (O'Hara, 7). Myers, accompanied by young James Malloy, began to treat European immigrants, most of whom were miners, and many of whom did not take public health advice very seriously, as exemplified in their house call to Mr. Wisniewski, an inebriated, flu-stricken miner (O'Hara, 26–27).

The ironic undercurrent of O'Hara's story is that, despite the valiant struggles of doctors and other public health workers, little could be done to stop influenza's deadly course. It spared no segment of the population, spreading most widely in rundown, overcrowded dwellings, amidst a poorly-nourished population, already subject to contagious diseases, such as diphtheria and polio. One's social status offered no immunity. Mr. David Evans, Doctor Malloy's good friend, was district superintendent of a large mining corporation, an important businessman in Collieryville, Pennsylvania. The Malloys learn of his unexpected death from influenza. He died within one week of their having seen him in good health. Once the epidemic had subsided in November 1918, James recalled how his relationship with Edith Evans, David Evans' daughter, simply faded away (O'Hara, 32). The infection abated in November, only to reappear as a third wave of misery.

Wallace Stegner, The Big Rock Candy Mountain *(1938)*

Wallace Stegner is said to have used the pandemic "as an incidental factor" in his best seller, *The Big Rock Candy Mountain* (1938) (Crosby, 316). Although the pandemic scene is, indeed, one incident in the tragic saga of the Mason family, more can be said about its relevance to the central theme of the moral character. Stegner explores the human experience of the outbreak and focuses on the idea of how members of a community can cooperate with each other during a medical crisis.

The influenza scene in the novel conflates three semi-autobiographical aspects of the author's life. The first was the blizzard of 1916, in which the temperature dropped to 51 degrees below zero Fahrenheit, and winds were clocked at 80-miles per hour. Wallace who was seven years old, found himself trapped with his fellow students and teachers in a school house, where they remained for over 24 hours until his father George and others rescued them (Benson, 30, 32).The second element is the persona of Harry "Bo" Mason, modeled, in part, on George Stegner who had bootlegged whiskey between Montana and Saskatchewan; the family had moved to Great Falls, Montana, in the spring of 1920, as the pandemic receded, and lived there until June 1921.

The third element, of course, is the 1918 pandemic itself, which also appears in Stegner's novel, *On a Darkling Plain* (1940). In *The Big Rock Candy Mountain*, the disease fills the fictional schoolhouse with sick and dying townsfolk in a matter of two days. Stegner writes that the crisis affected everyone, "either as a patient or victim or helper. A tenth of the town died, besides a lot of farmers who had crowded in to be of help. The cemetery was a lonesome place thereafter, and the bonds between the survivors were stronger" (quoted in Benson, 30). Benson observes that trials such as these turned the town into a community, in the fullest social sense of the word (30). Profound instances of social interaction, of selfless courage, charity, and moral responsibility, impressed nine-year-old Wallace. These three recollections are fused in the pandemic scenes of *The Big Rock Candy Mountain* (1938). Bo Mason, like George Stegner in the midst of a blizzard, puts the welfare of another person before himself, and the town which has transformed the schoolhouse into a hospital works together for the common good.

Unlike many of their neighbors who understandably shunned contact with each other during the second pandemic wave of October-November 1918, the Masons, Harry ("Bo"), his wife Elsa, and their sons Bruce and Chester, reach out to their neighbors during the crisis, and they do so at great peril to themselves. In the 1986 article, "*The Big Rock Candy Mountain*: The Consequences of a Delusory American Dream," Kenneth C. Mason characterizes Bo as a social outlaw, "a misfit and malcontent," as one who recognizes "no law or order that restricts or threatens his own best interests." In this critic's view, Bo is a creature of appetite, one who is not only socially irresponsible, but also "careless of family," stubbornly defiant, and consumed by his materialism (Mason, 35). These pejoratives fit a character who physically abuses his children, who abandons his family, and who runs a bootlegging business. But in the sometimes glossed-over chapter on pandemic influenza, the reader may find a more redeemable figure, one who puts the welfare of his family and of a relative stranger before profit and his own well-being.

In late–October 1918, the residents of Whitemud, a town modeled on Stegner's boyhood town of Eastend, southern Saskatchewan, hear rumors that the flu is moving westward. Bo overhears farmers in a pool hall expressing their fear, which is intensifying because of their rural isolation. One man says: "Suppose ... a whole family got sick with this flu, and no help around, and winter setting in solid and cold three weeks early?" (Stegner 246). Valid medical information is sparse and rumors are rife; for example, Bo hears "how the disease turned you black as ink first before it killed you, and how people in the last stage rose from their beds and ran screaming and gibbering through the streets, foaming at the mouth and biting anyone who got in their way" (Stegner, 246). The rumors originate from clinical realities, one physiological and the other psychological. The first reference ("black as ink") is to cyanosis, from the Greek *kyanosis* ("dark blue color"), describing the bluish or purplish discoloration of the skin resulting from deficient oxygenation of the blood. John M. Barry writes that, "In 1918 cyanosis was so extreme, turning some victims so dark—the entire body could take on color resembling that of the veins in one's wrist—it sparked rumors that the disease was not influenza at all, but the Black Death." The psychological disturbances brought on by the disease ranged from mental inertia to frenzy. At the most frenetic extreme is "maniacal frenzy" (*Influenza*, 187–189, 378–379). The image of paroxysmal flight is, therefore, a possible effect of the disease. Dr. O'Malley, the local physician in the novel, outlines reasonable preventive measures: avoid drafts and cold weather, stay indoors when overheated, and stay out of crowds. The doctor's advice is intended to maintain one's immune system while minimizing the possibility of contagion. O'Malley also informs Bo that towns in northern Montana, just south of the Canadian border, were already under quarantine (Stegner, 249).

Needing money to support his family in the coming spring, Bo decides to bootleg liquor into Montana and to sell it for its supposed medicinal value. Expecting the flu to reach them soon, since it is already reported in Regina, Saskatchewan, Bo sees a window of opportunity; but he must act quickly, for once the quarantine is fully in place, getting in and out of Montana will be nearly impossible. He is determined to cross the border and to return "like an old St. Bernard with a keg around [his] neck" (Stegner, 251). Predictions about the arrival of influenza are accurate: that very day, old Mrs. Reiger comes down with it (Stegner, 254). Seeking a quick profit, Bo promises his family that he will return in one day's time. Should anyone ask where he had gone, he instructs his wife Elsa to say that, "He was being sent for flu medicine" (Stegner, 257).

Traveling by car in a blizzard, Bo stops at the isolated farmhouse of Ole Pederson, an elderly recluse who is showing signs of illness. Aware that the flu is in the area, Pederson is reluctant to allow Bo to stop in and warm up, ironically fearing that the visitor is a carrier. Despite the recluse's anxious inhospitality, Bo feeds him and urges him to accompany him to town where he can receive medical care (Stegner, 259). Ole refuses to go, so Bo proceeds on his way. Crossing the border, he enters Chinook, Montana, to find the town under quarantine, the hospital full of flu patients, and the few residents out and about donning masks (Stegner, 200). Purchasing a good supply of liquor and still on schedule, he prepares to return to Saskatchewan—in the midst of a blizzard and with influenza around him.

On the way up north, he stops at Ole's again to see how the old man is fairing. When he finds him prostrate with the disease, he faces a moral dilemma—one that he resolves without any inner debate or hesitation. Instead of leaving the old man to certain death in order to ensure both his own safety and profit, Bo cares for him, loads him in his vehicle and heads north in search of medical care. Though he has placed himself in direct contact with the flu, risking contagion, Bo nevertheless puts Ole's welfare above his own (Stegner, 266–267). The humanitarian gesture is complicated by serious difficulty, as the car crashes and becomes stuck in a snow drift; during the crisis, Ole is a helpless burden. The crash destroys the bulk of the liquor, and Bo's profit leaks into the snow bank. But eventually, after freeing the car, he gets home. His family tends to Ole, who by this time is febrile, cyanotic, and critical, and arranges to have him transported to the quarantine infirmary.

Elsa, Bo's wife, is also a humanitarian. She assists the Van Dam family when the husband, Jim, falls ill. She brings coal and kindling for the fireplace and arranges for Jim's transport to the schoolhouse, now a makeshift infirmary. Mrs. Van Dam exclaims that Elsa's charitableness has exposed her to contagion: "Oh Lord ... now you've come too close to him [Jim]" (Stegner, 272). To the question of contagion, Elsa replies stoically and knowledgeably: "I'd have got close, one way or another.... None of us can hide away, I guess." At the time, Elsa was unsure of Bo's fate. Later, she reflects on an ironic fact: that the flu killed healthy young men before other segments of the population: it "took the strongest first, the ones with deep chests and wide backs" (Stegner, 280). For Elsa, "shaken by utter panic," the schoolhouse, now a place of intensive care and quarantine, had become "a symbol ... of plague and death because it housed in its four square rooms dozens of sick men and women" (Stegner, 281). Wallace's seventh-grade classroom was the Death Ward. Both Bo and Elsa contract the disease but recover, as does their son Bruce. The Armistice was signed on 11 November 1918, at which time the pandemic began to diminish in intensity, only to recrudesce in the winter of 1919.

The Recovery corpus consists of short stories and scenes embedded in larger works. So, in that sense, one can call the post-pandemic writings a composite of imaginatively rekindled memories. These writings complement each other and form a coherent survival account of how ordinary Americans endured the worst pandemic in human history. Because the medical survey in the first chapter is a record of scientific discovery and technology, it functions both as preface and background to the Recovery corpus. The desire for emotional recovery motivated authors to record what the pandemic had done to them, and their stories are testimonies of survival. The medical corpus records a grudging struggle against a natural threat. Together with the contemporaneous fiction, it constitutes the first phase of the influenza narrative.

3

Fiction of the Recursion Period: 2005–2006

In their imaginative recursions to 1918–1919, Myla Goldberg, Reina James, Thomas Mullen, and James Rada, Jr., explore important ethical, social, and public health issues of the period. While the Recovery writers memorialize their experiences in fiction, the Recursion writers, with the exception of Reina James whose grandparents were victims of the pandemic, are concerned foremost with biomedical dilemmas and controversies (James, Dust Jacket). A Recursion novel resembles the scenario, a subgenre discussed in chapter 5: both are dramatic renditions of a biological emergency; both reveal human foibles and institutional vulnerabilities and strengths; and both predict outcomes from existing conditions. Like the attack scenario, the Recursion novels focus on difficult public health and social welfare problems. Both forms incorporate defensive strategies: the scenario, against terrorism; and the Recursion novel, against the 1918 pandemic. The comparison also extends to the notion that defensive strategies against either natural or manufactured threats are not fool-proof. Thus, the Recursion authors highlight the tragic lessons of 1918–1919: the violation of human rights in life-or-death situations; unprepared governments and medical systems overwhelmed in a crisis; and the imperative that medical research meet the challenges of emergent disease.

Recreating the crisis of 1918–1919, Recursion writers depict medical personae who, undeterred by repeated failures or difficult conditions, labor in hospitals, in clinics, and in the field. But too frequently, under untenable conditions, their best efforts fail. These novels recognize that public health inadequacies, in 1918–1919, were exacerbated by the demands of war. In fictional portrayals of government-funded human trials, as in Goldberg's book, we find inspired investigators and self-effacing volunteers. Goldberg's well-researched story presents human trials aimed at isolating the pathogen and eventually at devising a vaccine; however, nothing meaningful is achieved since the experiments are based on the spurious assumption that *H. influenzae* (Pfeiffer's bacillus) rather than a filter-passing agent caused the disease. From an historical perspective, this misallocation of time and effort in the campaign against the bacillus is perplexing in light of the fact that, in 1918–1919, the virus was not an esoteric concept. As mentioned in the introduction, S. B. Wolbach, in 1912, lists 30 possible viral diseases ("The Filterable Viruses"). In 1912, Drs. Peyton Rous and J. B. Murphy demonstrated that filterable agents caused tumors in chickens ("On the Causation of Filterable Agents"). And, in 1918, Drs. Nicolle and Lebailly, followed by Gibson, Bowman, and Connor, argued from strong evidence that influenza was caused by a filter-passing virus. Because research was geared to Pfeiffer's claim and employed methods appropriate to bacteriology, the actual cause of influenza remained elusive until the early 1930s.

Medical personae in most Recursion novels practice in multiple roles rather than as specialists. Instead of teamwork and cooperation, we find them in some stories practicing in isolation, acting as family practitioners, microbiologists, and immunologists, trying in vain to identify the pathogen and to develop a vaccine. This is especially true in James Rada, Jr.'s novel, where a vaccine of questionable efficacy is created from a convalescent's blood serum. Ironically, although Goldberg's story features a well-staffed, government-funded installation, without the biotechnological progress of the late 1920s and 1930s, including animal models and egg-culturing techniques, the vaccine trials of 1918 are futile. Reina James dramatizes a moral paradox in the UK: limitations in resources and in medical care mean that the critical demands of the war and of public health cannot both be satisfied. The idea of the quarantine as a means of inhibiting the spread of disease has proven its worth, but only if conducted according to legal and medical guidelines; in unprofessional hands, as Thomas Mullen shows, it amounts to an exercise in futility. The theme of determination and futility links the four Recursion novels.

Myla Goldberg, Wickett's Remedy *(2005)*

The biomedical focus of Myla Goldberg, in *Wickett's Remedy*, is on clinical trials conducted at the quarantine station on Gallops Island, located off the coast of Boston, Massachusetts, in Portsmouth Harbor. It was used as a hospital to treat immigrants who were too sick to enter the city (Goldberg, 194). Dr. Joseph Gold, the director of the human experiments planned for the island, announces that they are taking part in a "quest" to "penetrate the innermost mysteries of this affliction" and to pierce the veil of ignorance (an allusion, perhaps, to Somerset Maugham's 1925 novel, *The Painted Veil*), which has "allowed the epidemic to spread with such alarming speed" (Goldberg, 200). Despite his enthusiasm, they will fail.

The influenza trials Goldberg describes are based on actual medical procedures, conducted in the autumn of 1918, to test recent claims, by above mentioned Japanese and French investigators, that the pathogen had been isolated. From December 1918 to March 1919, Japanese researchers, Yamanouchi, Skakami, and Iwashima, who were on the right track, conducted five procedures and claimed to arrive at relevant findings (Kolata, 60–61; Taubenberger & Morens, "Historical Context," 585). They inoculated flu sputum filtrates into the noses and throats of 12 healthy volunteers; introduced blood from influenza patient into healthy persons; and, as a control, instilled into the noses and throats of 14 healthy subjects cultures of Pfeiffer's bacillus, pneumococcus, streptococcus, staphylococcus, and many other strains of harmful bacteria, harvested from the sputa of influenza patients. The experiment was compromised at the outset in that many of the volunteers, who were medical workers, had already been exposed to influenza, an oversight Rosenau and Goldberger, the actual Gallops Island researchers, had tried unsuccessfully to avoid. The 14 persons in the Japanese trial who received the bacterial cocktail did not develop influenza. The Japanese researchers construed this to mean that the germ was a submicroscopic, nonbacterial agent; however, doubts were raised over their claim that a filterable virus had positive results in volunteers 100 percent of the time.

The United States Public Health Service also wanted to test the validity of experiments that Nicolle and Lebailly had performed at the Pasteur Institute, in Tunis (Taubenberger & Morens, "Historical Context," 585). On 15 October 1918, Lebailly announced that he had found initial proof of a virus as influenza's cause (Nicolle & Lebailly, 607–610). The assumption that Pfeiffer's bacillus was the inciter had been made in 1892, as mentioned in chapter 1, when the German bacteriologist Richard Pfeiffer announced that he had isolated the organism from decedents. This theory gained support at Camp Devens when Leslie Spooner and colleagues in the medical corps, reported finding the bacillus in the noses, throats, sputa, and pleural fluids of pneumonia patients (Spooner, Sellards, and Wyman, 1310–1311). However, the presence of this microbe, investigators would point out, was insufficient to qualify it as the cause.

The experiment of Nicolle and Lebailly is revealing. They performed a three-step procedure: (1) attaining unfiltered sputum from febrile, three-day-old human influenza cases, they inoculated this material into monkeys' nostrils and conjunctiva. Five days later, a macaque got sick with a high fever. On the sixth day, another sickened. Both recovered, and it was irrefutable that the secretions were virulent; (2) filtered solutions taken from human secretions and diluted with salt were injected into two volunteers from a local army base. Both got influenza (headache, backache, a fever of 102 degrees Fahrenheit, and were convalescing in 12 days). The investigators realized that influenza weakened a patient to the degree that a secondary bacterial infection could set in with devastating effect. Pfeiffer's bacillus, streptococcus, and hemolytic or red blood cell–destroying bacteria present in the secretions of the dead were proof of opportunistic infections; however, no particular strain of bacterium was *always* present and in sufficient abundance to identify it as the probable cause; and (3) they began a series of injections into healthy volunteers, using human secretions as filtrate mixed with three cubic centimeters of infected bonnet monkey blood, and with the blood of influenza patients in the second day of illness. Although the bacterial tests were negative, through the process of elimination they surmised that the cause was not bacterial. On 15 October 1918, Nicolle and Lebailly attained more positive results. Once the infected secretions were cleared of bacteria through filtration, the remaining fluid caused influenza in volunteers. The logical inference of the French scientists, corroborating the Japanese trial, was that a sub-microscopic, filterable agent had caused the infection.

Experiments conducted by the British Medical Corps at hospitals in Étaples, France, from June 1918 to February 1919, during the third wave of the pandemic, were also revealing. J. A. Wilson, John R. Bradford, and E. F. Bashford, whose work is surveyed in chapter 1, performed human and animal studies. They obtained and filtered the sputa of human flu patients and then inoculated twenty animals with both the filtrate and pure cultures. The results, reported on 19 February 1919, were astounding: 19 of 20 animals developed influenza-like lesions in lungs, liver, kidneys, and heart. On the basis of this result, they claimed to have isolated and cultured the cause of influenza, but it turned out that bacterial contaminants had skewed the test and invalidated their claim.

The United States Public Health Service carried out joint experiments on influenza etiology in Boston and in San Francisco (February–March 1919), and these experiments are the basis of Goldberg's novel. Milton J. Rosenau, J. J. Keegan, Joseph Goldberger, and G. C. Lake were the medical personnel conducting the Boston experiments on Gallops Island, in November 1918. Influenza donors for the Gallops Island experiment were presumably sick with flu and hospitalized at the U.S. Naval Hospital at Chelsea and at Peter Bent Brigham Hospital (Rosenau, 312). Using pure cultures of Pfeiffer's bacillus (the main suspect), secretions from the upper-respiratory passages of influenza patients, and blood from typical cases of the flu, they introduced infectious material into the volunteers. The Pfeiffer's bacillus in suspension was instilled into the noses of three non-immune volunteers (presumably, those who had never been exposed to the disease), and into three controls who had a history of an attack in the present epidemic. No reaction to Pfeiffer's microbe occurred. The second experiment (no date recorded) involved a suspension of *different* strains of Pfeiffer bacilli. Ten presumably non-immune volunteers received these strains but had no reaction.

Since pure bacterial isolates had no immunological effects, the second step was to use filtered and unfiltered secretions drawn from the upper-respiratory tracts of cases in the active stage of influenza. Thirty healthy men were inoculated with sprays, swabs, or both in nose and throat. Time intervals between attaining and inoculating the secretions, a point Myla Goldberg includes in the novel, were progressively shortened to a mere thirty seconds, to see if the specimen degraded over time to produce a false negative. Once again, the results were negative for influenza transmission.

In the third experiment, members of one group of volunteers that had been inoculated with secretions were then exposed to active influenza cases to simulate transmission conditions. Each of the ten members of the volunteer group came into close contact for a few minutes with *each* of ten selected cases of influenza in the wards of Chelsea Naval Hospital. Four volunteers were exposed less than 24 hours after onset of the disease in infected cases. Each volunteer breathed on, and shook hands with, ten different infected cases. No infection was transmitted.

In the final experiment, secretions from five typical cases of influenza were secured and filtered. The filtrate was then inoculated subcutaneously into each of ten volunteers. At the same time, blood from the same cases, was pooled, mixed, and injected into each volunteer in another group of ten men; 45 minutes passed between the drawing of blood and the inoculations. Patient-donors came from two epidemic foci, the majority from the USS *Yacona*, on which 80 of 95 crew members had been stricken between 17 and 29 November 1918.

The San Francisco experiments, conducted concurrently with those on Gallops Island, took place at the Angel Island Quarantine Station, on Goat Island, and the volunteers were from Yerba Buena Naval Training Station. These experiments were carried out jointly by Drs. G. W. McCoy, of the United States Public Health Service, and De Wayne Richey, United States Navy.

The results of a number of experiments testing disease transmission and attempting to isolate the influenza pathogen were foregone failures since they mistakenly began with the erroneous premise that bacteria caused influenza.

The Yerba Buena volunteers, unlike those selected from the Deer Island

Naval Training Station, had not been exposed to influenza in the immediate epidemic and, therefore, were presumed not to have acquired immunity. The experiment began with the introduction of bacterial cultures into their systems to see if they caused influenza. All of the men were vaccinated with large doses of bacterial inoculum (Pfeiffer's bacillus, three types of pneumococci, and hemolytic streptococci). Second, a group of ten volunteers were divided into two five-man squads. One group received via the nose heavy suspensions of emulsified cultures of eight strains of unfiltered Pfeiffer's bacillus. The other group received the same material after it had been passed through a Berkefeld filter. The results, after seven days, were negative. An editorial note appended to the 10 January 1919 report prudently advises that, "For the present the sanitarian will do well to continue to apply the general principles of control that are based on the justifiable assumption that the disease is a droplet infection.... It would seem to be wise to give renewed emphasis to the importance of going to bed at the very earliest stages of the attack."

Myla Goldberg preserves historical accuracy while veiling events and characters. The chief investigator, Dr. Joseph Gold, for example, is modeled after Dr. Joseph Goldberger, M.D. (1874–1929). Leaving the Public Health Service, in 1899, for medical research, by 1918 he was assigned to work on influenza. With a team of Navy researchers, Goldberger, as described above, initiated a series of experiments to determine influenza's cause and pattern of spread. In November 1918, at the height of the second wave, he and his colleagues tried to infect healthy volunteers with influenza secretions taken from sick patients and with pure cultures of Pfeiffer's bacillus, the presumptive cause. The purpose was to identify the responsible microbe, which was erroneously believed to have been a bacillus. The trials did not succeed in isolating the pathogen.

Myla Goldberg's Dr. Gold, though portrayed as an idealist, is still pragmatic about their twofold purpose: to understand the workings of the disease and to find medical and immunological ways of preventing future suffering and death. His hope is for complete eradication (Goldberg, 200). Though his long-range goal may be unachievable, his words are, nevertheless, rousingly noble, and his emphasis on research is justified: sound method and acute observation, he avows, will bring positive results. Teamwork, essential to biomedical research, is stressed: "Together, we will function as one mind" (Goldberg, 201). The volunteers whom Dr. Gold praises are serving a higher cause; in truth, their incarcerations, though not for serious infractions, are to be commuted and their combat duty waived if they participate. Their personal risk is unambiguous in that they will be placed "directly in the epidemic's path" (Goldberg, 201).

The prisoners, shackled and attired in prison gray uniforms, arrive from the United States Naval Detention Camp on Deer Island (Goldberg, 206). All of the men are healthy. But, according to an official report of the actual experiment, their medical histories with respect to influenza vary: 68 had been exposed to an epidemic of influenza before coming to Deer Island; 47 men had had no history of attack during the recent epidemic; and 39 "were without history of an attack of such illness at any time during their lives." This epidemiological breakdown of the 154 volunteers is significant: the 39 with no lifetime history of attack would theoretically be the most susceptible to the causative agent. Having no immunological memory of it, they would be the ideal cohort for the trial because the microbe, once introduced into their systems, would ostensibly be present in blood and secretions and then cultured. In the fiction, however, only two general groups are described: those who had no history of exposure to influenza patients *during the pandemic*; and those who were not carriers, though they could have been asymptomatic—but, as it turns out, there was no reliable way to make certain either was the case upon their arrival (Goldberg, 207).

Gold continues to hyperbolize and propagandize. The medical team identifies the disease with German tyranny, and he makes it clear that whoever has second thoughts about participating can simply return to Deer Island (Goldberg, 226–227). Opting to participate rather than to be re-incarcerated and ultimately deployed to Europe, the men learn about the procedures they are to undergo. Each test will last one week, during which time the subjects will be quarantined, their physical conditions carefully monitored. Should anyone contract influenza as a result of the experiments, that individual will receive the best of care (Goldberg, 227).

Gold introduces his protégé and an assistant surgeon, Dr. Percival Cole, whose name is appropriated with slight variation from that of Dr. Rupert Cole, a prominent researcher on flu-related pneumonia. After preliminary lab tests, Percival Cole administers Mather's microbe intra-nasally and orally to the first group of ten men (Goldberg, 230–234). This microbe was one of many suspected as causing influenza. Mathers, we recall from chapter 1, was one of Pfeiffer's critics. Once in quarantine, the first ten are observed and their vital signs recorded periodically. Myla Goldberg introduces into the main text a newspaper article that reflects the premature conclusions of one group of influenza researchers who, based on incorrect evidence, began to manufacture vaccines. Goldberg interpolates background material such as this to enhance the historicity of the central narrative. One interpolated article, entitled "New Serum Bars Pneumonia," claims unjustifiably that a vaccine had been formulated to prevent the disease, which indicates that, in the public consciousness, influenza (the prequel responsible for viral pneumonia) and bronchopneumonia (the sequel or bacterial complication) were being used synonymously, as doctors had complained, and that the ambiguity stemmed from the medical profession itself, as researchers frantically scrambled to come up with a reliable way of controlling the disease (Goldberg, 238). The article criticizes the illogicality of the proceedings. The inclusion of a vaccine advertisement in the context of the trial reveals that unproven vaccines were in production *before* clinical trials were even commenced.

Goldberg emphasizes the crudity with which the on-site trial is conducted, especially with respect to biological safety and the treatment of infectious substances, and this claim is borne out by historical research (Eyler, "The Fog of Research"; Bresalier, "Fighting Flu"). By 15 November 1918, men in the East Ward who had received doses of Mather's microbe were still healthy (Goldberg, 247). On 15–16 November, a second test began: ten more volunteers received inoculations of bacterial isolates, but this time the material was taken directly from the noses, throats, and respiratory tracts of three acute cases of influenza, the specimens having been transported from the naval hospital to the island. The specimens had been mixed in saline suspension and administered (Goldberg, 248–249). Younger doctors on staff question the soundness of these procedures. Referring, in particular, to the acute-case secretions just administered, one doctor reasons that the specimen was taken from a patient some 30–70 hours before use on Gallops. In light of an additional two hours of transport time, and the fact that the cultures were moved in an insecure glass bottle, the doctor is all but certain the microbes are dead (Goldberg, 252). In all likelihood, the culture is useless, and nothing was to be gained by giving it to the men (Goldberg, 252). Any infectious agent in the transported samples had, in the elapsed time, been rendered inactive; yet in the control cultures live bacteria were present. Another physician who subscribed to the bacterial theory of influenza reacts strongly to these implications: "Next you'll be saying that influenza isn't even bacterial!" (Goldberg, 253)—an intended irony—although bacteria of various species, it would be determined, could cause respiratory disease in the sequel. Another doctor theorizes that *B. influenzae* (Pfeiffer's microbe) could still be the cause but that it had lost potency in transit. By the second day, it becomes clear that the experiment had failed: the ten who received the acute-case specimens were still healthy (Goldberg, 259).

On 17 November 1918, direct-transmission experiments begin. Influenza patients from the Chelsea Naval Base are brought to Gallops in order to determine if casual contact or airborne transmission is the route of contagion (Goldberg, 260–261). Certain that this test will yield results, the investigators expose ten apparently healthy men to the four bed-ridden influenza patients: they shake hands with each other, the Gallops volunteers inhale the sick men's respirations, and finally contaminated nose swabs are dabbed into the volunteers' noses (Goldberg, 261–264). The results are negative.

An unforeseen event occurs. Dr. Cole contracts influenza, presumably from the transported patients (Goldberg, 287)—precisely how is undetermined. Unethically, the researchers take blood from Cole, with the intention of inoculating it subcutaneously into volunteers. This action, to which Dr. Peterson demurs, contravenes experimental protocols, as Goldberg's marginalia state (Goldberg, 287). The test, Dr. Gold is assured, will have positive results, but blood-inoculation ultimately fails, and Dr. Cole dies of pneumonia (Goldberg, 289). At the autopsy, Dr. Gold, shocked to see his colleagues' sodden lungs, declares (in a paraphrase of Dr. William Henry Welch's prescient words): "In thirty years in this profession, I have never seen anything like this. This must be some new kind of infection ... or plague" (quoted by Crosby, 9; Goldberg, 303–304). The volunteers and all others lose faith in the Gallops Island experiments, and the newspapers repudiate any premature claim that medical science has found a cure (Goldberg, 315, 319).

Goldberg's protagonist also has a historical analogue. The probable source of the Lydia Wickett persona is Lydia Phillips, a would-be nurse who, in early October 1918, had found herself in the midst of the second wave. Richard Collier, whose book, *The Plague of the Spanish Lady*, is one acknowledged source of *Wickett's Remedy*, describes Phillips as "symbolic" or representative of the spirit of volunteerism that emerged during the crisis (90). A petite, naïve, and compassionate 23-year-old (just like Wickett), Phillips wanted to become a nurse, but unlike the fictional persona, she had yearned to be a nurse from her youth (Goldberg, 157). Wickett, on the other hand, tested this vocational path at 23, after her one-day stint as a volunteer in Carney Hospital. Phillips, on the other hand, had applied unsuccessfully to the nursing program at St. Thomas's Hospital, London. Unlike Lydia Wickett who was raised in South Boston and was not well off financially, Phillips was the daughter of an established umbrella manufacturer. Phillips had not given up on nursing and on St. Thomas's, despite the rejection. Her fortunes changed with the outbreak of war in 1914 when, on a holiday voyage to South Africa, she and her mother were confined to Johannesburg for the duration; apparently, no shipping was available to return home. Despite this turn of events, Phillips remains both "resourceful" and "self-willed." She also had a strong work ethic, offering to sell her "trinkets" to finance her own education in a business college. Although Phillips worked briefly as a shorthand typist for wholesale merchants in the suburb of Malvern, the dream of becoming a nurse persisted.

In the first week of October, Phillips responded to an advertisement in the now-defunct *Rand Daily Mail* which announced the need for volunteers during the epidemic. The most urgent call came from the Twist Street School Emergency Hospital, where help was needed four hours each day. Like Lydia Wickett at Carney Hospital, Phillips had decided to volunteer at Twist Hospital and then to tell her mother about her decision (Collier, 90–91). Lydia Wickett hopes to quiet her family's anticipated objections about volunteering at Gallops Island, describing "the imperative to volunteer and the nobility and purpose of her labor," but she would hide the fact that, for months, she would be caring for influenza patients and in direct contact with the disease (Goldberg, 162). Considering the fact that her mother had just experienced the loss of a son, of a son-in-law, and of a neighbor's child, her reaction to Lydia's ingenuous nobility is predictable: "If you love us half as much as you loved him [her husband Henry], you would not be throwing yourself into his grave" (Goldberg, 178–179). Phillips, too, had to muster a cogent enough argument to convince her mother who, at the same time, tried adamantly to dissuade her from this hazardous decision (Collier, 90–1).

Unlike Lydia Wickett who arrives at Gallops Island alone, an excited Phillips had entered at Twist Street Hospital "with a motley group of volunteers" (Collier, 91). Like Wickett, she entertained altruistic ideals of immediately caring for the sick and dying, and as meriting the trust conferred on Florence Nightingale (1820–1910) at Scutari. Nightingale's career in the Crimea, as J. N. Hays states, "assumed mythic proportions in the English-speaking world" (221). Revered as the "Lady with the Lamp," she cared for soldiers, was a sanitary reformer, but was not known for being a compassionate nurse (Hays, 148; 221–222; Collier, 91). Both Wickett and Phillips seem to be neither aware of, nor concerned with, the practical difficulties of nursing, its drudgery, low wage, and the ingratitude with which they so often treated, but they are cognizant of the staff nurse's uniform (Goldberg contrasts Nurse Foley's spotless, elegant uniform with Lydia's plain attire). Phillips is disappointed that, instead of a uniform, she receives only an apron and "a piece of white cloth twisted to resemble a nurse's cap" (Collier, 91).

Phillips and Wickett are disappointed when they find that their duties are not living up to their expectations. Phillips is assigned to cramped accommodations, and the atmosphere is fetid, while Wickett is equally dismayed with her lonely quarters and by the strange sounds of the night and crashing surf. In a reflective moment, while lying "on a small, narrow mattress in a draughty room," Wickett self-incriminates: her vocational decision, now felt to be a selfish rather than selfless choice, amounts to "the crime of deserting her family, [a] callous act that more than justified her current solitary confinement" (Goldberg, 204). Both Phillips and Wickett draw consolation from the prospect of contributing to the war effort. Phillips places herself in the tradition of Florence Nightingale in the Crimea, whereas Wickett sees the flu as a national foe, on par with Kaiser's Germany (400,000 Germans, it is important to note, also died of influenza in 1918 [Hochschild, 350]). Wickett's identification of the flu as a mortal enemy of the nation was certainly not far-fetched, since the disease would account for more American combat deaths than were cumulatively suffered in 1914–1918, in 1941–1945, in 1950–1953, and in 1964–1975. Whereas Wickett's patients are healthy and amiable volunteers, elected to participate in the trials, Phillips' patients, all of whom were in various stages of influenza, were "frightened and alone, made savage and resentful by fear and by pain" (Collier, 91). One wonders if Collier is editorializing here in regard to patients' savage resentment or if Phillips had had a bad experience. Presumably, Collier relied on archived periodical sources such as the *Rand Daily Mail*, but more than that cannot be said with any certainty (Collier, 318).

Phillips' duties contrast with Wickett's. While the latter had to assist with rudimentary assays, tend to patients' basic needs, and to record vital signs, Phillips recoiled when the staff nurse brought her into a room to care for a filthy, unkempt vagrant. Phillips was assigned to foot massage duty, ostensibly to improve circulation. Despite the unpleasantness, she struggled and completed the treatment. Collier writes that, as a result of this experience, she had serious vocational doubts; thus, "in shame and blind despair," she told herself that she could never be a nurse (92). The doubts arose simply because nursing practice under bad conditions did not correspond to her unrealistic notion that Florence Nightingale somehow did not get her hands dirty. As it turned out, Phillips reconsiders service. At 8 a.m. on the second day Phillips learns that the vagrant had passed away during the night. Shocked by his death, she finds herself "torn between compassion for a human being who had passed on unfriended and a feeling, almost, of affront" (Collier, 127). She decided she would not betray the profession she had desired to join. The work was far from glamorous. She took temperatures, pared finger- and toenails, changed soiled linen and pajamas. Her experiences were heartbreaking and stomach-wrenching, but she was determined to persist (Collier, 129). Phillips believed that all of her time at Twist had been a test of courage. Subconsciously she drove herself to see how much she could endure (Collier, 181–182). Phillips became a patient herself. Collier lists her among the survivors and the address as "Twist Street School Emergency Hospital, Johannesberg (Transvaal), South Africa" (364). The inference is that she had contracted the disease, perhaps because of her volunteering there, and that she survived.

Lydia Kilkenny Wickett, as a dynamic or evolving character, matures through experience. When she had arrived at Gallops Island, she felt as if she were on a mission to fight disease in the tradition of Nightingale in the Crimea, and she saw Nurse Foley, in her elegant uniform, as the nurse she herself was meant to be (Goldberg, 195). Her self-effacing altruism has a deeper, psychological motive, and, this introspective element recalls the real-life situation of Lydia Phillips. But Lydia Wickett's psychological burden is much heavier than that of Lydia Phillips. In South Boston, Wickett was unequipped to mourn the influenza death of her brother Michael who had died at Camp Devens (Goldberg, 195). Her emotional conflict was that she desperately needed to mourn her brother but could not do so fully without him at her side, suggesting that she was overly dependent upon him (Goldberg, 196). Part of the reason for volunteering, as it is suggested in the novel, was to find closure by attending to young military personnel who were like her late brother, and who also faced the threat of influenza. Since she cannot be transformed into a nurse through on-the-job training, she is dejected, and Nurse Foley does not hide her own disappointment over Lydia's lack of professional training (Goldberg, 177).

In Lydia Wickett's mind, the war had been projected onto the bodies of the volunteers, and her brother Michael or her husband Henry seemed to occupy every quarantine bed (Goldberg, 241). It is reasonable for her to dread seeing the men sicken and to see them turn into "enervated forms too weak to raise their heads, muddy-chested creatures struggl[ing] for breath" (Goldberg, 243). Moreover, she realizes that once influenza appears in their ranks, there would be time neither for self-indulgence nor for mourning. An important landmark in the development of her personality emerges through suffering and reflection when she acknowledges that "she had come to Gallups [*sic*] in pursuit of oblivion. Now she dreaded her wish's fulfillment" (243). Once she forgets her past and finds closure, the narrative trajectory suggests that she can discover a purpose in life.

Once the Florence-Nightingale fantasy is dispelled, Lydia realizes the implications of her decision and can express her emotions freely, though she remains ignorant of how biomedical trials work. Appalled that the men are to receive infectious secretions, she expresses a legitimate revulsion for human experimentation and an ethical concern. She raises these concerns with Dr. Percival Cole who sympathetically responds that the stated purpose of the study is to identify the initiating microbe and its mode of transmission, not to kill volunteers. In fact, they had been apprised of the risks, and they willingly participated. Yet Wickett is unconvinced; she cannot deal with the possibility of being complicit in the deaths of one or more volunteers (Goldberg, 250). Ironically, despite Cole's statistical assurances that less than 10 percent of flu patients succumb to the disease (actually 2 percent), and despite Dr. Gold's guarantee that the best medical care will be extended to any volunteer, it is Dr. Cole himself who contracts influenza and dies from secondary bacterial pneumonia (Goldberg, 251, 296–297). This is another experiential landmark in Lydia's emotional life. She recalls Cole's grandiose claim that the Gallops Island project was going to make history, but his physical deterioration and suffering render this a hollow pronouncement: "If this was what history making required, then Lydia was content to remain outside history's reach: a nameless clerk in a department store, a childless woman who would be forgotten after her death" (Goldberg, 296–297). The tone of self-pity is transient: she must now make sense of the entire project, which has amounted to multiple failures, and of her role as a medical worker, whether credentialed or not.

An important change occurs in her attitude, amounting to a kind of adaptation to circumstances. She begins to treat her day, "as a complex mechanical contrivance in which she was a smallish cog. She filled her mind with the clicks of a cog; she moved with the steadiness of a cog, travelling her designated circuit in Dr. Gold's machine" (Goldberg, 298–299). This cognitive method reflects neither self-deprecation nor hopelessness. To the contrary, it adverts to an emotional mechanism, essential to the health-care worker's efficiency: she focuses on her delegated tasks without questioning their significance or her importance in the process. The cog metaphor has two meanings, of course, as a tooth on the rim of a wheel or gear and as a subordinate but vital person. Wickett was distressed by her subordinate role, but, at once removed from self-pity, and after seeing the futility of the medical machine and the death of one of its operators, she has recognized the vitality of her role as record keeper and assistant—as a cog without which the mechanism could not work efficiently.

Wickett's memories still haunt her because her trauma was profound and its effects persistent. She will not visit Percy Cole because he will remind her of those whom she has lost (Goldberg, 299). Cole's final wish was to have Wickett witness his autopsy, an experience that sickens her. But her education as a front-line care provider is humbling and effective. She agrees to attend, thinking in practical terms that, "After weeks of foundering, she would leave [Gallops] with a bit more medical knowledge, something concrete and incontrovertibly true" (Goldberg, 300). The incontrovertible truth that Goldberg so artfully conveys through Lydia is that the physicians are not immune to the diseases that they confront. Thus, Cole's corpse is cyanotic, the skin blistered, and the 700 gram lungs so sodden that even the veteran surgeon (echoing Welch again), Dr. Gold, is aghast at the effects of "some new kind of infection ... or plague" (Goldberg, 304). What has become incontrovertibly true to Wickett is that Cole, under dissection before her, "is a dead animal." All present were "nothing more than animals, bloated by vanity, into wearing clothes and ascribing lofty purposes to their actions, when in reality they all died the same dumb death" (Goldberg, 304).

Wickett's experience has not hardened her to the present situation. When she learns that Harry Bentley, one of the volunteers, has become symptomatic, she is said to have overreacted considerably and can barely maintain her composure. According to the marginalia, which provide an alternative perspectives on the narrative action, she was so nervous that the patient had to take his own temperature; and a second marginal notation has it that, upon learning of Bentley's fever, she became hysterical and sounded like "a crazy woman" (Goldberg, 316–317). Bentley's fever will turn out not to presage influenza; nevertheless, the experience is another turning point in the psychological development of the Lydia Wickett persona. Bentley's illness causes a change in outlook and behavior in regard to her daily routine. She now is fully aware of herself as "a small cog in a large machine" but must work to control or suppress her raw emotions (Goldberg, 318). The cog metaphor reveals that, when faced with the possibility of Bentley's impending medical crisis, Wickett makes a sincere effort to adapt to her position as a health care provider. The most efficient way to optimize the patient's care, Wickett understands, as if through a revelation, was emotional distancing between the health care professional and the patient. She, therefore, must apply herself, self-effacingly, to her limited but necessary role on Gallops. As a cog in the machine, she is a diminutive but necessary part of the mechanism.

Nurse Foley becomes aware of Wickett's dread regarding the volunteers—that influenza would be induced in them and that some may die in the process. Consoling and educating her at the same time, Foley reminds Wickett that to study disease transmission requires healthy subjects. Over a five-day period, the medical personnel at the station would have to make certain that the volunteers had not brought the flu with them (Goldberg, 209). This information stays with Wickett, although she retains it superficially. Her vocational disappointment and psychological confusion are burdensome. Aiding medical science, she learns the hard way, is not the same as aiding medical practice. She continues to fault herself for abandoning her family and for leaving the ill at Carney Hospital, where practical medicine can be put to good use. To resolve her conflict she embraces her statistical duties, determined to improve Nurse Foley's professional opinion of her, which, at this point in the story, is low (Goldberg, 217).

Reina James, This Time of Dying *(2006)*

The connection between World War I and the pandemic raises several questions: where did the influenza pandemic begin? Were the conditions of war conducive to its development and continuation? And did the end of the war hasten the end of the pandemic?

On 2 November 1918, the British medical establishment was aware that the autumn 1918 second wave was extremely virulent and that war conditions were making matters worse. The Council of the British Medical Association (B.M.A.) reported that "the congregation of [a] large number of men in huts and billets, and in crowded transports," has allowed influenza to spread widely among military personnel who carry the infectious agent to other places ("Work of the Council," 494). The Council understood the mode of contagion as well: "infection is disseminated by personal contact under conditions in which good ventilation is difficult or impossible"; the "extreme contagiousness of the disease has been proved to be due to its aerial convection ... by means of the 'drop-infection' from person to person and not by transportation of the virus through the air at large," that is, miasmatically (494). All of this was known in November 1918.

The etiology of influenza (its origin and cause) was still hazy. A compiled 1918 review by the Medical Research Committee of the B.M.A. pointed out that, although many still adhered to the belief that Pfeiffer's bacillus was the infective agent, there was no certainty as to the real nature of the *virus* (used generically for infectious agent). The bacteriological theory, in their opinion, was questionable: "[Pfeiffer's bacillus] was not found in widespread localized outbreaks," and, when detected, it was accompanied by other organisms. The Director-General of the Army Medical Service had doubts about "the etiological significance of Pfeiffer's bacillus, and considered that the existence of some yet undiscovered virus must be regarded as possible" (494). Laboratory cultures showed, furthermore, that the organisms chiefly responsible for "secondary pulmonary complications," were "pneumococci and streptococci" (494). They even cite the recent research of Nicolle and LeBailly as providing "good evidence that a filter-passing virus does exist" (495). Although the identity of the nonbacterial organism would be discovered fifteen years later, the B.M.A. accurately summarizes the state of medical research on influenza in November 1918.

Ironically, the pandemic swept the globe despite the British health establishment's lucid realization that overcrowding helped to spread the disease; that infected travelers carried it far and wide; that the infection was spread largely by aerosolized droplets and not by atmosphere; that secondary pneumonia, caused by pneumococci and streptococci, was the most dangerous aspect of influenza; that Pfeiffer's bacillus was the unlikely source of primary infection; and that a filter-passing agent could be the inciting cause, as demonstrated by contemporary experimentation in France. All of these insights, of course, were fundamentally important to the history of influenzal research but ineffective at a time when the war and the pandemic had intensively coalesced.

To this day, we are uncertain as to where the pandemic started. It certainly was not in Spain. The microbiologist John S. Oxford and his colleagues have studied from a biomedical standpoint what I call the war-pandemic interaction. In 2001, Oxford and co-workers looked at medical documentation of the period from 1917 to 1918 suggesting that the 1918 virus had spread eastward, from Europe to China, although contemporary avian outbreaks have consistently been concentrated in China and Southeast Asia (*Royal Society*, 1857–1859). In 2002, Oxford et al. reiterated the idea that the 1918 pandemic originated on the Western Front; that "World War I was a contributor"; that the pandemic broke out in a European country other than Spain, as early as the winter of 1916 or 1917; and that early respiratory disease outbreaks before 1918 are documented in army camps located in France and in the UK. To illustrate the zoonotic possibility, Oxford includes photo insets showing a piggery at Étaples camp, in France, ca. 1918, and one of soldiers handling geese at a market in 1919. The third paper in the series stresses that influenza might have had an ideal environment in northern France for its development and for genetic interchange with other viruses, especially where thousands of soldiers were exposed to lethal gases such as chlorine and mustard gas, and lived in close proximity to livestock and other animals, namely pigs, ducks, geese, and horses. This unsanitary, overcrowded, and toxic environment, Oxford et al. hypothesize, was conducive to "the emergence of the 'Spanish' influenza pandemic of 1918–1919." The notion that earlier outbreaks in these locations adumbrated the Great Pandemic is also borne out in the medical literature. Illustrating the continuity of the investigation, Oxford et al. studied pathology reports from the army barracks at Étaples and Aldershot. They found that the disease outbreaks of the winter of 1917 were the same as those of the first infection of influenza in 1918. The authors maintain that the return of infected soldiers to their European and North American homelands, in the autumn of 1918, "catalyzed the pandemic" (*Vaccine* [2005]).

Other interpretations exist. Epidemiological evidence, according to John M. Barry in 2004, indicated that a new influenza virus had sprung up in Haskell County, Kansas, early in 1918. The virus had traveled eastward to Camp Funston, took its toll there, and then was carried via troop transports to Europe (*Influenza*, 92). Camp Funston, therefore, could have been the starting point for the U.S. epidemic, the epicenters of which were the crowded military camps. Stating that the war and the pandemic were "inextricably related," Anton Erkoreka, in 2009, offers a third variant of the war-pandemic interaction. The origin of the pandemic was Asian, and the virus had been transported to Europe after all: "links between the Spanish influenza and Asia can be established in terms of the Chinese workers at Camp Funston and the Indochinese soldiers of the French Army affected by the Annamite Pneumonia." Erkoreka suggests the possibility that, in European army camps, viruses from Indochina and China recombined, increasing the virulence of the 1918 autumn wave (190–194). Modern researchers of the war-pandemic interaction, despite their differences over point of origin, consider the possibility that cessation of the war foreshortened the influenza crisis.

The war-pandemic interaction is central to Reina James' 2006 novel, *This Time of Dying*. The ethical and epidemiological problems in the novel are related not to the origin of the disease but rather to public health strategy in the UK. The dilemma involved the allocation of vital resources in a crisis having two interdependent fronts: one was the war in France and Belgium; and the other, the pandemic in the UK. For UK policymakers, in 1918, matters of public health hinged on three questions: (1) should vital resources be expended on a national campaign against influenza even though medical and social interventions were known to be ineffective? (2) Even though victory over Germany was in sight but not guaranteed, should overcrowded British factories and troop transportation be curtailed or halted in order to control the spread of the disease? And, (3) since the conditions of the war were theoretically responsible for the origin, intensity, and protraction of the pandemic, would an impending Allied victory bring an end to the pandemic?

Reina James' fictional rendition of this historical debate is implicit in her characters and in their situations. She presents two diametrically-opposed positions: one, represented by the actual Principal Medical Officer of the Local Government Board (L.G.B.), Sir Arthur Newsholme, M.D. (1857–1943), and the other by a fictitious doctor, Thomas Wey. Ironically, neither character says a word in the novel. On the one hand, Dr. Newsholme is represented, in absentia, as being grossly malfeasant; and his inaction during the pandemic, the cause of many deaths. On the other hand, Dr. Thomas Wey, whose death from influenza is described omnisciently on page one (Monday, 14 October 1918), is portrayed as a courageous physician who tries unsuccessfully to communicate the gravity of the pandemic directly to Dr. Newsholme, through epidemiological data compiled while treating patients in army camps at the onset of the pandemic. Though Dr. Wey's corpse is found on the pavement, his ambiguous data and dire warnings, preserved in his writings, come into the hands of a London undertaker, Henry Speake.

The tragedy of influenza in Great Britain, as *This Time of Dying* has it, arises from a recalcitrant medical establishment in Britain, disconnected from overseas medical institutions and (if Wey's plight is meant as an example) oblivious to epidemiological communiques from field hospitals. Wey's predicament, moreover, suggests that in-theater military hospitals were dysfunctional, since the doctor appears as a solitary clinician/epidemiologist with neither institutional nor collegial support nor basic medical care. The chief medical officer of the new Ministry of Health, Sir George Newman (1870–1948) also stands in historical contrast to Newsholme. Having the dual advantage of hindsight and peace, he would propose improvements in communication systems and in other essential services. A public health physician, Newman, in 1920, would publish a comprehensive 26-point analysis and health prospectus on the influenza pandemic. The document outlines (1) the clinical character of influenza (paragraphs 4–9, vi-ix); (2) its cause (paragraphs 10–12, ix-xii); (3) its epidemiology (paragraphs 13–20, xii-xix); and (4) means of investigation and prevention (paragraphs 21–26, xix-xxiii) (Newman, *Report*). Newsholme, in contrast, was stuck in an ungovernable situation.

Reina James' imaginative reconstruction of the war-pandemic interaction blames the L.G.B. for its failure to address the medical crisis adequately. On this point, her imaginative dramatization of these events corresponds to that of social historians, such as Sandra M. Tomkins, who tries to account for the paradox that Britain's "highly developed public health establishment" responded so ineffectively to the pandemic. Tomkins argues that medical professionals and public health administrators dismissed the danger and advised that the public live with the ordeal. Institutional obstacles and scarce resources paralyzed local administration, rendering their dedicated efforts ineffective ("The Failure of Expertise"). I hope to revise this position by taking a closer look at the facts.

Contemporaneous literature gives us some understanding of where Newsholme stood in this controversy. With the pandemic raging into its second month, as medical officer of the L.G.B. he was criticized by the Central Council of the British Medical Association (B.M.A.). The council did not intend to impugn his expertise, past achievements in public health, or proposed innovations in research and care, but rather to point out that the L.G.B. was out of touch with local public health agencies throughout Britain and that its influenza initiative was late. In the Annual Report of March 1917–March 1918, Newsholme states that he had instructed local authorities to take "precautionary steps" against influenza, the first wave of which began in the spring and summer, and he assures the B.M.A. that he "will not allow red tape to tie his hands, but will take immediately any remedial measures that may be recommended" (quoted in, "The Etiology of Influenza," 494). To that end, he promises to hold a conference of medical authorities and bacteriologists, on

Monday, 4 November 1918, to research the cause of influenza and methods of cure.

The Central Council was surprised that Newsholme did not appear to be familiar with research and development already well underway, including advances in military medicine, and that he had not already coordinated the L.G.B.s program with these institutions. His critics reiterate that the L.G.B. was unsynchronized with, and disconnected from, local agencies that worked directly with communities. Local authorities, they explain, had already taken precautions. What they (and the B.M.A.) so urgently needed was "better information." Newsholme, they implied, lacked foresight, for the spring epidemic had given ample warning of "what might follow"; in addition, the history of influenza epidemics showed that the disease tended to flare up in winter. The criticism of Newsholme's office and leadership is acerbic: "The [L.G.B.] has not made use of the opportunities during the last six months" to learn anything about the nature of the disease in the laboratory, clinic, or through "the collation of statistics" (a dig at Newsholme who was a biostatistician), whereas the Council of the B.M.A. has done just that ("The Etiology of Influenza," 494).

Newsholme's culpability hinges on four questions: (1) a brilliant physician and biomedical scientist, was he simply ill-suited to administration? (2) Was the system in its present state dysfunctional? (3) Can its ineffectiveness be ascribed to poor leadership and to systemic failures? And (4), in the context of the war-pandemic interaction, did the lassitude of the L.G.B. during the second wave contribute to the high mortality rate? There is reason to believe that the L.G.B., however dysfunctional it was in 1917–1919, could not have altered the course of the pandemic. The war-pandemic interaction was the source of the problem.

To make sense of this complicated issue, we need to review the literature further. Newsholme argued his own case in the same issue of *The British Medical Journal.* He highlights improvements in the state of public health in England and Wales, 1917–1918, since the 1871 inception of L.G.B., and suggests further strides. He admits to what was common knowledge: the board itself was, indeed, out of touch, adding that "the administrative machine" needed to be simplified, while "public health and medical work" required extension ("The Etiology of Influenza," 497). Communication between the board and both local levels of administration and community programs had to be improved if the people were to know about influenza and what was being done to control it. To improve public health on the local level, he proposes a more integrated system with satellite agencies from the board in close contact with the local communities: "a combination of smaller authorities is needed to avoid in future redundant small schemes and Lilliputian administrative arrangements" (497). Newsholme outlines three initiatives: (1) to expand research on the causes of disease; (2) to initiate more complete training of the medical profession for this work; and (3) to simplify and strengthen the administrative machinery (497). To the Ministry of Health and the Council of the B.M.A., however, such measures had to have been in place before the second pandemic wave recrudesced. Newsholme's ambitious, short-term projects could do nothing in the present, although his successor, Sir George Newman, M.D., would call for and enact similar programs (*Chief Medical Officer's Introduction*).

Let us now turn to James' protagonist, Dr. Wey, an officer in the British Army and Medical Corps, who lives out his last days as a flu victim in a cheap London hotel (James, 4–5). We learn through indirect evidence that, while in the military, he had cared for flu victims in army camps in France or Belgium and had compiled epidemiological data indicating that the disease threatened world health. At the outset, it seems that Wey's predicament is implausible. Discharged because of his ailment, his homelessness and lack of medical care are difficult to square with the fact that, in 1918, British medical and nursing officers "were part of a well established and relatively stable organization" (Shanks et al., "Nurses and Physicians"). Nor was Wey's information revelatory. Though influenza's etiology was as-yet undefined, it had been clinically recognized in the British Expeditionary Force (B.E.F.), as early as April 1918 (Crosby, 25). Its impact on the conduct of warfare was headline news. King George V got it in May, the British fleet could not set sail for three weeks since 10,313 men were sick, and the British 29th Division postponed its attack on La Becque on 30 June (Kolata, *Flu*, 11, 291). On 9 November 1918, an Influenza Advisory Committee working for the director of the General Medical Services, though aligned with Pfeiffer on the inciting cause, had no doubts about how severely influenza was affecting the British Army, and some among them speculated on the virulence of the pathogen: the organism of the first wave, according to the Advisory Committee, "may have become more virulent"; or "there have arisen some conditions favouring its growth and producing a very large increase in its numbers" ("The Etiology of Influenza," 505). Knowing that the current manifestation of the disease was more virulent than its summer predecessor, they asserted that it was spreading globally at a fast rate, and, due to environmental and demographic conditions peculiar to the war, that it was devastating the army: "these conditions seem to be almost world-wide, as the disease has spread itself in Europe from Spain to France, Italy, Germany, and England, and there was an epidemic in the United States a year ago" ("The Etiology of Influenza," 505). It was undeniable that army camps were foci of infection and that troop movements spread the disease. The problem was how to control its spread in time of war without losing the military advantage and without protracting the conflict and, inadvertently, the pandemic. The content of Wey's papers, in the final analysis, was well known by October.

One could argue that, had the L.G.B. kept the population informed about the pandemic, Wey's dire predictions and obscure notations would not have been so alarming. Composed on cheap paper, in indecipherable handwriting, and dated 13 October, Wey's posthumous warning is that a plague had descended on the people that "may well leave the earth to the animals." (James 5–6). The writer implores Newsholme to stop the transport of ships and to close the ports, virtual impossibilities in time of war. And the urgent message ends with the assertion that the writer can prove what he says and that he is "a man of science" (James, 6). Wey had obviously experienced the destructive synergy of war and pandemic in field hospitals. Once in the stranger's apartment, Speake reads at the top of page one the underlined phrase, "*Particular Circumstances.*" Below this heading is a list of dates and descriptions of the weather (James, 7–8). On 15 October, Speake mentions having inspected columns of initials, figures, and temperatures (James, 11). Among the more legible sentences are notes Wey had made for his official letter to Newsholme. Although the information tabulated on these pages appears authentic, Wey's figurative language is distracting. He writes, for instance, that "the world's body" can barely breathe, that the world's wounds open and young lives spill out, and he reiterates the injunction that only peace and quarantine could afford some hope for mankind, as "Death is crossing every sea." "This pestilence," he accurately declares, "will not be confined. I have examined the dead in France and I have seen the young men die in London. I fear we are lost" (James, 12). Wey cryptically observes that the world has been made sick by young men; the disease had, indeed, struck the 20–40 year old male population the hardest and that the troops in transit were carriers. Wey obviously died of influenza (his color is heliotrope blue) (James, 12). It appears that Wey had been doing epidemiological work regarding morbidity and mortality rates in the military and that his incomplete work was related to the war-pandemic interaction.

Wey's frantic call for port closings and for troop extraction, though epidemiologically correct in principle, were logistically impractical and historically naïve (James, 32). He dies on 14 October 1918. In all probability, he was lucid in mid–September and would have known that it was the beginning of the end for Germany. On 21 October, Speake recognizes that Wey's message does not take the war into account: "The very idea that the ports could be closed! And would we leave our armies where they stood? Or bring them home and surrender to the Germans?" (James, 64). From mid–September to late

October, the course of the war had turned sharply in favor of the Allies. From 18 September to 10 or17 October, the Allies had won the pivotal Battle of St. Quentin Canal, as a combined Anglo-American and Australian force breached the Hindenburg Line; from 22–27 September, the British won a series of Transjordan battles; the Meuse-Argonne Offensive began on 26 September; the Hundred Days Offensive would continue throughout October. In that month talks were going on between Germany and the Allies regarding an armistice ("Timeline of World War I"). The *coup de main* came when the German navy suffered an unsustainable loss, not at sea to Allied fire, but through a mutiny that erupted on 29 October in the German fleet at Kiel, spreading to Hamburg and Bremen. The mutiny is reported to have involved 20,000 German troops and submarine crews in all harbors (Lutz, 140–141; "Unrest in Germany," 4–5; Stumpf, "Diary"). The Kaiser's government and war machine were grinding to a halt just as the pandemic was intensifying. The Allies, therefore, were winning the war against the Germans—but not against influenza.

Wey's call for mass withdrawal of land and sea forces is an understandable reaction to the second wave and to the realization that troop movements were spreading the pandemic, but it fails to acknowledge the war-pandemic interaction. Gradually, Speake gets some sense of the conundrum: de-mobilization, an absurd thought, could seriously jeopardize the war effort, even though it might improve the health crisis.

Before assigning blame to Newsholme, it would help to understand the situation better. During the war, the chief medical officer had to decide how meager resources should be allocated. In the autumn of 1918, since the top priority was to feed medical manpower and materièl into the war effort, Newsholme had to make difficult choices. The medical community had resigned itself to the fact that influenza could not be cured and could only be prevented through social distancing; but, because of the war, the latter remedy was not implementable in overcrowded industrial sites, on troop transports, and in cantonments. In addition to limited resources and crowded factories, Newsholme had to contend with the risk of nationwide panic if he went public. The only feasible way out of this situation was to win the war quickly. In that way, the conditions fueling the pandemic—industrial crowding, the lag in research, and the movement of troops and refugees—would desist. In effect, defeating the Germans would defeat influenza, and this could be accomplished if resources were strictly rationed.

In a sense, Newsholme is reduced to a straw man in the novel: an imagined adversary. He may not have been cut out for the job as L.G.B. medical officer, the system was out of touch with local boards, and at his hearings he was trying to control the damage. But much can be said in his defense. His professional competence cannot be questioned. The author of voluminous studies on biostatistics and infectious diseases (smallpox, diphtheria, tuberculosis, influenza, and others), he developed an "eclectic epidemiology" (Eyler, *Sir Arthur Newsholme*, 27, 50); hence, he understood the importance of interdisciplinary research in modern medicine. He also comprehended how the war and the pandemic interrelated. In an introductory address to the Royal Society of Medicine, on 13 November 1918, he defended his decision *not* to enact a public health initiative, first, on the grounds that influenza was uncontrollable. "I know of no public health measure, which can resist the progress of pandemic influenza" ([1919], 3). In *Public Health and Insurance* (1920), he reiterates that: "we have to confess our continuing relative helplessness in preventing ... influenza when ... it makes its devastating swoop on the entire world, and secures a larger number of victims than the World War itself" (23). He knew that, to control the spread of influenza, nothing short of a comprehensive program of eradication would suffice; thus, he writes in 1920, that the "failure to prevent the spread of [influenza] infection from a portion of the total cases must necessarily nullify attempts to check the general progress of an epidemic" ("Some Considerations," 486). A tried-and-true method of controlling infection, social distancing called for the avoidance of crowds. Newsholme knew this but found it to be impractical during the war. He reflects, in a dejected tone, that the high rates of morbidity and mortality among munitions workers and armed services personnel could have been lower had "the known sick ... been isolated from the healthy; if rigid exclusion of known sick and drastic increase of floor-space for each person [had] ... been enforced in factories, workplaces, barracks, and ships, [and] if overcrowding could have been ... prohibited." The manpower and industrial requirements of the country, along with the need for medical personnel in overseas hospitals, however, had to be met if lives were to be saved in the long run, and if the war were to be brought to a swift and favorable end. Newsholme faced the fact that industrial, military, and hospital crowding could not be helped in time of war. The nation's survival depended on production, despite the risks at home. In his capacity as chief medical officer, Newsholme was powerless: (1) neither medical nor immunological interventions existed to thwart influenza; (2) social distancing would imperil the nation if enforced in the military industry at that crucial time; and (3) in view of the collective emotional state of the nation, the risk of panic was unacceptable.

Under the circumstances, Newsholme could neither have foreseen the virulence of the second wave, nor should he be blamed for lack of foresight. In his Whitehall Office, he is portrayed by some as having to render a life-and-death decision affecting a population of more than 34 million people (Snodgrass, 280). This is untrue. Here are Newsholme's own observations as he undertook a kind of national triage. His major premise was that, "the relentless needs of warfare justified incurring the risk of spreading infection" ("Discussion on Influenza," 13). To issue public warnings of a possible recrudescent wave of influenza "would be useful if a prophylactic were available (none except one in the early experimental stage has been suggested [the vaccine was useless]), or, if by issuing advice the progress of the epidemic could be stayed" ("Discussion on Influenza," 12–13). Neither could be done. To make matters worse, "the spread of influenza cannot be halted by 'communal means' either: it is impossible to stop its spread in "the domestic circle" ("Discussion on Influenza," 13). He acknowledges, in July, having authored an official memorandum for public use, "but on the balance of considerations its distribution was not considered expedient at that time" ("Discussion on Influenza," 13). These considerations pertained to the war-effort, to industry, to battlefield logistics, and to the impossibility of social distancing in time of war: "There are national circumstances in which the major duty is to 'carry on,' even when risk to health and life is involved" ("Discussion on Influenza," 13):

> This duty has arisen ... among munitions workers and other workers engaged in work of urgent national importance; it has arisen on a gigantic scale in connexion with the transport during 1918 of many hundreds of thousands of troops to this country and to France overseas. In each of the cases cited some lives might have been saved, spread of infection diminished, great suffering avoided, if the known sick could have been isolated from the healthy; if rigid exclusion of known sick and drastic increase of floorspace for each person could have been enforced in factories, workplaces, barracks, and ships; if overcrowding could have been regardlessly prohibited. But it was necessary to "carry on," and the relentless needs of warfare justified incurring this risk of spreading infection and the associated creation of a more virulent type of disease or of mixed diseases ["Discussion," 13].

It is impossible to speculate what could have happened had he chosen to deploy resources in an all-out preventative campaign. Had he delivered a public service message, what could he have said, other than to require masks, to proscribe expectoration, and to be inoculated with a dubious vaccine? If carrying on with the business of national defense ended the war, then it could possibly have hastened the end of the pandemic (its third wave would extend to the winter of 1919). Though the Armistice brought a cease-fire, the overcrowding in factory and barracks continued and would only be eased gradually. It is entirely conceivable that more than one-quarter million British citizens could have died if the war had not ended in November 1918, and if the war-pandemic interaction had continued on unabatedly.

To a degree, the political civil war at the center of the story distracts from the complex biomedical drama, since culpability is directed at the L.G.B. rather than at a natural disaster and at the unsolvable problems the coincidence of war and pandemic had produced. Had Reina James considered Dr. Newsholme's burden—a broken system, a world war, and a lethal, untreatable disease—his struggle would have appeared more like the stuff of Greek tragedy than of bureaucratic inefficiency. In place of the conventional opposition between Newsholme the stereotypical bureaucrat and Wey the undaunted physician (or Newman the public health innovator), this novel could have explored the epidemiological and geopolitical paradox of the milieu: that, in 1918, humanity was at war with itself *and* with nature. Of this reality, Newsholme had no doubt.

Thomas Mullen, The Last Town on Earth *(2007)*

In the historical context of "quarantines" (understood in the generic sense) during the 1918–1919 pandemic, Thomas Mullen's fictional mill town, Commonwealth, is not unusual.[1] Alfred Crosby cites one example of how a community, in the autumn of 1918, resisted the advancing pandemic. Mountain Village, a small town located in the Yukon Delta, Alaska, escaped the effects of the pandemic completely, an eventuality Crosby attributes to good leadership (Crosby, 248). When Mountain Village learned of the approaching danger, continues Crosby, the village's local teacher took the initiative, informing community leaders who, in turn, educated the population as to how to avoid and to treat the disease. In public meetings, residents discussed all matters pertaining to influenza, including the proposed closure of town. Crosby uses the concept of quarantine not in the strict CDC sense, but rather broadly to mean barring non-residents from entering, and residents from returning to, an uninfected area until the crisis is over. Mountain Village's apparent success stemmed from the cooperation of all those who lived there and from an active leadership that provided the latest information, offered guidance, and maintained a forum for discussion.

John M. Barry, in *The Great Influenza*, Mullen's chief historical sourcebook, describes towns in the San Juan Mountain area of Colorado that fared rather well in preventing the incursion of disease, an outcome Barry attributes to the work of a well-informed town that had sufficient time to prepare. In one town, Lake City, armed guards prevented nonresidents from entering. In Silverton, social-distancing measures were put into place: all businesses closed; but somehow the virus was brought into town anyway, and 125 persons died. In the town of Ouray, armed guards, positioned at the borders, stopped miners from Silverton and Telluride from trespassing; however, for unclear reasons, the infection penetrated these barriers. In early October, the railroad town of Gunnison, Colorado, to which Mullen refers explicitly, quarantined itself well before anyone contracted the disease and banned social gatherings. Lawmen blocked roads, and anyone disembarking from a train at Gunnison station was arrested and held for five days—that is, sequestered as if the person were an asymptomatic carrier (Barry, *Influenza*, 345–346).

Contemporary epidemiological studies on quarantine practices in 1918 demonstrate that social distancing, isolation methods, and legal checkpoints allowed several jurisdictions to resist the pandemic. Markel and colleagues (2006) studied six U.S. communities that had reported relatively few cases of influenza, in 1918–1919, while nonpharmaceutical interventions were in effect. Of the six interventions, archival data show that the U.S. Naval Base at Yerba Buena Island in San Francisco Bay and the mining town of Gunnison, Colorado, were the most prepared. Under the direction of the Public Health Office at Yerba Buena Island and at Gunnison, almost no cases of infection were recorded for two and four months, respectively. Several factors contributed to these successful outcomes: one was geographical (both locations were "essentially cut off from all contact with the outside world to shield themselves from the incursion of influenza"). The investigators in this study helped to define the policy of closing a town, using the serviceable phrase "protective sequestration," meaning to bar ingress into the town. This phrase distinguishes the kind of closure found in Mountain Village and in Gunnison from the CDC's definitions of quarantine (i.e., to restrict the movements of healthy or asymptomatic persons believed to have been exposed to flu) and of isolation (i.e., to detain, examine, and eventually release). Protective sequestration prohibited community residents from leaving the area; and any visitors, from entering. Anyone who manages to get past the barriers was quarantined (i.e., in CDC terms: isolated). Once the quarantine period had ended, and after medical examination, healthy individuals could move about the village freely. A remote mountain town, Gunnison had a geographical advantage. Strict public health measures were initiated there, the local population cooperated fully, and civic leaders informed and prepared the population. Gunnison also kept track of the pandemic's westward movement, from August to September, and unlike East Coast cities, was prepared before people fell sick (Markel et al. [2006]).

In several related studies investigators concluded, from a study of 43 cities over a 24-week period, 1918–1919, that quarantine, isolation, sequestration, and social distancing reduced mortality (Markel et al., [2007]). McLeod et al. (2008) report that, in 1918–1919, maritime quarantine, the interdiction and observance of ship traffic and passengers in Continental Australia, American Samoa, New Caledonia, Tasmania, and along the Pacific Rim, successfully prevented contagion. The data suggest that, for these islands, maritime quarantine delayed or even prevented influenza's arrival. These islands also recorded lower excess death rates than jurisdictions not controlling maritime borders. The effect on commerce, they note, could be mitigated if this situation were to arise in future: plane crews, passengers, and cargo handlers had been detained temporarily for medical observation.

The combined use of several modes of nonpharmaceutical control during an influenza pandemic could be an effective deterrent against infectious spread. Nishiura et al. (2009), examining the effectiveness of quarantine as a border control measure, predict that quarantine (in the CDC sense) would be 95–99 percent successful in preventing infectious individuals from entering a community. To determine if an asymptomatic person were carrying the virus, 4.7 to 8.6 days (if not longer) were required before the incubation period expired (Doc Banes in the novel enacts a four-day quarantine [Mullen, 130]). If rapid diagnostic testing were available, the period of quarantine for suspected visitors could be reduced; but no such testing was available in 1918–1919. Nishiura's group concluded that, in the future, border quarantines for island nations could delay or prevent the arrival of pandemic influenza.

The research consensus surveyed here maintains that nonpharmaceutical interventions—e.g., public health leadership, information and communication, quarantine, isolation, social distancing, and protective sequestration—can work effectively, and the South Pacific jurisdictions exemplify the use of multiple strategies. Kelso, Milne, and Kelly (2009) emphasize that social distancing (the closing of schools, businesses, and entertainment centers) will play a crucial role "in the potential control of a future pandemic"; and such interventions can arrest influenza epidemic development if combined and maintained for a relatively long period.

In a 6 October 2009 interview, Thomas Mullen summarizes the extent of the research undertaken to write *The Last Town on Earth* ("An Interview") The "impetus" for the book had come from an article on virology that parenthetically mentions the influenza pandemic and how unaffected towns in the Rocky Mountain states and in the Pacific Northwest, fearing the disease, had blocked off roads and posted armed guards to prevent anyone from entering. These efforts, however, raised procedural, legal, and moral questions: what protocol would the guards follow if a stranger disobeyed them? Would armed force then be legally and morally justified? What should be done if the individual was nonviolent and needed care? How flexible should the guards be, given the possibility that the person was a carrier? This complicated issue and the crucial decisions the guards had to make inspired the most dramatic and action-packed scenes in the novel.

Mullen had tried to learn more about these isolated towns and about the methods they used to enact what he calls "reverse-quarantine." The phrase means the residents of the uninfected town, once gone, could not return until the pandemic had ended; nor would outsiders be allowed to enter. The phrase is congruent with the CDC's "protective sequestration" (Markel et al. [2006]). But his research turned up little information. Even John Barry's encyclopedic history of the pandemic treats this aspect of the story cursorily. Mullen reasons that these towns got very little publicity since, at that moment, the war was reaching a critical stage and demanded public attention, even though the pandemic was decimating large urban populations throughout the country, precisely the situation with which Newsholme was contending in the UK at that time. Mullen is correct in assuming that the montane northwestern towns were relatively small and geographically remote and that these factors contributed to their ability to fend off, or at least to delay, the onset of the disease. In addition, resistance strategies in remote areas were not front-page news and could not be compared to public health efforts in crowded cities where the morbidity and mortality rates were highest.

One other reason for the relative obscurity of the quarantine plan in Mountain Village, Alaska, or in Gunnison, Colorado, was that the flu moved with such devastating rapidity that news agencies and local historians of that period just could not keep up with events. Nearly a century later, we are learning how these inland communities in the Pacific Northwest used epidemiological information to their advantage. They were aware, for example, that the focal points of the pandemic were military cantonments on the East Coast, and that the virus flourished in these locations and inexorably moved westward in the respiratory tracts of rail, bus, and automotive travelers. Distance afforded the northwestern communities with some time to plan and, unlike the British government at the time, they used this reprieve wisely. With a historical sketch of the northwestern ordeal, Mullen imagines the diametrical opposition of two towns: Commonwealth (a study in incomplete public health planning) and Timber Falls (a study in no planning).

The town of Commonwealth, Washington, the epicenter of Mullen's epidemiological tragedy, was supposedly founded on utopian principles. To its founders, Charles and Rebecca Worthy, the civilized world is dangerous; and communicable disease and crime are the outgrowths and the burdens of industrial society. This small community closes itself off from the outside world because they disagree with the political, philosophical, and economic status quo. For Rebecca, "rejecting the world" is a doctrinal statement, intended to demonstrate "how it could be improved, so that others would follow their example" (Mullen, 23–24). As Philip Worthy learns, "the quarantine designed to block out the flu" has the ironic effect of "cutting off the town from its previous ideals of right and wrong" (Mullen, 287). When influenza invades Commonwealth, the adverse changes in human behavior are predictable; the ideals upon which the settlement rests are proven to be naïve. Under duress, the inhabitants of Commonwealth become fearful, suspicious, distrustful, selfish, dishonest, and violent. Mullen observes that, "The whole dilemma of utopian politics" in a perfect society cannot be realized since human beings are frail, imperfect, self-centered, and inconsistent ("Interview").

On the idea of "reverse-quarantining," there are two opinions in Commonwealth. Some reject sequestration as incommensurate with the idea of an open society. Moderates, on the other hand, support it as a survival measure. The quarantine's failure can be attributed, not to a conceptual misinterpretation, but rather to the inept way it was instituted. There appears to be no trained law-enforcement in the village, no public health system, no legal counsel, and no communication with neighboring towns to apprise them of their activities. Commonwealth's knowledge of the flu's westward onslaught is through word of mouth and from public media in Timber Falls where some mill employees live or visit regularly.

It is the Timber Falls connection and the movement of Commonwealth mill workers that will be the utopians' undoing. The Commonwealth checkpoints seem to have disregarded itinerant travelers who use porous borders routinely. The plan was foredoomed: it lacked professional supervision, equipment, and most of all humane flexibility: isolation wards were needed for those stricken with flu, whether they were insiders or outsiders; and quarantine facilities, with medical observation, were required for an outsider who seemed healthy. The only physician is a competent country doctor with only a rudimentary knowledge of influenza. There is no hospital, no clinic, no ambulance, little medicine, and unlicensed volunteer nurses. The level of medical care and preparedness in this progressive settlement is primitive. Commonwealth's quarantine plan, according to Mullen, is hastily contrived. If quarantine were mandated for a city or state today, Mullen observes, the barriers would be professionally manned; but, even then, the risk of human rights violations would still exist ("An Interview").

Graham, a guard who thinks in black-and-white terms, experiences an acute moral dilemma. He must decide whether to execute an obstinate outsider, a beaten and hungry conscientious objector who went AWOL because of the abuse other soldiers heaped upon him for his convictions. As Mullen notes, although men were permitted to declare themselves C.O.s because they had anti-war feelings, and although 65,000 men requested noncombatant roles, most were pressured into recanting, and 17 died for their principles (Mullen, "Author's Note," 391). The situation into which Graham has been thrust leaves no room for compromise, no middle path, no holding pen where the intruder could be accommodated temporarily and assessed medically during an incubation period. If healthy, the stranger could be permitted to stay. If unhealthy, the stranger would be sequestered. Without these alternatives, Graham ends up killing the forlorn soldier: "The sound and the force of the shot made Philip jump.... He saw the soldier's chest burst open, cloth and something the color of newly washed skin flying forward" (Mullen, 12). Graham's main concern, after delivering a second shot, is whether the dead body remains contagious and if so, for how long (Mullen, 13). He justifies homicide on the grounds of self-preservation: if the vagrant was a healthy carrier, a condition he could neither confirm nor deny, he threatened his family and the entire town, and the risk of that outweighed anything less than lethal force. Graham does not regret his action, but he acknowledges that both he and the soldier are victims of circumstance—of "the randomness of fate that had placed him on that path in front of Graham" whose decision would be haunting (Mullen, 70, 188). Reflecting on the occupational hazards of millwork (as evident in Graham's four-fingered hand) and on the present ordeal, Philip wonders, "if there was some end point, some line in the dust, some amount of pain and suffering beyond which one could never continue" (Mullen, 43). The motif of protective boundaries, both psychological and physical, resonates in the novel and was a fact of life during the pandemic when public places were off limits, and when human interaction of any kind was a risk.

Philip Worthy, Charles and Rebecca's adopted son, who had witnessed Graham's act while on barricade duty, would experience a similar trial when, after a brief gunfight with another intrusive soldier, Private Frank Summers, he imprisons him, committing both captor and captive to a makeshift quarantine period in a storehouse. Philip's moral decision is not appreciated by the townsfolk who think he has introduced a potential threat into their midst. Once the approximate 48-hour incubation period (a dangerously foreshortened period) had elapsed, Philip is released but publicly vilified and even scapegoated. The quarantined soldier, now baselessly suspected of being a fugitive German spy, is subjected to further indignities, and then Graham murders him, believing that, in so doing, he was protecting the town and serving his country. In fact, the second intruder, also an AWOL soldier, had earlier risked his life to save the recently-deceased conscientious objector. It is because Private Summers had killed the C.O.'s tormenters that the former went AWOL (Mullen, 269–284).

The moral confusion afflicting Commonwealth residents stems from their ignorance about the pandemic. More directly, it is the rebound effect of haphazard and porous sequestration, in which no provision for quarantine or isolation was made. Townsfolk, not militia, are enjoined as guards and given the authority to use lethal force if necessary—but by whose authority, and what constitutes a necessity?

Officials in neighboring Timber Falls, a more affluent and mainstream community, are less concerned with disease control than they are with challenging Commonwealth's sequestration. Bankers, law-enforcement officers, and others, as citizen-members of the American Protection League (APL), however, are federal officers, deputized by the Justice Department. According to the CDC information sheet, federal jurisdiction supersedes local auspices, but the APL is not concerned with public health.[2] Instead, the APL, which was sponsored by the Department of Justice, enforced conscription laws and tracked down un–American activity. Among its nationwide membership of 300,000 were "vigilante 'superpatriots'" who were known to violate the civil rights of immigrants (Mullen, "Author's Note," 391). The opportunity for the misuse of power was great. Timber Falls, a town with widespread influenza, chooses to follow its ideological impulses: hysteria, rumor, pseudo-patriotism, economic rivalry, labor disputation, political philosophy, and xenophobia motivate them to besiege Commonwealth. From the perspective of federal law, the APL, though it is legally sanctioned, could be unethical in practice. Conflicts over jurisdiction and authority make for tense moments throughout the novel.

As communal tensions increase, the town doctor, Martin Banes, M.D., makes house calls and acts as an epidemiologist when influenza finally appears in town. Gradually, he becomes aware of the growing crisis as he gathers information. A millworker named Yolen exhibits flu-like symptoms, is prostrate, has pulmonary edema, and 24 hours after the initial consultation is cyanotic (Mullen, 216). Banes suspects the worst and realizes that whomever Yolen had contacted must be examined. Dr. Banes visits the unaccounted-for millworker Leonard, whom he finds dead. Leonard had died of hemorrhages, consistent with influenza in its cytokine phase (Mullen, 217–218). The chapter concludes with the foreboding line: "It had begun" (Mullen, 218). As Dr. Banes knows full well, the quarantine had been breached.

Once Charles Worthy and Dr. Banes are reasonably certain that Yolen had indeed contracted influenza (no necropsy, no hospital, no mortuary), they decide to make the news public, an intelligent move. Yolen is then placed in isolation, with armed guards around his home (Mullen, 224). Meanwhile, Philip Worthy blames himself for Yolen's illness. He isolates himself, shirking human contact and considers himself an outcast. Believing unfoundedly that he has somehow picked up the germ from Private Summers and was an asymptomatic carrier and public health threat, Philip secludes himself emotionally: "He wished he could close himself off, a personal quarantine within the quarantined town" (Mullen, 218).

The fragmentation of Commonwealth society and the alienation of its citizens is a result of the war-pandemic interaction. Mullen points out that, "Fear of spies, the loss of loved ones overseas, and the sense that the country's very way of life was under attack combined to form a volatile environment" (Mullen, "Author's Note," 391). Philip imagines that this is the price that must be paid for acting mercifully, for, like Graham, the consequences of his decision weigh heavily on him. Since Graham believes that Philip is the carrier, he unjustly criticizes Banes for mistakenly assuming that the incubation period is 48 hours or less; Graham has a point, although Philip was not the carrier (Mullen, 229). Furthermore, Graham's suspicions, fueled by ignorance, fear, and guilt, convince him wrongly that the imprisoned soldier is not only a disguised German spy, but also a source of disease whose every breath threatens him and his loved ones. In his embittered and narrowed mind, he is convinced that murdering the soldier is both an act of patriotism and a moral obligation. To Graham, Private Summers is a dangerous interloper, a carrier of influenza, "and now it's coming out of him. The longer he stays here, the worse it'll get" (Mullen, 230). Graham even entertains the seemingly absurd notion that Private Summers is a bioterrorist who has purposefully transported a German-engineered toxin to Commonwealth (Mullen, 230). German scientists and the military, in World War I, had indeed used biological weapons but on a limited scale aimed primarily at horses, mules, sheep, and cattle, which they infected by saturating feed with bacterial cultures (Bristow, 77; S. Harris, 217–218). Private Summers, on the other hand, has become the scapegoat of dystopian Commonwealth. He is not an agent of Dr. Anton Dilger (1884–1918), the infamous German-American bioterrorist and saboteur.

Although Dr. Banes isolated Yolen, he also suspects that doing so might be a futile gesture since Leonard and others have contracted the disease from him. Thus, Banes has been "forced to acknowledge that the flu was already spreading uncontrollably," and that soon "there would be more infected homes than the town could possibly quarantine" (Mullen, 237). The principle of social cooperation and of community spirit that Commonwealth professed at its founding has given way to uncompromising survivalism. No one, Dr. Banes realizes, will help Yolen's wife to nurse or feed him. Nor is there a Lydia Wickett anywhere in town: "the women who ordinarily served as [Dr. Banes'] nurses [in the most practical sense of the term] in extreme times had all steadfastly refused to do so now—they didn't want to risk bringing flu home to their families" (Mullen, 237). The pandemic reduces the once-altruistic, gregarious residents of the town to a reclusive colony.

The index case and pattern of infection come to light, thanks to Dr. Banes' epidemiological discovery that Yolen had had a few drinks with two shingle weavers, Otto and Ray (Mullen, 240). Ray became ill the same day as Yolen and was in the same condition. Otto had reported to work the previous day but became incapacitated and left for home. When Banes checks on Otto, the patient is delirious and coughing. How Leonard had contracted the disease was as-yet unclear. Banes, despite his limitations, is a dedicated physician, visiting everyone listed as Leonard's friends, along with family members and collateral contacts. When the store proprietor Flora Metzger develops symptoms, Banes is greatly disturbed since the general store was always crowded, and patrons signed in at a ledger, using the same pen (Mullen, 240). It was too late for social distancing. Like Dr. Rieux in Camus' *The Plague*, Banes could be little else than a witness to the events that were fast growing "beyond his skill and reckoning" (Mullen, 241). As the morbidity rate rises, Banes could only get to work identifying patients, offering advice, and treating patients with the remedies he had.

Public safety deteriorates. Once the Metzgers are ordered to close their store to contain contagion, supplies, already low, dwindle to a dangerous level. The Worthys' private vegetable garden is ransacked (Mullen 248); and the Metzgers' store, broken into and robbed of goods (Mullen, 304–305). Panic becomes palpable (Mullen, 249). Millworkers whose family members had died or who were sick themselves taunt Philip whom they blame for the pestilence (Mullen, 254); ironically, the men who berate Philip were among those whom he had served while on watch. It was abundantly clear that "the fear of the flu had changed everyone" (Mullen, 255). They blame Philip; he blames himself; and, in turn, the innocent Frank Summers (Mullen, 267). The quarantine, implemented to preserve the town, ironically overshadows it. For Philip Worthy, Commonwealth is "a town in full eclipse" (Mullen, 287).

Banes concedes that isolation is not working as more households are stricken. Nor is sentry duty of any use since the disease spreads too quickly. It is at this point that Graham decides to kill Private Summers, as if the soldier's death would somehow end their plight (Mullen, 297–300). Graham rationalizes his behavior, justifying homicide in the name of imperatives inapplicable to the situation. Because Graham conceives of himself as a patriot, a defender of town and country, and a sentry who never leaves his post, he justifies the killing of Private Summers.

The pandemic's impact on Commonwealth terrifies its residents to the point that they are "no longer interested in communal sacrifice" (Mullen, 303). The real cause of the breach comes to light through Dr. Banes' investigation. Instead of cooperating for the common good, millworkers visited Timber Falls clandestinely to see girlfriends and for liquor and then, in flagrant violation of civic regulations, returned to Commonwealth, ready for work and carrying the influenza virus. Emergency measures are contemplated for the sake of survival but difficult to implement. Once the Metzgers' store closes, and since no goods are coming in, basic nutrition becomes a problem (Mullen, 306). Charles Worthy considers radical measures after consulting the magistrates, quite contrary to the ethos of Commonwealth. The thought of a house-to-house search, however, is quickly dismissed, even in desperate times (Mullen, 307).

Once the quarantine is officially lifted, Commonwealth's inhabitants cannot resist the APL whose members had weathered the flu, had convalesced, and were now robust. These men arrested anyone who had failed to register for the draft (Mullen, 368–369). But the shock of the APL raid and the cessation of the flu brought people out of seclusion. When the population of Commonwealth learns the truth about Leonard and his friends, vigilantes hunt them down, but the millworkers are all found dead before retribution is exacted (Mullen, 382). When Graham's deeds come to light, people shun him. Philip, who shoots a policeman in the midst of a federally-sanctioned raid becomes a fugitive. His father's hope is to find a way "to justify Philip's actions" since the sheriff had invaded Graham's home and was using unlawful force. In Philip's mind, killing the sheriff saved lives (Mullen, 383), a rationalization ironically akin to Graham's.

The constructive potential of the quarantine in Commonwealth had been undermined from the beginning, and the failure to implement it in conformity to legal and medical guidelines leads to the town's destruction. When the war ends and the second wave recedes, the utopian legislators of Commonwealth revive their ingenuous worldview: "they were free to reimagine the lives they had pursued before it began. Charles was confident there would be a way to justify Philip's action" (Mullen, 383). Apparently, the Commonwealth utopians will become further acquainted with harsh reality. First, the Armistice of 11 November had been signed the day of the APL raid, which means that its aftermath would extend into late autumn and the winter snows, when the third wave of the influenza virus would arrive. Second, Philip Worthy who had killed a federalized law enforcement officer is a fugitive felon who will be tracked down and apprehended. And, third, the notion that the Worthys will "reimagine" their social vision suggests a retreat to fantasy. The war-pandemic interaction was an invaluable lesson in psychology and human behavior, from which they learned nothing.

James Rada, Jr., October Mourning *(2006)*

During the second wave of the pandemic, physicians worked feverishly to halt the spread of the disease and to protect the population from infection. Laboring under the mistaken belief that bacteria were primarily, if not solely, responsible for the crisis, they hastily devised and administered vaccines that were untested and of questionable value. The unknown dangers and false hopes raised by hasty vaccine production drew criticism. In no uncertain terms, the *JAMA* editorial board declared, in the 26 October 1918 issue, that the medical community neither had a tested serum, a means of curing influenza, nor a "specific vaccine or vaccines for its prevention." This was the current state of influenza medicine, "all claims and propagandist statements in the newspapers and elsewhere to the contrary notwithstanding." Practitioners and researchers, they stress, had to keep in mind that "efforts at treatment and prevention by serums and vaccines, now hurriedly undertaken, are simply experiments in a new field." For the editors, there is no substitute for the scientific method, for the gathering of salient data, for thorough evaluation, and for the conferral of experts over time: "exact results can be determined ... only after a time, in most cases probably not until the epidemic is past and all the returns canvassed" ("Serums and Vaccines," 1408).

The editors' advisory did not dampen the enthusiasm of those who had been working on vaccines made from bacteria. This is amazing in view of the fact that, in the midst of the second wave, medical scientists, as surveyed in chapter 1, had real doubts about a bacterial cause of influenza. Drs. Spooner, Sellards, and Wyman, for example, could not account for a major inconsistency: "clinically atypical pneumonia" was present in influenza patients but Pfeiffer's bacillus was not ("Serum Treatment," 1310–1311). Drs. McGuire and Redden, advocates of using convalescents' serum as vaccine, began to question Pfeiffer's claim and entertained the co-pathogenicity idea ("Treatment of Influenza Pneumonia," 1310). Also in the bacterial-causation camp, Dr. Benjamin S. Paschall, in reply to the 26 October editorial cited above, considers the board's position as extreme, while at the same time acknowledging that no proven serum exists against influenza (1602). The case against Pfeiffer's bacillus would become incontrovertible by March 1919: bacteria other than Pfeiffer's, Paschall acknowledges, were largely responsible for complications. Ernest W. Goodpasture, Peter K. Olitsky and Frederick L. Gates, in late autumn 1919 and winter 1920, confirmed that bacteria were implicated in the secondary effect in the disease process, while the "essential effects were produced by a substance wholly unrelated to bacteria"—that is, by the unseen pathogen (Goodpasture, "Bronchopneumonia, 724–725; "Experimental Study." 1497–1499).

The *JAMA* editors who had collated British and German abstracts on influenza in early November summarize what was known and not known at the time: (1) "we do not understand the true nature of the condition now being called epidemic influenza"; (2) there is not sufficient evidence to regard any one of the different forms of bacteria found in the respiratory tract in the cases of the disease as the primary cause"; (3) bacteria, including Pfeiffer's microbe, "may be secondary invaders, transmissible from person to person with almost the same ease as the supposed, but unknown, primary cause" ("Observations," 1580). As far as the *JAMA* editors were concerned, an unknown agent caused the initial attack and could be followed by pneumonia-causing bacteria. These tentative conclusions would be vindicated, in 2008, when Morens et al. discovered that the majority of deaths in 1918–1919, "likely resulted directly from secondary bacterial pneumonia caused by common upper respiratory tract bacteria" ("Predominant Role of Bacterial Pneumonia").

Even though the efficacy of bacterial sera was in question, the pharmaceutical industry produced vaccines on a large scale. In October 1918, C. Y. White, chief bacteriologist of the Philadelphia General Hospital, oversaw the manufacture of 10,000 three-shot dosages of vaccine that were freely disseminated to physicians and to thousands of Philadelphians. The vaccine was compared to one that was recently used against an outbreak of polio in the city. This multivalent preparation containing deadly strains of several bacteria had no effect on influenza (Crosby, 84; Barry, *Influenza*, 356).

Influenza vaccines, produced at this time in Boston, New York, and Philadelphia, did have a psychological benefit, heightened by coincidence: their placebo effect coincided with the natural recession of the second wave, and the vaccine was credited with the results (Crosby, 84). Dr. Timothy Leary, of Tufts Medical College, shipped his vaccine to beleaguered San Franciscans, claiming it arrested influenza and prevented pneumonia and death. Once again, by early November as the disease subsided, the vaccine was again thought to have been effective (Crosby, 100–101, 105). Without evidence, William Henry Welch extolled the use of gauze masks in a 10 August 1918 *JAMA* issue (Barry, *Influenza*, 211). A San Franciscan law requiring masks was so controversial that an Anti-Mask League, composed of "public-spirited citizens, skeptical physicians, and fanatics," had been organized to enforce it (Crosby, 112). Ironically, neither vaccines nor masks made any difference (Barry, *Influenza*, 358–359, 375).

As John M. Eyler argues, in "The Fog of Research: Influenza Vaccine Trials during the 1918–1919 Pandemic" (2009), reports of the preventative benefit of multivalent bacterial vaccines were ambiguous, inconsistent, and contradictory. Ensuing debates showed that the medical profession did not even agree on what constituted a proper vaccine trial. To remedy this serious deficiency, the American Public Health Association established standards that would remain in place for a quarter century. Even though the bacterial vaccine campaign did not contribute tangibly to health care during the pandemic, the value of this research belongs to the history of bacteriology (Eyler, "The Fog of Research"). In 1880, while pioneering vaccination development for bacterial infections, Pasteur "had an instinct that a process akin to vaccination might hold for other diseases," by which he meant submicroscopic organisms or viruses (Bulloch, 241–242). Pasteur's instincts were certainly correct.

James Rada, Jr.'s *October Mourning* revisits the medical context of the second wave, and in particular, the debate outlined above. His medical personae express the frustrations of actual physicians who, in September 1918, had no protocol through which they might help their patients. Once again, scientific acumen met only with futility. The protagonist, Alan Keener, M.D., (perhaps a nominal conflation of actual researchers, Drs. J. J. *Kee*-gan and Simon Flex-*ner*) has nothing more than aspirin to offer, and its overuse would be toxic: "So many cures seemed to be within the grasp of medicine and yet just out of reach. Influenza was one of those things. Researchers knew what caused it, in theory, but they hadn't been able to stop it so far" (Rada, 9). Actually, they thought they knew but did not.

Despite the fact that Keener subscribes to the bacteriological hypothesis, he still imagines that an etiological breakthrough in influenza research is imminent (it was, in fact, less than fifteen years away). In a debate with his supervisor, Dr. Hyatt, Keener asserts that the germ theory is "the basis of the influenza contagion." In saying this, he is following in Pfeiffer's line of argument. Keener is familiar with then-current theories on pathogenesis, as he speculates on a genealogical connection between the causes of the 1889–1890 and current pandemics. But molecular genetics would disprove the idea that the 1918 strain was a lineal descendant of its 1890 antecedent. In 2006, the year of the novel's publication, viral sequence data from the reconstituted H1N1 genome suggested "that the entire 1918 virus was novel to humans in, or shortly before, 1918, and that it thus was not a reassortant virus produced from old existing strains" (Taubenberger & Morens, "1918 Pandemic"). Keener's purpose in the novel is not to argue the merits of the Pfeiffer-Kitasato theory; rather, his intention is to alert Hyatt to the early stages of a second influenza wave, he believes responsible for the recent death of his patient, Sarah Jenkins (Rada, 19). Keener astutely warns his colleague that the first wave subsided on its own and not through medical interventions, so a second wave might be imminent (Rada, 20).

Authorial prolepsis occurs in the chapter of 26 September, when Keener describes the cause of Jenkin's pulmonary inflammation as an immunological overreaction. At Sarah Jenkins' autopsy, he tells Dr. Jack McCullough that, "Her body tried to fight off the flu in her lungs, but it reacted too strongly to the disease and wound up doing more harm than good" (Rada, 26). Keener's insight reflects Rada's careful research; however, in terms of the history of medicine, Keener's co-pathogen theory, set forth in 1918, is too far ahead of its time. In 1997, when the H5N1 avian flu virus had moved from poultry to people, World Health Organization investigators discovered in postmortem examinations of two victims' high serum levels of cytokines, proteins "that regulate the intensity and duration of the immune response" (Webster & Walker, 124–125). The H5N1 virus, precursor of the 1918 virus, induces excessive cytokines, leading to "toxic-shock syndrome" which kills the patient or causes pulmonary damage, predisposing the influenza patient to bacterial colonization (Webster & Walker, 125). Apparently, Rada invests Keener with extraordinary talents: etiological insight and pathophysiological foresight.

Drs. Keener and Peter Markwood, a pathologist at Western Maryland Hospital, examine lung tissue specimens taken from Sarah Jenkins, who had recently died of influenza. Her body revealed cyanosis, sodden lungs, and bloody fluid in the lungs: "The aveoli and capillaries in her lungs had burst" (Rada, 32). Among the abundance of microscopic debris in the lung tissue, Markwood discovers "the bacillus" (Rada, 32). Rada is fully aware of the debate surrounding Pfeiffer's claim, and he has Keener point to a significant discrepancy: "the spring cases of the Spanish flu didn't have Pfeiffer's Bacillus," whereas the deadlier fall cases did, "as was reported in Philadelphia" (Rada, 32–33). Acknowledging the anomaly, Markwood understands its implications: if Pfeiffer was wrong, then the only reputed indicator of influenza's presence had been negated, and, as a result, medical intervention might be reduced to trial and error.

Keener questions other basic assumptions. One is that the so-called *Spanish influenza* was not a form of influenza at all; nor was it Spanish in origin (Rada, 33). Gina Kolata points out that, in February 1918, influenza mildly afflicted the tourist town of San Sebastian on the northern coast of Spain, infecting young adults more than the elderly and children. By April, however, Spain was in the midst of the second wave, and eight million Spaniards became ill, including one third of Madrid's population. The disease then spread widely, becoming a global disaster. Conveniently, it was labeled *Spanish* flu, perhaps because Spain, unlike other European countries, had not censored its news reports (Kolata, *Flu*, 8–10).

On 27 September 1918, Keener, like the pensive Dr. Rieux in Camus' *The Plague*, urges that sera and vaccines be developed: "The problem is you need to find someone who has immunity against the disease and compare that person's blood to everyone else. No one seems to have found such a person yet" (Rada, 34). Four basic definitions are useful at this juncture: (1) *innate immunity* refers to bodily defenses, present since birth and not involving "specific recognition of a microbe"; (2) *adaptive* or *active immunity*, to the body's production of specific types of cells or antibodies in response to an antigen (Tortora & Derrickson, 432, 440); (3) *passive immunity*, to resistance against harmful microbes, conferred when antibodies are either naturally or artificially transferred from one organism to another (e.g., natural passive immunity is when a fetus receives antibodies from its mother) (Campbell and Reece et al. G-27); and (4) *passive immunization* or *vaccination*, to which Rada is referring in this context, is acquired from the direct transfer of antibodies through blood serum, as in the inoculation of antibodies taken from someone convalescing after a bout of flu; or it could involve the injection of inactive or attenuated pathogen, that induces "B and T cell responses and immunological memory" (Campbell, Reece, et al., G-27). Vaccine producers, in 1918, were harvesting antibodies from flu convalescents under the assumption that their blood contained cells with immunizing properties.

The paradox of influenza in 1918–1919, is that *innate immunity*, in some patients, caused more damage to the lungs than did the virus. Cytokine proteins and other cells which inflamed the lungs, causing edema, high fever, and Acute Respiratory Distress Syndrome—the 1970s acronym ARDS—referring to how viral infection impaired breathing; as the infection weakened the immune system, the release of interferon and of related antiviral proteins would be inhibited (Barry, *Influenza*, 247–48). The cycle concludes as respiratory bacteria invade debilitated lungs.

Keener's 27 September 1918 comment about inducing passive immunity is timely (Rada, 28–34). Rada's research is historically accurate. Polio vaccinations in 1910, involved the inoculation of antibodies from convalescent patients into sick ones. L. W. McGuire and W. R. Redden tried this procedure in 1918, on influenza patients at Boston's Naval Hospital. The experiment, though it had promising results, proved to be methodologically flawed ("Treatment of Influenza Pneumonia," 1311–1312; Barry, *Influenza*, 283–284).

Keener is also an innovator. His immunological method, at this point, steers away from bacterial causation. Instead of injecting sick patients directly with unfiltered convalescent blood sera, he decides to use a convalescent's *bacteria-free filtrate* for immunization vaccine. In other words, he abandons the bacterial hypothesis as the initiating cause and joins the avant-garde Japanese and French scientists: namely Yamanouchi et al. and Nicolle and LeBailly, respectively. The Yamanouchi-Skakami-Iwashima experiments, carried out from December 1918 to March 1919, used filtrates (bacteria having been removed), instilled into the respiratory tracts and bloodstreams of healthy volunteers. The aim was to induce influenza using presumably *bacteria-free* suspensions. They announced resoundingly positive results, but, since their experiments were flawed in several respects, their findings (as noted above) were invalidated (Crosby, 282; Kolata, 60–61). Keener's idea of late September adumbrates the Japanese experiments, commencing in December 1918.

Rada's description of public health measures instituted at the time is historically accurate, even down to the controversial issues. In regard to public health and hospital measures to contain the pandemic, however, Keener is somewhat short-sighted. At the height of the emergency, Hyatt enunciates a reasonable social-distancing policy for his overburdened hospital: he proposes limiting the number of admittances to control contagion. Flu sufferers are to be sent home, and doctors will make house calls. Keener objects to this policy on the grounds that not sequestering patients in the hospital will only spread the disease publicly, causing more deaths. Hyatt, however, argues persuasively against blanket admittance: he has no proof that anyone turned away from the hospital had died as a result; he will be protecting not only convalescing patients but also hospital staff; no hospital-based treatment has been shown effective; and most people survive the flu. Keener's judgment is questionable with respect to the Cumberland Board of Health's issuance of a public health directive on 4 October. This directive ordered the closing of public locations, required ventilation on all public transport, proscribed public expectoration, and required the use of handkerchiefs for coughs and sneezes. Keener, however, is not in favor of these precautions which actually were commonsensical and effective to some degree (Rada, 86–87). He is justifiably concerned about a proposed employment policy: to replace one-sixth of the sick workforce, men from Baltimore and Philadelphia were being recruited, a problem at the heart of the Commonwealth crisis in Mullen's book. Since they were to commute to work, this would spread the virus more widely (Rada, 88). The Keener-Hyatt dialogue reflects a historical verity: measures to control the pandemic had not been standardized.

Rada's understanding of the morbidity and mortality rates is accurate, as is evidenced by Keener's comments on infection: 40 percent of the population gets flu, less somewhat in rural areas, meaning that 10,000 cases would be expected in the immediate area. Of the 10,000, however, only 2 to 3 percent will die (200–300 fatalities). Though this germ is far deadlier than the seasonal variety, its mortality potential is relatively low in proportion to the number of infected, 98 percent of whom recover (Rada, 93). Yet statistics and ratios are meaningless when a loved one is involved. After Keener loses his daughter to influenza, his disaffection with the public health strategy and his helplessness are made known: "It frightened him that so many people were dying. It meant that the Board of Health warning had come too late. The flu had already spread wildly throughout the city and was now beginning to make itself known. Now it was simply killing many of those people it had already infected before the Board of Health had taken action" (Rada, 97).

Keener and Markwood, acting as immunologists, collaborate on an experimental vaccine. Learning how to develop it, presumably from recent biomedical literature on "the harder- and earlier-hit communities," they gather a biological mixture from the biological mixture from secretions of flu victims in Cumberland, filter it to eliminate large cells and debris, and hope that the filtrate contains the active pathogen. In the autumn of 1918, to use bacteria-free filtrates in the hope of isolating a submicroscopic organism responsible for the disease was not the norm. Their work, which was concurrent with the avant-garde French and Japanese, had earlier precedence. The German researcher Walther Kruse, in 1914, had collected nasal secretions from cold sufferers, filtered out bacteria, and then re-introduced the filtrate intra-nasally to healthy volunteers, who developed colds (Crosby 279). This line of research went cold until 1918, when Keegan and Rosenau, replicating Kruse's method, tried to isolate flu virus and transmit the disease to healthy volunteers; however, the possibility of pre-exposure to influenza negated the experiment (Crosby 277–279; Kolata 55–62). If we recall, Gibson, Connor and Bowman, historical correlatives to the fiction, were conducting experiments of this kind on primates.

With diphtheria in mind (a bacterial disease), Keener and Markwood assume that the pathogen, once inoculated into patients, would stimulate an immune response neutralizing the germ. On this, they are aligned with Emil von Behring's discovery that only the serum of immune animals neutralized the diphtheria toxin (de Kruif, 192; "Immunity to Diphtheria in Animals" [1890], 141–144). Keener loads 10 syringes with the filtrate, as Markwood prepares additional dosages. They began testing in the patients' rooms (Rada, 107–108). Early results on 7 October are inconclusive. One patient, Lorene Sears, claims that she had begun to recover when receiving the vaccine, so the patient considers the vaccine a precautionary measure (Rada, 110). Keener's assessment of the results from 20 patients, however, indicates that the vaccine failed; two of the worst cases die, while cases like Sears' are ambiguous (Rada, 112).

Undeterred in his search for a way of fighting the disease, Keener reapproaches the problem epidemiologically. Although the flu is highly contagious, he realizes that few die from it; that is, only about 25 out of every 1,000 who are sickened (2.5 percent). Although this is an encouraging (and historically accurate) statistic, the problem is that one out of every two people comes down with it (Rada, 113). It seems even more likely, therefore, that a blood-borne property is responsible for natural resistance (Rada, 113). A viable vaccine cannot be made unless the pathogen is known. That is the crux of the problem in October 1918, and it remained so into the 1930s.

James Rada situates the narrative squarely in its historical/biomedical context and places his energetic physician, Dr. Keener, at the forefront of viral immunology with respect to influenza. On 8 October, while studying blood samples, Keener realizes that the answer to the vaccine problem lies in serology. He works through the night, "trying to come up with significant differences between the infected and healthy that could be distilled into a vaccine" (Rada, 124). The failure of his filtrate experiment is procedural and not due to the incorrectness of the hypothesis that directs his experiment. Ironically, a manic salesman-turned-street preacher/bioterrorist believes he can intentionally spread the disease. The irony is that the perpetrator, Carson Riley (also known as Kolas), has survived the flu and presumably carries antibodies that could be used as vaccine (Rada, 159–160). This is the opportunity for which Keener had been waiting: "He had a sample from someone who was immune to flu. Now he could study the blood sample and compare [it] to samples from patients who had died. The differences would be the answer he needed" (160).

Despite using the Riley vaccine on 100 flu patients, Keener cannot claim success. He remains unsure of the vaccine's efficacy, "since the flu had already been on the decline throughout the country when he developed the vaccine"; once again, Rada is historically precise. Keener hopes, on 25 October, that the vaccine will at least hasten the flu's recession. Early in 1919, a third less virulent influenza wave appears and runs its course. Ironically, the vaccine is useless, but the struggle to produce it, like Lydia Wickett's determination, is nothing less than heroic. In the counteroffensive against influenza, medical science and practice met with futility because research and technology, in 1918–1919, had not yet acquired the capacity to understand its cause. The Recursion literature, in the aggregate, is an imaginative correlative to the history of influenza in 1918–1919.

Part Two

The Characterization Period (1995–2005)

4

The Characterization Project: 1995–2005

From the 1930s to the 1940s, influenza research would become a multidisciplinary field, involving serology, immunology, animal experimentation, and vaccine production (Taubenberger & Morens, "Historical Context," 587). To the lengthening roster of big names in virology and influenza research were added Thomas Francis (1900–1969), Sir Charles Stuart-Harris (1909–1997), Sir Frank Macfarlane Burnet (1899–1985), Anatoli Smorodintsev (1901–1986), Maurice Hilleman (1919–2005), and Jonas Salk (1914–1995). These investigators would contribute to our understanding of the causes, mechanism, and effects of influenza. Johan V. Hultin, M.D., who is today a retired pathologist, joined their ranks in 1951. In 1949, Hultin, then a doctoral student in microbiology, overheard Dr. William Hale (1898–1976) suggest that permafrost-interred tissue from 1918 influenza victims might contain traces of viral RNA. From that day forward, Hultin's professional life and the history of influenza research would be profoundly changed.[1]

Hultin proposed an ambitious dissertation project: an Alaskan expedition that would attempt to retrieve samples from the remains of influenza victims, buried for over three decades under permanently frozen layers of earth. The thought of exhuming tissue samples to discover what had caused the 1918 pandemic was put into action. Hultin managed to get approval for his project from a faculty adviser who had worked in Alaska, during the summer of 1949. With the assistance of the paleontologist Otto Geist (1888–1962) and others, Hultin contacted several Alaskan missions to research their influenza histories.

According to a published account, three sites along the coast of the Seward Peninsula were possibilities: Nome, Wales, and Brevig Mission (in 1918, called Teller Mission). Nome turned out to be unsuitable because a river had changed course, melting the permafrost.[2] A bush pilot flew Hultin to Wales on the Bering Strait. The mass grave was plainly in sight, but the bluff had fallen on the beach, leading Hultin to assume that no permafrost was there. After an arduous trip by air, boat, and on foot, the expedition arrived at Brevig. Conferring with the matriarchal village council, Hultin met three survivors of the pandemic who recounted what it was like, in November 1918, when 90 percent of the villagers had died. Hultin explained that finding genetic remnants of the virus could possibly allow modern scientists to reconstruct the organism and eventually to develop a vaccine in case it returned in some form. The villagers who had been inoculated for smallpox understood the practical importance of the expedition, so they granted permission to exhume bodies.

At the gravesite, Hultin's party dug down one foot below the surface until they reached permafrost which they melted with a bonfire.[3] On the second day, at the depth of four feet, they found the well-preserved body of an adolescent girl and, farther down, 72 more bodies. For three days they dug to a depth of six feet where they found three more perfectly preserved corpses from which they took lung samples. Eight biopsied specimens were taken, placed in thermal mugs, and preserved with carbon-dioxide snow from fire extinguishers. They took precautions, crude by today's standards, sterilizing instruments in boiling water, and donning surgical masks and gloves. Transporting the specimens to the University of Iowa microbiology laboratory, they began work in negative pressure hoods, culturing the samples in chicken embryos. While samples of lung material yielded bacteria, the ferrets receiving intranasal instillations of the culture remained healthy, and repeated negative results led to the discarding of the specimens. Nothing more could be done at the time since molecular biology was a new science. But a great discovery was imminent: the development of the double-helix model of DNA in the early 1950s, by Pauling, Watson, and Crick.

In the mid–1990s, the search for viable remains was resumed in cooperation with Dr. Jeffery Taubenberger, of the National Institute of Allergy and Infectious Diseases. Molecular pathology is the medical specialty Taubenberger employs to understand the 1918 virus. As he explains, these pathologists use the methods of molecular biology and genetics for the purpose of medical diagnoses.[4] Taubenberger and his colleagues thought it was possible to find fragments of 1918 viral genetic material from preserved autopsy tissues at the Armed Forces Institute of Pathology (AFIP), in Washington, D.C. The specimens, fixed in formalin and enclosed in paraffin blocks, might contain traces of RNA from the 1918 novel virus. Two basic problems prompted their work: why was this virus so virulent? And where did it come from? If they could answer these questions, medical researchers might then be able to plan for a future pandemic through the development of effective vaccines and antiviral drugs. If genetic material could be found in these minute tissue samples, the 1918 virus could possibly be reconstructed so that further research might answer these important questions.

The work began in 1995. The National Tissue Repository at the A.F.I.P. had 100 1918-autopsy cases on file.[5] Only 13 of the 78 finger-nail-size tissue samples, however, were determined to have recoverable genetic material. The investigators were particularly interested in decedents who had succumbed to influenza rapidly—those, in other words, who had died from what would later be revealed as the cytokine storm *preceding* secondary bacterial colonization. Of the 78 cases under scrutiny, most had died from secondary bacterial pneumonia, but 13 candidates appeared to have died within a week and from respiratory-tract edema and hemorrhage. In 1996, the investigators considered the case of a soldier who had died on 26 September 1918, at Fort Jackson, South Carolina, of acute pulmonary inflammation and edema. His right lung showed pathology consistent with viral pneumonia; therefore, the sample was more likely to have fragments of influenza RNA.

In 1997, through genetic sequencing of these fragments, Taubenberger and colleagues were able to identify the pathogen as a Type A/H1N1 influenza virus.[6] That year, they found a second archival case, of a soldier who had also died on 26 September 1918, at Camp Upton, New York. He had passed away in three days from acute pulmonary edema, again consistent with influenza's prostrating onset. RNA fragments, once analyzed, supported the 1995 findings. The Camp Upton soldier, like his Fort Jackson counterpart, had been stricken by a Type A/H1N1 influenza virus. Initially, it was thought that the virus belonged not to an avian group, but rather to a subgroup of strains that infected both humans and swine. Confirming experiments performed in the 1930s, the retrieved 1918 material seemed most closely related to early swine influenza strains. Phylogenetic tests of all influenza genes, however, would eventually suggest that both human and swine flu H1N1 lineages had a common avian ancestor. On this basis, they theorized that an ancestral virus might have entered the mammalian population at some time before 1918.

At this juncture, Hultin's 1951 expedition and the Taubenberger group's 1990s research fortuitously converged. After reading the 1997 paper cited above, Hultin was encouraged to return to Brevig Mission, Alaska, forty-six years after his initial trip, with renewed hope in finding viable tissue samples in the same permafrost graves. Hultin contacted Taubenberger, told him about the failed 1951 expedition to Brevig Mission, and proposed that they collaborate on a second expedition to retrieve and analyze permafrost specimens.

The proposal was enthusiastically received, and Hultin's expedition returned to Brevig Mission in August 1997.

According to the account, after receiving permission to exhume bodies, and with four young Eskimo villagers assisting them, Hultin's team returned to the gravesite.[7] By the second day, they had reached a depth of seven feet. There, they found the body of an obese woman, whose well-preserved, dark red lungs showed pathology consistent with viral pneumonia. The lungs of the unearthed permafrost corpse were preserved well enough for Hultin to obtain substantial tissue samples to ship to Taubenberger at the AFIP. Compared to the minuscule archival samples with which Taubenberger and his co-workers had been working, Hultin's samples were substantial (even though the extracted genes were fragmentary). Thirteen thousand tissue samples made it possible, eventually, for the Taubenberger research team to sequence the viral genome, a painstaking job that would take nearly a decade to complete.

The Brevig (Teller) Mission tissue had RNA fragments and, upon comparison, were all considered to be genetically identical.[8] Theorizing that the 1918 influenza virus was likely of avian origin and that the ancestral virus had undergone mutations adapting it to man, the investigators turned their attention to the problem of zoonotic infection. Along with vaccine and antiviral development, they considered how this information could lead to ways of inhibiting mutations responsible for antigenic shifts and pandemics.

In the March 2006 paper, "The Origin and Virulence of the 1918 'Spanish' Influenza Virus," Taubenberger et al. made the long-awaited announcement that "the complete genomic sequence of the 1918 influenza virus has been deduced from the use of archived and frozen lung tissue."[9] They hypothesized not only that the virus contained genes that had originated from avian-like strains, but that the 1918 virus was "the common ancestor of human and classical swine H1N1 influenza viruses." However, molecular analyses of the retrieved 1918 hemagglutinin and neuraminidase genes—the protein responsible for viral binding to a host cell and the enzyme facilitating the extrusion of new viruses from it, respectively—did not exhibit the kind of mutation accounting for the deadliness of influenza strains. But they did learn that the reconstructed 1918 virus was virulent in mice, while another gene, called non-structural NS, was sequenced completely and tested for its capacity to increase virulence. In sum, sequence analyses of the 1918 pandemic influenza virus had allowed researchers to determine the origin of the 1918 virus and to help them identify genetic features responsible for its virulence in humans. Research is ongoing.

The lines of viral descent soon became distinct. The 1918–1919 pandemic, scientists conjectured, had spread from humans to swine in 1918. The two viral lineages, at that point, then diverged from one another into two phyletic lines, one human and the other porcine. The 1918 swine lineage has been continually evolving ever since 1918, but the human lineage, after 1918, became endemic and remained so up until 1957. In 1957, human H1N1 apparently disappeared. In 1977, however, it suddenly *reappeared,* some propose, because of a laboratory-freezer release in Russia; as a result of this purported breach, H1N1 is now circulating endemically in a mild form (Taubenberger & Morens, "1918 Influenza," 15).

The Characterization project, from 1997 to 2005, elicited its share of supporters and critics, the latter being justifiably cautious about experimentation of this kind. Dr. Peter Palese, Horace W. Goldsmith Professor and Chair of the Department of Microbiology at the Mount Sinai School of Medicine in New York, contributed to the Characterization project and in 2012 recalls the controversy it had precipitated in 2005: "News stories around the globe debated the merits of our research and television pundits argued opposing viewpoints" ("Life-saving Science"). In the early 1990s, Palese's lab had developed the method by which mutations can be inserted into viruses to render them "more easily transmissible" ("Life-Saving science"). Terence M. Tumpey and collaborators, in a landmark 2005 paper, recount how, with the complete 1918 influenza virus coding sequence in hand, they were able to produce an influenza virus through reverse genetics, one that had all eight of the gene segments of the 1918 virus ("Characterization" [2005], 77–80). The live construct allowed them to investigate the organism's high level of virulence. Tumpey's group concluded that its virulence, revealed in its ability to kill mice and proclivity for bronchial epithelia, was derived from "the coordinated expression of its genes."

Despite government reticence over publishing the methodology and results of the reconstruction experiments, Palese and colleagues maintained that this achievement was important from the standpoint of public health. Having a live version of H1N1would permit scientists to learn why the virus was so dangerous and how it could be neutralized. Publication of the 2005 paper in *Science Magazine* paid scientific dividends: the 1918 virus, virulent though it was, turned out to be sensitive to the seasonal flu vaccine and to common antiviral medications. As a consequence of these breakthroughs, by 2005, the H1N1 strain responsible for 1918 Spanish flu was no longer viewed as an unmanageable threat.

5

Terrorism and the Biological-Attack Scenario

Pandemic influenza has been a popular subject in novels, published from 1998 to the present. Situating these novels in historical context will give us an idea of how much these writers owe to contemporary events, especially to biomedical science. We can begin with two key historical events of the modern period of pandemic literature: one is scientific and the other is legislative. At the center of several novels is the genomic characterization of the H1N1 influenza virus, described in chapter 4. From 1997 to 2005, teams of scientists worked tirelessly to identify the genetic makeup of the virus that caused the 1918 pandemic. They isolated its genes: neuraminidase in 2000, the nonstructural gene in 2001, the matrix in 2002, the nucleoprotein in 2004, and the three polymerase segments in 2005 (Taubenberger et al., "Discovery and Characterization," 587). One major aim of the project was to learn which genes control virulence, transmissibility, and other important factors; understanding the genetic mechanisms of the influenza virus will allow scientists to create medicines and vaccines against it. This great scientific achievement defines the Characterization Period.

The ongoing international research on influenza has been complemented by government efforts to optimize public health and social services. In 1997 avian influenza, a dangerous form of the disease that could threaten humanity, emerged in China and has since appeared sporadically there, in Southeast Asia, and along the Pacific Rim. Recurrent outbreaks prompted the United States government, in May 2006, to publish the *National Strategy for Pandemic Influenza Implementation Plan/Homeland Security Council*. This document sets forth ways to prepare the nation for such a pandemic (*National Strategy*). Appraising the capabilities of federal, state, and local agencies to manage an influenza emergency, its authors recommend that attention be given to U.S.

borders and transportation systems to monitor and control the movement of infected persons in and out of the country; to strengthen international partnerships and to open lines of communication in case of an emergency; to foster inter–Agency cooperation here at home, coordinating public health agencies, all departments of government, the private sector, and local communities; and, during an outbreak, to contain infected animals, reducing human exposure to zoonotic pathogens. The latter provision is important in that it would inhibit viral interchange between species and the possibility of subsequent mutations leading to human-to-human transmission.

The threat of bioengineered microbes being used against civilian populations complicates the problem of how to manage an emergent disease. Novelists who are interested in the theme of pandemic influenza, and who are cognizant of the natural and unnatural threats just described, have written catastrophic thrillers on the subject. For a novel of this kind to be successful, research into the history of biomedical science is a must, and this prerequisite extends to readers and to those who comment on these stories. Because this fiction is so topically allusive and intellectually informed, and because a critical reader needs a glossary and background, I will preface the literary discussion with authoritative information on bioterrorism. The most important questions historians have tried to answer are: who are these people? And why do they use germs as a weapon?

Profiles and Motives

The biological activities of rogue operatives and cults have preoccupied government surveillance agencies since the 1960s. In a 1999 CDC paper, Dr. Jonathan B. Tucker—who is a biological and chemical weapons expert—documents the history of recent bioterrorism. Tucker concludes that, from 1960 to 1999, incidents of biological terror were actually quite rare. In recent years, although the number of these events has increased somewhat, as have hoaxes, historically they amount to relatively few cases. Of these few cases, even fewer have succeeded. Actual terrorist attacks using these weapons, before 2001, had caused no fatalities. The Rajneeshee cult's 1984 use of *Salmonella typhimurium* to contaminate food in The Dalles, Oregon, for example, sickened 751 persons but killed no one (Osterholm & Schwartz, 85). Investigators, in 1985, searched the cult's compound, including the Pythagoras Medical Clinic, the Rajneesh Medical Corporation, and an underground lab. They found that a nurse, Ma Anand Puja (Diane Ivoinne Onang), had stored glass vials of salmonella disks in the lab which had been ordered from a Seattle medical supplier; the CDC determined that the salmonella strain in the disks was identical to what had been used in 1984 (Miller et al., 24). With sufficient funding and basic know-how, the cult was able to produce a biological weapon, but fortunately conventional detective work was able to neutralize their activities.

As to the social identity, the political orientation, and the motivation of bioterrorist groups, the Database of the Monterey, California Institute of International Studies (Tucker's source) shows great diversity. Whereas left-wing radicalism was a common orientation in the 1960s-1970s, the trend since then has been in the direction of "national-separatist groups and individuals or ad hoc groups bent on revenge" (Tucker 6). An interesting, more recent development in this cohort has been the increase in the activities of "violent sects or cults that believe in apocalyptic prophecy." These groups often claim to have an exclusive revelation of the world's end, of their privileged position in a regenerated world, and of the need for violence as a means to that end (Tucker, 6).

Although these groups or individuals might have desired to cause mass casualties, Tucker points out that, up to 1999, they had neither the technological know-how nor the scientific resources to use a biological agent in a large-scale attack. The Japanese cult, Aum Shinrikyo, is a case in point. Despite having financial resources and a degree of scientific expertise, it failed on ten occasions to conduct an aerosolized anthrax or botulinum toxin attack in a city, although their chemical terrorism using sarin in the Tokyo subway was successful. Tucker extrapolates from the data that future bioterrorism alerts will most likely be either hoaxes or limited operations. Nevertheless, the potential danger persists for a serious incident because not all bioweapon technology is sophisticated; and unemployed, unscrupulous scientists are always looking for work.

Tucker enumerates traits common to modern bioterror groups that figure prominently in the corresponding fiction. Writers whose fiction I discuss in chapters 5 and 6 were well aware of these typical traits and profiles. Comparing bioterror incidents and perpetrators to each other, in the period from 1970 to 1998, Tucker finds six distinguishing features: (1) these groups often had a charismatic leader; (2) some groups belonged to, or were affiliated with, "an outside constituency"—a global organization or a sponsoring state; (3) a doctrine portending the end of the world and the cult's elected role in a final dispensation often appears as a manifesto and inspirational resource; (4) either an individual or a splinter group performs the bioterrorist act; (5) the cohort or lone perpetrator was psychologically imbalanced, either paranoid or given to grandiose imaginings of historical purpose; and (6), when threatened, organizations aggressively defended themselves.

According to the Monterey Database, the majority of the terrorist groups under review had a charismatic leader. The Rajneeshee Cult, for example, was led by a charismatic guru, Bhagwan Shree Rajneesh. Aum Shinrikyo's leader was the blind Japanese religious figure, Shoko Asahara. Terrorist cells professing a radical social doctrine in which violence is a sanctioned means to that end adhered to an array of doctrines: some subscribed to ecological terrorism; the Weather Underground (1970) and the Red Army Faction (1980) were Marxist revolutionaries; the Minnesota Patriots Council (1991), a right-wing movement, opposed government taxation; Aum Shinrikyo (1995) envisioned doomsday and the establishment of a theocratic state in Japan; and Larry Wayne Harris (1998), though prosecuted as an individual, had links to white supremacist and separatist groups. With the exception of the Weathermen and the Red Army Faction, who professed Marxist ideology, the other major bioterrorists in Tucker's survey, from 1970 to 1998, were either individuals (as in Harris' case), or splinter groups, or autonomous cells. We shall see that the imaginative writings of Crane, Case, and Kalla, discussed in chapter 6, appropriate much of this information.

In the late 1990s, for most Americans (the present writer among them), the subject of bioterrorism may have appeared as an exclusively international concern. That sense of insularity disappeared for most Americans on the morning of 11 September 2001. It did for me as I witnessed acrid black smoke billowing out of Tower One at The World Trade Center and saw people falling, one after another, from the gaping furnace on the upper floors. By this time, both towers had been struck. Bystanders seemed riveted to the asphalt, as the NYPD tried unsuccessfully to move the gathering crowd behind the illusory safety of police lines on West Broadway. The illusion of insularity was gone.

The worst bioterrorism event in U.S. history followed the destruction of the Twin Towers. In October 2001, inhalational anthrax killed a tabloid editor in Boca Raton, Florida, two postal workers at a Washington, D.C. facility, and several other people whose mail had been cross-contaminated by invisible anthrax spores that, during processing, had wafted out of contaminated letters, addressed to U.S. Senate majority leader, Thomas Daschle. By 22 November, at least eleven cases of pulmonary and seven cases of cutaneous or skin anthrax infection had been confirmed. At the time, U.S. intelligence suspected a connection between the anthrax letters and the perpetrators of the 9/11 attacks, but no direct linkage between Al Qaeda and the anthrax terrorist could be found. Eventually, it was determined that home-grown, rather than international, terrorism was responsible. Evidence for this theory was that the anthrax bacillus identified in the letters turned out to be the virulent Ames strain. Originally discovered in Ames, Iowa, in 1957, this strain had been widely used in American bioweapons and vaccine development; so it was from American soil (Kohn, 354–355; Preston, *The Demon*, 161–202).

On Wednesday, 23 March 2011, *The New York Times* reported that a panel of psychiatrists had analyzed the medical records of Dr. Bruce E. Ivins, a microbiologist at the U.S. Army's biodefense center at Fort Detrick, Maryland, and concluded that the FBI's case naming Ivins as the bioterrorist was "persuasive." Ivins had committed suicide in July 2008. The panel based its finding on Ivins' behavior and history of psychiatric care. According to the panel, Ivins had sent the anthrax letters to gain revenge against imagined enemies, including the news media. Another reputed motivation was a desire "to elevate his own significance," as a way to win funding for his research, ironically, on anthrax *vaccines,* funding for which had been threatened in 2001. Ivins and colleagues, from 1990 to 2004, ironically had churned out papers on immunization *against* inhalational anthrax in prestigious journals, including *Infection and Immunity*, *Journal of Infectious Diseases*, and *Vaccine*. So his expertise was unquestionable. The motives ascribed to Ivins—the desire for revenge and to elevate his status before his peers—correspond to Tucker's motivational factors, namely a "sense of paranoia and grandiosity," along with defensive aggressiveness. The Ivins case, in general, illustrates the convergence of several factors: emotional imbalance, the need for revenge, and technical expertise with, and direct access to, a dangerous pathogen (Shane, "Anthrax Letters": A19; *Amerithrax Documents*; "Amerithrax").

But questions have lingered. *The New York Times* later reported that the psychiatric panel, along with a toxicologist and two Red Cross officials (where Dr. Ivins had been a regular volunteer), had not examined the records of other suspects. Furthermore, scientists dispute the FBI's Closing Inquiry and verdict on Ivins, arguing that the anthrax spores used in the crime were coated with silicon-tin, a technique that Ivins could not have used with the equipment he had. To cast even more doubt on the verdict, a National Academy of the Sciences' panel contended that the scientific basis of the FBI's genetic linkage of the attack-anthrax and Ivins' lab supply was "inconclusive." A conceivable source for the anthrax, other than Ivins, might have been someone having access to classified government research on anthrax that the military and the Central Intelligence Agency had conducted. The National Academy of the Sciences called for further investigations of the attacks focusing on the government's classified work (Broad & Shane, A1, A13; Willman; Hugh-Jones et al.; Engelberg et al.).

Biological-Attack Scenarios

As we move from recent history to imaginative writing, it may be surprising to find that bioterrorist fiction, whether on influenza or another disease, can take two closely related forms, distinguished from one another by their respective formats and purposes. One is the *scenario*, and the other is traditional fiction. The first part of this chapter is devoted to the scenario: an outline "of actions making up the plot and the appearances of the principal characters" and "a provisional acting-out of possible situations" (Holman and Harmon, 469; *OED*, Vol. 15, 107).

A pandemic or bioterrorist scenario in which enemies unleash an infectious disease on a civilian population reveals vulnerabilities in current medical, local, and state systems and provides a forum in which mitigative strategies can be discussed and tested. A biological-attack simulation, experienced through role-playing, as a table-top simulation/discussion, as a real-time exercise in the field, or as a literary text (Schoch-Spano, "Bioterrorism"), is meant to instruct government leaders and national-security analysts about whether the public health system and social infrastructure, in its present state, could withstand a biological attack, the outcome of which depends not only on the mode of dispersal but on the kind of agent used.

Dr. Monica Schoch-Spano describes four such scenarios. In a February 1999 simulation, an audience of federal and national leaders in public health participated in a hypothetical smallpox attack targeting a crowded auditorium, attended by the U.S. vice president. The disease spreads rapidly, as models predicted: in less than three months, 15,000 Americans were expected to have contracted smallpox, and 500 were projected to have died; and, in less than nine months, the disease would have reached fourteen countries (Schoch-Spano, "Bioterrorism," 9–10; O'Toole, "Smallpox"). In an October 1999 "Biowar" docudrama, aired on TV's *Nightline*, a second scenario has terrorists releasing anthrax spores in a city subway. Inhalational anthrax, estimated to have struck 65,000 people in eight days, kills 52,000 people. A third scenario, the June 2001 "Dark Winter" exercise, is a role-playing drama. The U.S. National Security Council's twelve senior officials, meeting in closed session, have to enact ways of dealing with a smallpox attack. In three cities, 16,000 are projected as having died in less than two weeks (Schoch-Spano 9; "Dark Winter"). The BBC's production, "Smallpox 2002—Silent Weapon," the fourth scenario cited, was broadcast in February 2002. Dr. Schoch-Spano believes this to have been a very effective demonstration because it reached a large international audience. The drama, set in 2005, chronicles a smallpox attack that had been ongoing since 2002. An unprecedented, realistic feature of the drama was to allow the public to participate in it. For a bioterrorism scenario to be meaningful, it has to be authentic, technically accurate, and designed to protect the public (Schoch-Spano, 11).

Bioterrorist scenarios have common elements: a targeted environment, the attackers' declared or inferred motives, *modus operandi* and tactics, a highly-infectious microbe, epidemiological implications and psychosocial effects, and a combined local, state, and national response. The aftermath of the simulation is then critically appraised. Scenarios have important, practical uses beyond government policy. A fictional narrative such as this, beyond suggesting the probable outcome of an attack, is also a training tool, and a model for anticipating a real emergency. Along with public reports and articles, the scenario is, therefore, a *literary* component of the public health strategy. In terms of genre, the biological-attack scenario is a cross between expository and fictional narration. An imaginatively constructed story based on historical evidence, it exposes dangerous possibilities and suggests real remedies.

Although both the scenario and creative fiction can communicate public health messages about infectious disease and terrorism, in certain obvious respects these subgenres differ from each other. Characterization is one area of contrast. Fictional characters operate in both forms. Because fictional characters are ideally, "extended verbal representations of a human being, the inner self that determines thought, speech, [and] behavior," their development does not fit the pragmatic aims of the scenario (Roberts & Zweig, 279). More appropriately, characters in a scenario are stock figures: they behave and think according to their strictly prescribed roles. There are perpetrators, officials, medical personnel, and a faceless, victimized population, identified largely in terms of morbidity and mortality statistics. A writer producing an epidemiological scenario is narrowly focused on cause-and-effect events in a staged emergency. In this drama of ideas and outcomes, pre-set behaviors are assigned either to an open-ended drama or to one with a foregone conclusion. Readers, viewers, or participants are the critical thinkers, delegated the task of finding systemic weaknesses and of proposing emendations.

The scenarist might just as well as have been writing the plot to a novel or movie. Faced with a number of possibilities, he or she can begin with the likeliest mode of attack or choice of pathogen, how the characters will perform, and to what illustrative end. Each persona and agency, scripted to behave according to the plot, will expose disconnections to the readers/participants who will, in turn, work to improve management efficiency.

The scenarist and participants are aware that, in large cities, the network of surveillance, the quality of intelligence, and the ability to react efficiently can be optimized but never perfected. They know that the scenario is an approximation. That is why professionals in relevant disciplines are the participants. If a scenarist is a medical professional, for example, he or she knows the system, is familiar with its chronic problems, with gaps in preparedness, has routinely wended through chaotic ERs, and is familiar with typical lapses or delays in diagnoses. Seeing the system from the inside-out permits the scenarist to scrutinize existing conditions acutely, to anticipate weaknesses a terrorist event will exploit. Studying past responses to similar emergencies, such as those involving natural disasters, can suggest how, for example, a panicked population might or might not behave or how an ER might improvise to accommodate a surge of sick patients. Although the scenario is a pre-conceived story, it is credibly based on past events and on current knowledge; it has the potential to expose unanticipated vulnerabilities. Although imperfect, it is nevertheless a useful planning device.

The scenarist must have a plot or a series of plots—each with a beginning, middle, and end. Otherwise, the reader/participants will have difficulty tracing the chain of events. Both scenarist and literary fictionist, therefore, will have rising action, orientating information about time, place, characters, and actions (Roberts & Zweig, 271). Whereas in literary fiction this information is needed if the reader is to be artfully introduced to character, setting, and milieu, for the scenarist it is used only if it contributes factually to a desired effect. Since the simulated narrative is configured to analyze a complex system of events and to instruct readers, the biological activities of the terrorists, population density, environmental factors, incubation time-frames, transmission metrics, knowledge of index cases, and other technical factors are all interwoven in the exposition. As errors are compounded, the situation worsens.

Both fiction and scenaristic prose contain a point at which the conflict develops, and where the protagonists face antagonists, both human and microbial. A crisis is reached in each form where the conflict is most intense (e.g., when morbidity is at its highest), and where the narrative reaches a turning point. This is the juncture, in either expository or imaginative writing, at which correct decision-making and effective action must proceed sequentially, resolving the complication and avoiding catastrophe, both literary and literal.

The climax of a scenario, as it is for the short story or novel, is the turning point in dramatic action; and the crisis is the point at which "the rising action reverses and becomes the falling action" (Harmon & Holman, 102). The final phase of both literary and scenarist writing involves a resolution or literary catastrophe, marking the end of the dramatic conflict (Harmon & Holman, "Catastrophe," 84). The scenarist reacts, expeditiously, to arrest an attack or to minimize and reverse its effects. If this is not achieved, a scenario can be open-ended, the problem left unresolved but open to later discussion.

A novel can present a central idea and embody values and characters. If personae are realistic, they will embody both strengths and weaknesses and be imperfect. But, in bioterrorist fiction, the line between good and evil is often boldly drawn, even if protagonists may sometimes be flawed and antagonists, in some ways, appealing. The bioterrorist, however characterized, is execrable. Antagonists such as these, consistent with historical profiles, are motivated by a destructive ideology or religious doctrine, a mania, vengeful obsession, self-aggrandizement or mendacity. The protagonists—more often, medical heroes and heroines or law enforcement and military figures, or some combination thereof—embody democratic values and humanitarian principles, oppose this destructive force relentlessly, momentarily fall victim to, or are directly threatened by, the pathogen or its creator(s), but eventually find a way to overthrow the deadly scheme or to play an important part in the resolution.

Government decisions in the early stages of the scenario's crisis can initiate a cascade of effects, creating the impression of impending chaos. In this way tension rises and is sustained as in any drama. A premature public disclosure by a governor, for example, may cause public unrest and panic, leading to absenteeism in municipal employment, to breakdowns in communication, public safety, transportation, and commerce, and perhaps even to restrictions in the shipment of medicines to a beleaguered region. Delayed disclosure, conversely, could set into motion a series of equally deleterious effects: if the disease is highly contagious, and if a warning is delayed, personal precautions will not have been taken, front-line physicians will not have had the early warning required as patients arrive, are misdiagnosed, and then leave the hospital or clinic and spread the disease to new contacts. All of these possibilities are true to life. It is amazing to see that the injection of a seemingly minor event or a precipitous decision can cause a situation to spiral out of control. A covert microbial attack in an unprepared city—the adversary unknown and the weapon unseen—can get out of hand rapidly.

Since the aim of the scenario is to show what could happen in a bioterrorist crisis and to reveal the ramifying effects of misjudgment, of a wrong policy, or of either overreaction or inaction at a crucial moment, the emphasis is on decision-making and on the subsequent progression of events, not on character development. Whether a governor is an ideal statesman, a mixture of conflicting traits, or highly unethical, has no bearing on the scenarist's primary aim: to display the hypothetical event realistically, to map out a series of cause-and-effect reactions, to test the effectiveness of various countermeasures, to improve pre-emptive defenses, and to highlight ways of protecting the public better. The emphasis in this fictional subgenre is on corporate judgments and actions, not on individual motives or proclivities.

Characters in a bioterrorist novel, however realistic, dynamic, and evocative, are also pre-conditioned and assigned a set of traits and roles to play in the story. But here the writer's emphasis is not exclusively on the progression of events, as it is in a scenario with its demonstrative purpose; rather, it is on creating an imaginary world peopled with realistic and interactive characters facing life-threatening problems that must be solved. These characters, if they are representatively human, will have physical, emotional, intellectual, spiritual, and social lives. If we look at the physician-as-hero in popular bioterrorist fiction, it becomes apparent that the authorial goal is to create a believable protagonist who, under the pressure of circumstance, lives up to high professional standards, providing optimal health care under the worst conditions or treating a mysterious disease rapidly. The fictional writer in this genre, however, has to be especially wary that the round personality being cultivated does not flatten out. Under the duress of a bioterrorist event, the medical protagonist may be inflated into a superhero or heroine—not a doctor-without-borders but a doctor-without-limitations, one who plays multiple roles.

In both literary and scenarist fiction involving bioterrorism, the writer has to find a point of equilibrium, as far as characterization is concerned. The scenarist, on the other hand, does not develop a fictive personality unless motivation and personal information are salient to the plot. If the focus of attention is on the attack, on its effects, and the reaction, excessive characterization may distract attention from the intricate web of events and the unfolding exemplum. The character could be an efficient professional whose behavior is meritorious, but his or her actions are subordinate to the pragmatic thrust of the scenario: to stress the system in all essential service areas—public safety, health and hospital, pharmaceutical, food and water supplies, mortuary, power grids —to see what breaks, what needs to be fixed, and what needs to be upgraded.

An Anthrax Scenario (1999)

In the paragraphs below, I focus on a possible case-history of anthrax dissemination in an urban environment. Specifically, I will be looking at complementary texts: Dr. Thomas V. Inglesby's "Anthrax: A Possible Case History" and at Dr. John G. Bartlett's "Applying Lessons Learned from Anthrax Case History to Other Scenarios" (1999). A bioterrorist scenario, such as Inglesby's, is a model or simulation: it takes into account a number of complex factors, such as the nature of the pathogen(s), terrorist tactics and modes of dissemination, and the quality of the emergency response. As an epidemiological model, it necessarily includes factors pertaining to the targeted environment (time and duration of exposure, wind direction and speeds, demographics) and the capacity of the public health system to recognize, and to react to, the unfolding threat in a timely manner. A comprehensive and informed scenario such as this one helps the reader to visualize how terrorists, armed with dangerous pathogens and simple delivery systems, could perpetrate an attack; what the likely epidemiological effects would be; how long it takes for the public health system to confirm a diagnosis; how the medical response is put into effect; and what weaknesses in the public health system are revealed; in addition, it considers the psychological impact an attack of this magnitude could have on the civilian population, on first responders, and on the government.

Unlike in literary fiction, the interpretation of an epidemiological scenario will consider whether the course of events described in the primary text conforms to actual circumstances. From an eight-hour training course on bioterrorism held at The Johns Hopkins School of Medicine, in 1999, doctors proposed a chain of events in which terrorists released anthrax spores into the air in a densely populated urban center. Inglesby narrates this terrifying event and outlines complications; in the secondary text, "Applying Lessons Learned from Anthrax Case History to Other Scenarios," Bartlett conducted interviews and communicated with agencies in order to test the premises in the fiction.

As Bartlett inquired about protocols and procedures at The Johns Hopkins University Hospital, he discovered gaps in the system, many of which corresponded to those illustrated in Inglesby's account. The physicians with whom Bartlett spoke, for example, acknowledged that early-stage anthrax symptoms would, most likely, be mistaken for flu and that patients would be sent home; that the emergency room at JHUH, already filled to capacity, could not accommodate the sudden influx of patients expected in a terrorist attack; that a radiologist would most likely not be able to identify anthrax from a chest X-ray alone; that a laboratory technician would be able to identify a bacillus in infected blood cultures but, initially, would not be able to differentiate it as *Bacillus anthracis*—although, should three or more cases coincide, a speedy diagnosis would be ordered and expected in 48 hours; but, even in that eventuality, communication with other agencies would be problematic. Bartlett found, however, that antibiotics were available in greater quantities at university hospitals and were more accessible state wide than in the scenario, but he agrees with Inglesby's supposition that local, State, and federal agencies, along with medical professionals, need to work together more effectively. To remedy these real deficiencies, Bartlett calls for the establishment of training and planning programs, as requirements in medical education and in hospitals, and for the federal government and private sectors to be supportive.

Read in sequence, Inglesby's scenario and Bartlett's Application have a fourfold, complementary purpose: to imagine a bioterrorist attack; to expose conditions in the public health system and in government that could seriously hinder the response, resulting in greater loss of life and social unrest; to compare issues raised in the scenario to actual conditions; and, through this contrast, to isolate specific problems that genuinely need to be solved. Thus, fiction based on present conditions is used as a means to improve future circumstances. To demonstrate how the scenario and test-case findings contribute towards a pragmatic end, I will consider the role of inter-agency communication in this particular emergency.

The terrorists themselves are made to issue a warning in the scenario: unless certain demands are met, they tell the FBI, aerosolized anthrax will be released in five northeastern cities. Although the threat is credible, inexplicably, "no information was relayed to city officials in Northeast [i.e., Baltimore] or elsewhere," a major gap in intelligence and communication. On 1 November, a 30-second emission of aerosolized anthrax spores from a truck travelling on Interstate 95 drifts upwind of a stadium housing 74,000 fans; the wind is said to have deposited spores on the stadium in nearby areas. Two days later (on 3 November), as patients begin to appear at various clinics and at emergency rooms, the prevailing diagnosis for the early respiratory symptoms is flu. As the caseload gets heavier, blood and sputum cultures reveal a Gram-positive bacillus, but this is not specific for anthrax. At this point, seeing frequent cases but still suspecting flu, nurses and physicians communicate with the city health department. By 4 November, when patients begin to die unexpectedly, local care-givers "urgently contact the state and city health department," who, in turn, alert the CDC. Despite the improvement in communication, by midnight, 4 November, 1,200 people have been infected and 80 have died.

Along with communication through official channels, word of the outbreak spreads between front-line clinicians in the state who are alarmed by the sudden appearance of "a rapidly spreading illness." The situation leaks out and is publicized on the morning news. News media trying to gather information interview families of the stricken and attending physicians, but the mistaken notion that the cause is flu persists. The mayor holds an emergency meeting of medical experts, health officials, and reporters outside city hall, many of whom continue to conjecture that a new strain of flu had emerged. During a news conference, a questioner in the audience raises "the possibility of bioterrorism." The scenarist has injected a volatile and believable element into the dynamic plot. Through this televised conference, the public is now alarmed. Ironically, as the communication network gradually is extended, conjecture, rumor, and misinformation hamper efforts to identify the pathogen. The scenarist, at this point, is showing that the public safety and medical networking goes on concurrently with other modes of communication, some of which are working at cross-purposes to the official conferencing.

In the early evening of 5 November, anthrax is definitively diagnosed.

That particular laboratory notifies city and state health departments, and these agencies, following the chain of command, notify the CDC and the FBI. In order to get a rapid diagnosis, one of these federal agencies sends the specimen to the U.S. Army Medical Research Institute of Infectious Diseases (USAMRIID). This move to the highest echelons raises the possibility that the responsible anthrax strain had been developed in a laboratory as a bio-weapon (chilling foresight). It took four days for all levels of government to interconnect. The mayor who, at this point in the ordeal, knows what the city is facing has direct access to relevant agencies at all levels of government. She expresses her anger at the FBI for not having informed her of the credible threat and is understandably upset over time wasted during diagnosis.

At this junction, the scenarist is pointing to two urgent problems: a communication breach between a federal law enforcement agency and local government, the latter being inhibited in its efforts to inform the public and to respond directly to local events. A second problem has to do with how long it takes to identify the pathogen: since the pathogen is being assayed by multiple agencies, from local hospitals all the way up to USAMRIID, the process is too time-consuming, which is especially problematic since antibiotic treatment for anthrax must be started as soon as possible.

When the lines of communication are fully open, the mayor learns about anthrax treatment. The news is not encouraging: antibiotic treatment works if administered early; however, since antibiotic supplies are insufficient (Dr. Bartlett found the opposite to be the case), a triage plan restricts their use as prophylaxis. Those who are already sick and likely to die will receive no antibiotics. State officials are now in constant contact with hospitals, warning them to expect a surge of patients and recommending how to care for them. Through news bulletins, the mayor regularly informs the public of the anthrax crisis, and she outlines recommendations for medical response (Inglesby, "Anthrax"). Lapses in communication persist, however, on the local level. Because of a disconnection between antibiotic suppliers, the distribution centers, and the mayor's office, and because no city plan was in place for mass distribution, some centers get no medicine.

As a result, by 6 November, the morbidity count having risen to 2,700, thousands panic, mob health clinics, and fear unfoundedly that they are infected. When false rumors emerge that medicine is in transit, mob violence erupts at distribution centers. Even though the population is told that the bacillus is not contagious, mass evacuations clog thoroughfares. Transit workers refuse to work, disrupting rail, bus, and air traffic. This action further impedes incoming supply routes. When the FBI admits publicly to having acquired intelligence one week in advance of the attack, the story is picked up on national TV as victims describe their ordeals and threaten legal action against the government. The scenarist's point here is that a communication disconnect at the local level, especially if it concerns medicines and health supplies, can trigger lawlessness, even if the government is fully informed and on the case.

In a postscript to the scenario, Inglesby raises a number of questions for further discussion, two of which emphasize the vital importance of communication: "Could the outcome have changed if state and local health had prior notification of the anthrax threats?" And, "How might health professionals and government officials interact with the media to best inform the public and avoid misunderstanding and panic?" Generally, the scenario shows that rapid, pre-set communication networks are essential since an effective response to a biological crisis depends on agencies working together to speed up diagnoses and to make treatment more efficient.

Bartlett's investigation of the Johns Hopkins University Hospital's preparedness in a biological-attack crisis keys in on problems related to communication. For example, it would take 72 hours to definitively identify the pathogen as anthrax, which could be a fatal waiting period for those with inhalational anthrax. Bartlett suggests a remedy: to call the Maryland Department of Health and Mental Hygiene directly. After reviewing statewide facilities and planning, he is pleased to find that one phone call to the State's Health Department would immediately enlist the aid of state epidemiologists who, after reviewing data and confirming the diagnosis, would then make multiple notifications to the Maryland Emergency Management Agency, to the FBI, to the Maryland Institute for Emergency Medical Services System; the latter agency could immediately contact emergency rooms statewide by fax.

A break in the circuit is found at this point. Bartlett observes that Emergency Management does not communicate with infection control programs and with practicing physicians. Communication, he suggests, has to be broadened to include front-line clinicians, perhaps through the press and "the medical society." Emergency Management could be a communication hub since it has worked this way in weather emergencies and could be adapted to a medical emergency, as "one point of contact that initiates the relevant cascade of events necessary for a response." Bartlett believes that such a communication network must be strictly regulated and have "a single voice for communication with the press and providers." The emergency response system would, in theory, facilitate open dialogue between all experts.

An important level of concern with respect to communication is not addressed in the *Application*: How should the government and medical profession communicate with the population? Inglesby's scenario shows how this is a significant concern since riots and mass exodus congesting Interstate 95 will exacerbate a crisis of this magnitude. Government representatives and media outlets need to find a balance when conveying information. Too little information raises suspicion. Disinformation raises legal issues and even greater suspicion and dread. Too much information can create confusion and a fertile bed for rumor. Misinformation can ignite social unrest. Media outlets, moreover, can intentionally complicate the problem if a measure of self-censorship for the public good is not exercised or if ratings are considered more important than civic responsibility, as in the example of TV interviews of anthrax victims being held while the crisis is ongoing.

Influenza as Ordnance

We will be looking at three novels in which influenza virus is developed into a weapon. Imtech, the bio-engineering corporation, in Dr. Leonard Crane's *Ninth Day of Creation* (1998), and a terrorist cult, in John Chase's *The First Horseman* (1998), employ the reconstituted virus as a weapon of mass destruction; the first, covertly for profit and ostensibly to secure United States' national interests; and the second, to realize an apocalyptic plan. To the novels of Leonard Crane and John Case, I add Dr. Daniel Kalla's *Pandemic: A Novel* (2005), in which Islamist extremists, compelled by theocratic dogma, bio-engineer an influenza strain into a weapon.

Tucker's outline of terrorist personalities, ideologies, and tactics, along with official CDC resources and WHO websites, will help us to understand if the influenza virus can be used as a weapon, and if its use in a bioterrorist novel would strain credibility. Before reviewing three schools of thought on the viability of an influenza weapon, we must, first, consider why certain microbes are thought to be the likeliest choices for biological aggression.

Let us begin with a fundamental question: is influenza virus a good weapon? According to the CDC, a pathogen is a bioterrorist threat if it satisfies these criteria: (1) it is easily disseminated or transmitted from person to person; (2) has a high mortality rate and is a public health problem; (3) can generate panic and social disruption; and (4) requires "special action for public health preparedness." Six pathogens belong to the highest priority group: anthrax, botulism, plague, smallpox, tularemia, and viral hemorrhagic fevers. Influenza, however, does not qualify for inclusion in Category A, even though it fulfills criteria (1) through (4). Nor does influenza have a place in Category B, the second of three groups. These agents are (1) moderately easy to spread; (2) result in moderate morbidity and low mortality; and (3) require special surveillance, along with "enhancements of CDC's diagnostic capacity." This group has twelve entries: brucellosis, the toxin of clostridium perfringens, salmonella and other food contaminants, glanders, melioidosis, psittacosis, ricin toxin, staphylococcal enterotoxin B, typhus fever, viral encephalitis, and cholera and other water safety threats. Emerging pathogens, such as hanta virus and Nipah virus that could be engineered for mass dissemination are in Category C, but influenza is not among them either (*CDC/Bioterrorism*).

When we compare what is known about influenza to the CDC criteria, discrepancies appear. Influenza certainly can have a high mortality rate; the technology exists to make strains transmissible from person to person through recombinant gene technology; it can cause panic, social disruption, and overburden the public health system; and it definitely requires, and is receiving, attention in terms of preparedness on every level of government. In view of these factors, and if the criteria are indeed imprecise, does influenza warrant a special category? Or should its potential danger if weaponized be reassessed? Would an influenza weapon in a bioterrorist novel be a realistic premise?

On the basis of four points, Drs. Zimmerman and Koch argue that influenza virus would not be the best choice for a bioterrorist agent ("Biological Weapons"). These scientists point out that the H5N1, avian Type A virus, would need to be genetically engineered to make it transmissible from person to person and highly infective. Even if the virus were stabilized for efficient transmissibility, however, a vaccine would then have to have been prepared to safeguard the developers. Further, if the virus were released in an unvaccinated, isolated population, there should be no risk of unwanted mutation that would subsequently imperil vaccinated populations (the attacker's country or people). An additional concern is zoonotic: the attackers would not be able to contain its spread via infected animals, especially migratory water fowl. Zimmerman and Koch maintain that technology necessary to identify the sources, and to prevent the occurrence, of unwanted mutations in H5N1 is unavailable. In view of the microbes listed in CDC Categories A and B above, the H5N1 influenza virus, though virulent, is highly unstable and a poor choice as a bioweapon.

Researchers at the Center for Civilian Biodefense Studies, at The Johns Hopkins University School of Medicine and School of Public Health, include influenza in their discussions on bioterrorism but only as an exemplum—that is, as a fully-documented public health emergency exhibiting the effects of a contagious disease outbreak on vulnerable populations. Two papers written by these researchers show that the influenza pandemic is important, not in and of itself, but rather as a *type* of catastrophic event, applicable to the study of bioterrorism and to disaster response strategies, generally. Monica Schoch-

Spana writes that the calamitous impact of the 1918–1919 pandemic in the U.S. "is an apt case to influence current bioterrorism planning efforts" ("Implications of Pandemic Influenza for Bioterrorism Response"). She then outlines principles intended "to assist medical, public health, and government leaders as they respond to the potential mass casualties and social turmoil initiated by a bioterrorist attack." In regard to the deadlier pathogens, such as smallpox, botulinum toxin, anthrax, or pneumonic plague, she suggests that influenza in its pandemic and inter-pandemic years furnishes a warning to the medical, public health, and political communities "about the potential frailty of populations and institutions in the face of an infectious disease emergency, particularly one initiated by a deliberately released pathogen."

Thomas V. Inglesby, whose anthrax scenario is reviewed above, along with Tara O'Toole and Donald A. Henderson, has written extensively on biological aggression. Donald Henderson led a worldwide campaign, beginning in 1967 and ending in November 1975, to eradicate variola major (smallpox) in the wild (Garrett, 42–45; Henderson, *Smallpox*). Inglesby, O'Toole, and Henderson suggest ways through which "the infectious diseases community might address the challenges of biological weapons and bioterrorism" (Inglesby et al., "Biological Weapons," 926). The 1918 pandemic's value is, therefore, that of a modern analogue, providing "insight into the potential ramifications of a major epidemic caused by one of the more serious biological weapons." The pandemic of 1918–1919 is, in their opinion, "the single event that might closely resemble the aftermath of a biological weapon." The influenza pandemic and a hypothetical bioterrorist attack, employing pathogens from the CDC categories above, have much in common: the pandemic caused social disruption and greatly burdened the health care system and civil infrastructure; and much the same is predicted for a bioterrorist attack. But the major difference between an actual and a hypothetical event is that the case-fatality rate for the 1918 influenza was low, ranging from approximately 2 percent to 5 percent. Thirty percent of those who contract smallpox will die, whereas more than 80 percent of those with untreated anthrax would not survive (Inglesby et al., "Biological Weapons," 926; O'Toole, "Smallpox"). For these authors, other than being an insightful analogue, influenza does not make the grade as a bioterrorist weapon.

Some are convinced, however, that influenza can be an effective bioweapon. Madjid et al., in 2003, urge that the possibility of "malicious genetic engineering to create more virulent strains" be seriously re-considered as a threat ("Influenza as a Bioweapon"). The terrorist attacks of 11 September (on The World Trade Center) and of 21 October 2001 (anthrax mailings) should raise the level of vigilance, as should the sequencing of the 1918 influenza virus (completed in 2005). With the sequenced H1N1, "unscrupulous scientists could presumably utilize candidate virulence sequences." Polio virus, for example, was synthesized from a written sequence (Cello, Paul, & Wimmer, 1016–1018). The fact that influenza virus is easily transmitted in aerosol spray and can be genetically engineered, "suggests an enormous potential for bioterrorism." In addition, Madjid et al. argue that influenza, unlike smallpox, is readily available. An influenza epidemic would not initiate an investigation because it occurs naturally; as a result, an outbreak of bioengineered H1N1 could have "a considerable head start on public health authorities." Since the incubation period for influenza is 1–4 days, whereas that of smallpox is 10–14 days, post-exposure vaccination for influenza would not be protective. Because influenza is widely present in the wild, persisting in avian, murine, and porcine reservoirs, it is harder to eliminate than other pathogens. Moreover, initial clinical screenings ("point-of-care tests") must be developed to differentiate between the early onset of influenza and smallpox.

Those who are alarmed about the bioterroristic potential of influenza research cite Dr. Ron Fouchier's and colleagues' recent experiments on ferrets, described in chapter 7, inducing mutations in avian influenza viruses. These mutations made the virus contagious between ferrets via aerosolized secretions, a capacity it does not naturally have. Ferrets, the experimental animals used in this study, are analogous to human beings in terms of their susceptibility to the virus; thus, if the avian virus can be made contagious between lab animals, there is the possibility that a mutation of this type in the wild could equally as well threaten human beings. The ultimate aim of these risky experiments was to engender a dangerous virus in a controlled lab setting so that new vaccines and antiviral medications might be developed should a similar event take place in the wild. Peter C. Doherty and Paul G. Thomas consider the bioterroristic risk this experiment poses ("Dangerous for Ferrets," 10). As a tactical or strategic weapon, they acknowledge, influenza "makes little sense." But that does not mean it cannot be a bioterror weapon: "the Fouchier mutations might be just what some made molecular 'greenie' needs to go forward with his dastardly plan of depopulating the planet." A "hypothetical maniac," according to Doherty and Thomas, would be able to duplicate the Fouchier experiment under crude conditions: all the mad scientist would need to do would be (1) to purchase "a few dozen ferrets and some cages at a pet store"; (2) acquire an "HPAI [Highly Pathogenic Avian Influenza] H5N1 virus from his source in an endemic country and do the experiment in a deserted farm or warehouse." The authors are not being facetious, in view of the fact that "virologists have known how to adapt flu viruses by serial passage or genetic reassortment for half a century."

6

Fiction of the Characterization Period: 1998–2005

In view of the scientific consensus, the influenza virus seems a poor choice for a bioterrorist novel. The CDC's exclusion of influenza from Categories A, B, and C, its instability, the sophisticated biotechnology needed to make it a deliverable weapon, and the epidemiological and the immunological precautions terrorists would have to take make a strong case against its use. Madjid et al. and Doherty and Thomas remind us, however, that the possibility of a biological attack with influenza is theoretically possible, especially if one considers attackers' motives or lack thereof. As a biological weapon in a nation's arsenal, the virus is ineffective and unwieldy. But criminality, insanity, and suicidal zealotry, as the commentary in this chapter will show, could provide the motive.

Leonard Crane, Ninth Day of Creation *(1998)*

Dr. Leonard Crane uses the reconstructed H1N1 virus as the bio-weapon of choice in the novel, *Ninth Day of Creation* (1998). Crane's synoptic book draws on contemporary biomedical resources, refers to the literature on microbial genetic engineering, and situates all of these elements in a fast-moving narrative.

One source of Crane's story is Philip E. Ross's 1993 *Scientific American* article, "Jurassic Virus?" (28). Ross reviews scientific opinions on whether or not it is possible to re-vivify extinct life-forms from genetic material, traces of which were found in naturally-preserved tissue. Crane's interest is not so much on the transformation of the virus into a weapon as it is on the idea of retrieving interred genes and on bringing an organism back to life. Ross describes the work of George O. Pomar, an entomologist, and Raul J. Cano, a microbiologist, who avow that it is possible to bring dead organisms to life through genetic engineering, and they had been working to that end with 40-million-year-old bacterial genes. According to Cano, one might gradually introduce ancient genes, via gene splicing and plasmids (reverse genetics), into an extant species until the modern DNA is entirely gone and the ancient organism reconstructed. Although scientists such as Michael A. Goldman, on the basis of DNA's molecular complexity, do not agree with their claims, Pomar and Cano remain optimistic that, in a matter of years, they will have successfully reconstituted the genome of the bacterium in their possession. Both virologists and microbiologists justify the need for the kind of work Pomar and Cano are undertaking, especially in regard to the virus that had caused the 1918–1919 pandemic. Drs. Peter M. Palese, Walter M. Fitch, and Robert G. Webster, at that time, were trying to reconstruct the ancestral form of H1N1 either from human remains or by extrapolating from the genomes of extant viruses. Crane even cites a 1976 article on the mapping of the influenza virus' genome (Crane, 661; Richey et al., "Mapping").

A second illuminating source for the book, which Crane credits, is Malcolm Gladwell's 28 July 1997, article in *The New Yorker*, "The Dead Zone." Among other issues pertaining to viral research and the Great Pandemic, Gladwell lucidly discusses a planned August 1997 expedition to the mining town of Longyearbyen, located in the Svalbard Archipelago, northwestern Spitsbergen, Norway (Duncan, *Hunting the 1918 Flu*, xi). Using ground penetrating radar and other technology, Dr. Kirsty Duncan, a medical geographer, and a team of scientists, hoped to retrieve tissue samples from the bodies of seven Norwegian miners who had died of influenza between 2 and 7 October 1918, and who were buried beneath the permafrost. There was a good chance that the bodies had been preserved at variable depths beneath the permanently frozen layer; however, the consensus was that the chance of finding live virus under those conditions was very low (*Hunting the 1918 Flu*, xi, 116–117). Nonetheless, extraordinary biomedical precautions were observed and legal, ethical, theological, and cultural considerations were also taken into account. Duncan describes the complexities of the expedition in her book, *Hunting the 1918 Flu: One Scientist's Search for a Killer Virus* (2003), and in her essay, "Biosafety at the Top of the World: Unearthing the Secrets of Spanish Flu" (2007). Despite their inability to recover the RNA of the virus, the expedition was professionally conducted. Her project brought public attention to Spanish flu and, like Dr. Schoch-Spano and others, she believes that the Great Pandemic "serves as a useful model for the potential ramifications of an infectious disease emergency or a bioterrorist attack" (*Hunting the 1918 Flu,* 280).

For historical context and background information, Crane consulted

Gina B. Kolata's 24 February 1998, *New York Times* article, "Lethal Virus Comes out of Hiding." This article would be expanded upon in a resourceful and readable book. Kolata sketches the history of earlier attempts to attain the genetic material of the influenza virus from tissue samples (*Flu*, 243–280). Both Kolata and Gladwell refer to the efforts of Taubenberger's team at the AFIP and of Hultin's northern expeditions, notably to the second one in collaboration with the AFIP. Returning to Brevig, in August 1997, Hultin and his co-workers, as pointed out earlier, found well-preserved bodies under the permafrost and were able to extract viable genetic material from lung tissues. While Hultin was working on the Brevig exhumations/biopsies, the AFIP molecular pathologists were collecting additional genetic fragments from archival specimens. As Kolata points out in the article, one sample came from Private James Downs who, while stationed at Camp Upton, New York, had contracted the flu, on 24 September 1918, and died from it on 26 September. Taubenberger's team was able to analyze one of eight genes, most significantly the gene that codes for the hemagglutinin protein that binds the virus to the host cell; the analysis showed, contrary to expectations, that this particular gene had not undergone mutation increasing the virulence of the virus. These investigators hope that analysis of the genome will reveal why the virus was so lethal and if it was of avian, of porcine, or of other origin.

The fourth and most authoritative source for Crane's fiction is the research of Jeffery Taubenberger and colleagues, specifically the landmark paper, "Initial Genetic Characterization of the 1918 'Spanish' Influenza Virus," which appeared in *Science Magazine* on 21 March 1997. In this paper, the researchers reported that RNA from an archived specimen (taken from the body of Roscoe Brown who had died of influenza in 1918, at Fort Jackson, South Carolina) contained nine fragments of viral RNA, sequenced from five coding regions: hemagglutinin, neuraminidase, nucleoprotein, matrix protein 1, and matrix protein 2. These sequences turned out to be "consistent with a novel H1N1 [Type] A influenza virus." Moreover, the data indicated that the 1918 strain, an H1N1 virus, was "distinct from all subsequently characterized strains." They conjectured that the 1918 strain was a novel form, an avian ancestor of both the human and the porcine H1N1 virus lineages. Although analyses of the 1918 sample genes correlated with mammals and not with birds, the investigators suggest that "at some point before 1918" an ancestral virus may have entered the mammalian population.

Against this background (and with 41 citations in the novel's *Reference* section), Leonard Crane constructs a complex plot. At the center of *Ninth Day of Creation* is the genetic characterization of H1N1, and the story unfolds in the context of contemporary scientific events. The protagonist, biochemist/

sleuth Richard Kirby, has discovered a third DNA helical strand. Scientists at Kirby's bio-engineering company, Imtech, illegally exhume preserved tissue samples from corpses buried beneath permafrost, in Juneau, Alaska. From these host specimens, they clandestinely generate "Swine Flu virus." The original strain is then altered in the laboratory. A synthetic Type A virus, designated BDM750A, it is "the first active strain to express proteins which have been totally redesigned" (Crane, 377). Intended for biological warfare, it has been genetically adapted to target Amerindians and to overthrow a Mexican regime hostile to the U.S. (Crane, 379, 404, 406, 408). The idea of an ethnically-targeted biological weapon is a theoretical possibility. In the 1950s, in fact, the U.S. Army was worried about enemy development of ethnically-selective agents that could be aimed at military bases (Miller et al., 42, 206).

Crane's knowledge of biological weaponry and of its post–World II history is evident in the literary characterization. In the late 1960s, the fictional Dr. Tulloch, an army general, is a biochemist in the United States Army Medical Research Institute for Infectious Diseases, at Fort Detrick, Maryland (USAMRIID), involved in the research and development of biological ordnance. In 1967, Tulloch is described as having had a role in weaponizing "what, at the time, was a newly-discovered virus going by the name of Marburg ... [one that appeared to be] both deadly *and* acutely contagious." Tulloch determined that, because the virus spread only through close contact, it was unsuited "for transmission amongst troops under battlefield conditions" (Crane, 424). Along with the Marburg research, he is given the foresight to know that the 1972 *Biological Weapons Convention* would only give the Soviet Union an opportunity to surpass the U.S. in biological weapons development; and he predicts Soviet experimentation with Marburg, which was clinically known in 1967 (Garrett, 53–60; *Convention*).

The fiction also alludes to later Soviet research on Marburg. Crane may have been thinking of the microbiologist William Capers Patrick, III (1926–2010), who was director of the U.S. biowarfare program at Fort Detrick, Maryland, and an expert on bioterrorism. In 1999, Patrick was shocked to see that the Soviets were annually manufacturing weapons-grade pathogens by the ton (Miller et al., *Germs*, 254–55; "Mr. Bio-Defense"). In the late 1980s and early 1990s, while the U.S. was no longer interested in Marburg virus, the Soviets were churning out 250 metric tons of this agent per year. A terrible accident in a Soviet laboratory had not been enough to dissuade them from the build-up; in fact, the victim's body became the source of an even more virulent strain of the organism. In the spring of 1988, the Soviets had assigned Dr. Nikolai Ustinov to develop Marburg virus into a weaponized strain. According to a defector, Ustinov had accidentally injected Marburg into his thumb while working with guinea pigs, and he died in three weeks. A more virulent and stable Marburg strain, called "Variant U" (named after the deceased scientist), was then made from Ustinov's autopsied organs, successfully weaponized in the Soviet's Vector Program, and was manufactured by the ton (Alibek, *Biohazard*, 123–133).

Crane is aware that chance and human error can affect biological experimentation of this kind. An epidemiological crisis erupts from a lab accident when the viral construct, in *Ninth Day of Creation,* is accidentally loosed. Once again, the author adeptly incorporates recent history into the story. A biological accident at Imtech results from the failure to replace laboratory filters and from building design flaws, two factors that bring to mind: (1) a Soviet accidental release of weaponized anthrax spores at Sverdlovsk in 1979 (Meselson et al.; Alibek, *Biohazard*, 70–86); and (2) the 1978 smallpox death of researcher, Janet Parker, a medical writer who, while visiting the University of Birmingham, in the UK, may have been infected due to laboratory design flaws (air duct C) in the animal pox lab one floor below her (Shooter, 38; Tucker, *Scourge*, 124–131) (Irene *Parker*, a newspaper reporter in Crane's novel, may be her indirect counterpart). Crane even refers explicitly to the Soviet accident: "A cloud of lethal anthrax spores was later confirmed by Russian sources to have drifted into the surrounding countryside killing hundreds of civilians" (Crane, 424–425).

The idea that weaponized influenza can be disseminated outside of a confined space, rather than tactilely or through droplet spray, is questionable. Weapons-grade anthrax which is particulate can be airborne, is so fine as to be invisible (for deeper lung penetration), and spreads like radioactive fallout. Smallpox virus, a hardy organism, is highly contagious in an enclosed environment, can be picked up from contaminated surfaces, such as soiled linen, and is viable in an open-air release: "The potential of aerosolized smallpox to spread over a considerable distance and to infect at low doses was vividly demonstrated in an outbreak in Germany in 1970" (Henderson, "Bioterrorism," 489; Alibek, *Biohazard*, 112–113). Even more alarming is the fact that smallpox virus can be turned into a dry powder that can be aerosolized like dry anthrax ("Scenario Planning Assumptions," *Atlantic Storm*). Another serious possibility is the asymptomatic carrier getting to a population center. D. A. Henderson recalls how, in the early 1970s, smallpox had been communicated by human carriers, border-crossing nomads in Ethiopia and Somalia or civil war immigrants in West Bengal, India: "many patients, even when ill, travelled long distances on foot, transmitting disease wherever they went" (*Smallpox*, 221, 227–228, 237–239).

Ninth Day of Creation is also interesting in the way chronological perspective is manipulated. Dr. Crane, a physicist, has penned a 658-page epic that spans less than two weeks in narrative time (late October to early November), the compressed time-frame chronologically replicating the Great Pandemic's second wave in mid-autumn of 1918, not in lethality, but in level of suspense and in breadth of action. The spatial and temporal movement in the narrative can be dizzying, and, for that reason, the novel may seem in need of editing. The author may actually have been experimenting with point of view. Somewhat like the historiographer Richard Collier, in *The Plague of the Spanish Lady*, the narrator in Crane's fiction is globally omniscient: scenes shift rapidly, from location to location, in order to suggest how concurrent human activities interact with each other and have far-reaching and unpredictable consequences. Crane's narrator captures the sense of absolute simultaneity. The reader can extract chapters related to a single persona and be able to experience events from that character's perspective. But the book consists of interwoven perspectives and experiences, all of which are described from a simultaneous viewpoint. In a single day, as many as a dozen scenic shifts can occur. Viewing this panorama through an omniscient lens, the reader sees what the narrator sees (and what the author has created): a moment in space and time. Within this Einsteinian world, space and time perception is "observer-dependent" (Park, 462). But from an omniscient viewpoint, converging lines of human activity and influence appear to move towards a coherent resolution. As the participants—individual, corporate, and national—pursue short-sighted goals, they are unknowingly participating in a conjectural history.

Another interesting historical aspect of the book is the lineage of Crane's bio-weaponry. Its tactical nomenclature belongs to the Cold War. "*Project Fail-Safe/Aztec Fire*" or BDM 750A is a product of genetic engineering, especially in its ethnic-targeting capability. It is explicitly a Fail-Safe or "positive control" asset. The concept recalls footage of B-52 crews scrambling to be deployed towards their targets in the warning phase of a crisis, to be recalled if the mission is cancelled (Kahn, 256). BDM 750A, if definitively a Fail-Safe weapon, must be equipped with a counteractive feature. But it is not clear in the book how this strain of influenza virus can be neutralized or recalled once released, unless the phrase Fail-Safe, in this context, is denotatively meant as having no chance of failure (Crane, 408, 426–28). A "fail-safe" viral weapon may be an oxymoron: for can the genetic stability of any virus be guaranteed? The Fail-Safe concept is tactically flawed. Dr. Herman Kahn pointed this out in 1960, in regard to the Strategic Air Command's idea of deploying air assets towards enemy targets pre-emptively. Doing so, ironically, could weaken defense or, in attempting to defend against a surprise attack, to set off a conflict accidentally: "unless plans are made to institute some form of continuous airborne alert, the calling back of planes may result in a reduction of capability ... a weak point in the system or a proneness to war by miscalculation" (258–259). In the Preface to their fictional best-seller *Fail-Safe*, co-authors Eugene Burdick and Harvey Wheeler grimly assess the danger and fallacy of the "fail-safe" principle: "The accident may not occur in the way we describe [in the novel] but the law of probability assures us that ultimately it will occur. The logic of politics tells us that when it does, the only way out will be a choice of disasters" (8). Crane's point seems to be that no bioengineered virus can be positively controlled.

Science and fiction, however, diverge from one another on an important point in Crane's novel: live virus cannot be directly extracted from eighty-year-old corpses (1918 to 1998). Crane's omniscient narrator observes that, "The retrieval from Juneau of two perfectly preserved host specimens had been remarkably straightforward, as had been the recovery from them of sufficient quantities of Swine Flu virus" (Crane, 377). The author's May 1998 e-mail interview of Dr. Jeffery Taubenberger clarifies the scientific facts. Taubenberger sees no possibility of survival for live virus: "Permafrost fluctuates between about -10 C.[+14 F.] and +4 C.[+39 F.], which is a temperature zone ideally suited to kill influenza virus. [Survival] would have required a sample to be frozen continuously in liquid nitrogen, or to be stored in a -70 C" ("Interview").

John Case, The First Horseman *(1998)*

John Case's influenza narrative, like Leonard Crane's, assimilates historical persons, events, and sources: (1) cutting-edge influenza research in molecular sequencing, which includes characters resembling real scientists (e.g., Drs. Fitch [34–36], Taubenberger and Hultin [33], Duncan [61], Ken Alibek [169], and even science writers like Gladwell [79], Kolata, and Richard Preston [176]); (2) the history of biological weapons research; and (3) the contemporary history of ecological activism. This author's methodology is to extrapolate to a plausible crisis.

The antagonist, consistent with Tucker's profilings, is a charismatic figure with dark messianic complex. Luc Solange (Light Sun-angel) envisions unleashing a revivified 1918 H1N1 influenza virus, the near-extinction of the human species, and survival of a cultic elect over which he will rule. The idea of a vaccinated remnant (1998) adumbrates Drs. Zimmerman and Koch's observation that an influenza terrorist would have to self-immunize before unleashing the virus or otherwise risk aborting the attack.

Solange's syncretistic doctrine loosely conflates apocalyptic theology and a form of radical environmentalism, portraying mankind as defiler of nature. The cult leader's organization, the Temple of Light, becomes an ordained instrument of natural restoration. For Case, the ideal weapon to create a pandemic is H1N1, the live genetic material of which is extracted from five dead Norwegian miners (Spitsbergen, in the Svalbard Archipelago, Norway, is the location of the Duncan Expedition). Since 1918, the miners had been interred in the village of Kopervik, beneath permafrost. The cult's notion is that the virus, once reconstituted, will be a natural counterforce to humankind. It will have a state sponsor in North Korea, where a laboratory accident had released a virulent influenza strain early in the novel, a product of a covert biological weapons program. This could be an indirect allusion to: (1) the suspected 1977 Russian H1N1 accidental release (Kendal et al., "Antigenic Similarity"; Taubenberger & Morens, "1918 Influenza," 15); and (2) to the Soviet's sprawling bioweapons industry, consisting of more than 40 facilities under the control of Biopreparat, 1988 to early 1990s (Alibek, *Biohazard*, 195; Case 38). U.S. scientists in the fiction who are investigating the incident suspect that the PDRK was experimenting with influenza on a molecular level to create a chimera, a monster arising from the melding of two organisms (Case, 41). Their suspicion is that, somehow, the North Koreans had acquired viable genetic material from an H1N1 descendant of the 1918 virus but that it had accidently escaped their labs, infecting the village of Tasi-Ko which had to be incinerated with air-fuel munitions (Case 43–45). The North Korean strategy, since the autumn of 1997, had been to employ an international cult to obtain genetic material from 1918 decedents buried in Norway. After the laboratory release, they supported the American-based cult in the development of the virus (Case, 176–77). Despite their radically different ideologies, the aggressors—the North Koreans and the Deep Ecology cult—pursue a "secret war" against the United States and the industrialized West (Case, 205).

The Hultin-Taubenberger and Duncan expeditions and laboratory work are central to Case's story. The Temple of Light had exhumed the bodies, on 9 September 1997, smuggling them into the U.S., using the names of five murder victims as cover (Case, 212). The North Koreans had been subsidizing the Temple with more than $50,000 for over two years (Case, 265). Once the North Korean biological accident and mitigation becomes an intelligence priority, The Temple of Light goes underground. With funding, with the RNA fragments, and with the expertise of Avram, a Russian refugee and unemployed Biopreparat technician or virologist, the operation is under way to create a consummate biological weapon (Case, 277–278). The fictional players are in place.

In two respects, however, the novel strains credibility. Bringing Biopreparat and the biological warfare industry of the Soviet Union into the plot is logical. But the influenza virus was not a microbe of choice in the Soviet biological arsenal. Biopreparat, in the Vector program, was more interested in anthrax, plague, tularemia, smallpox, Marburg and Ebola viruses, and chimeras, such as Venezuelan Equine Encephilitis combined with smallpox (Alibek, 259–260). The second incredible achievement is in molecular biology. In Case's novel, a Soviet Central Asian, Avram, boasts that he and his group had mapped the genome of Spanish influenza using the Kopervik tissue samples—an impossibility since it would take Taubenberger and his group a decade to do what Avram accomplishes in several months of narrative time. Not only have the Russian and his co-workers achieved this extraordinary feat, but through trial and error they reconfigure the virus to be resistant to natural immunity; rather than to increase its virulence or enhance transmissibility, they successfully bio-engineer the organism so that, 50 percent of the time, its antigens are shielded from antibodies, and it resists antivirals as well (Alibek, 278). They have, incredibly, induced an antigenic drift: through artificial selection the virus can elude antibodies half of the time; and resistant variants can then proliferate and gain dominance.

The plan is to transport the engineered virus to North Korea, probably so they could re-start their experiments. The Temple, meanwhile, has begun to test ways of disseminating the agent using U.S. Army methods, such as smashed light bulbs as containers. It uses an archival flu in its test run which spreads in California, Washington, Florida, and Wisconsin. The strain is identified as A/Beijing/2/82, the cause of a February 1982 Chinese outbreak. The fact that the identical strain had re-emerged indicates that it had come from an archive and was released intentionally. Authorities surmised as much because A/Beijing/2/82 was unchanged genetically. That means either that it had been on ice, static since 1982, or that it had been recreated in a lab (Case 294–295). Although A/Beijing/2/82 was a mild strain, the investigators speculate that these outbreaks were rehearsals for wider dissemination of a lethal virus, in this case, the immunologically-resistant influenza Type A virus (Case, 297). Testing proves this to have been the case and discloses that the virus had been genetically manipulated to resist antibodies (Case, 304).

The ultimate plan is to disseminate the virus throughout New York City, using tunnels, vents, the labyrinthine systems of electrical, water, and ventilation shafts and fans—a method the U.S. Army employed to test dispersion patterns of a benign bacteria using the plunger effect in the subway tunnels (Miller et al., 42). Given the environmental fragility of the virus, and the inability to wield it adroitly, a dispersion method relying on subterranean wind currents is implausible and more suited to anthrax dispersion. The terrorists' plan is foiled and their complicity with Pyongyang exposed. The Temple of Light is destroyed; its members, killed or incarcerated; and North Korean biological weapons activities are contained and deterred (Case, 364–373).

Case's research extends to environmental movements, a medley of doctrines, practices, and organizations (Eagan, 1–17). The terrorists' doctrine and motives align with the so-called Deep Ecology Movement. The philosopher Arne Naess (1912–2009), in 1973, articulated the basic doctrine of Deep Ecology. He called for a change of attitude towards nature, one in which the ecologist acquires "a deep-seated respect, or even veneration, for ways and forms of life" (96). A deeply ecological understanding of reality requires that one respects the intrinsic value of nature. Naess was convinced that not doing so would ultimately affect the quality of human life because it ignores or rejects the concept of man's interdependence with nature (96). That bio-diversity contributes to quality of life and ensures survival must not be forgotten. The struggle for life and the survival of the fittest really should be interpreted to mean learning to co-exist and cooperate with one's environment and with other forms of life (Naess, 96). Mankind, in Naess' view, must come to see itself as an integral part of the eco-system or biome, a district where life forms are environmentally adapted (Campbell & Reece, et al., G-5). Naess' basic premise—that the human species co-inhabits the biome—is valid and better understood when compared with similar points of view.

In the essay, "Infectious Disease as an Evolutionary Paradigm" (1997), Dr. Joshua Lederberg articulates a premise similar to Naess,' but in terms of humankind's relation to infectious disease. From Lederberg's standpoint, however, man and microbe exist in a host-parasite relationship, one in which man is more prey than predator. Lederberg differs from Naess on an important point. Humanity's survival depends upon wit and ingenuity when facing the relentless challenges of infectious disease. As Lederberg writes, disadvantageously "enmeshed in ecological circumstances," we must rely on medicine, vaccines, and technologies to keep up with ever-evolving microscopic parasites. Overcrowding, political, economic, and social stratification have exacerbated humanity's plight and increased susceptibility to contagious disease. International air travel can carry infections across the world. Condensation, stratification, and mobility uniquely define mankind as a species; but paradoxically, humanity remains vulnerable to newly-emerging diseases that can reach pandemic proportion.

Unlike Naess who seems to see natural selection as more of a power struggle than as a matter of evolutionary adaptation that, if achieved, fosters survival and procreation, Lederberg suggests that man must adapt in a "Darwinian fashion" to the microbial world, even though the human race cannot compete with microorganisms on an evolutionary level, the population growth of any one culture being measured in exponents of 10 to the sixth power. A new kind of symbiosis must be established in the human-microbe relationship. Parasitism does not work because the parasite (microbe) dies with the over-infected host (human being). Mutualism is a kind of interspecific equilibrium in which both species survive through their interdependence; through commensalism, a third form of symbiosis, one organism benefits while the other either benefits from, or is unaffected by, the relationship. At the very least, a commensal relationship between parasite and host is desirable; but, of course, given the diversity of infectious agents, the prospect of commensality depends upon many variables (Campbell, Reece et al. 1202–1203).

Richard Preston, in *The Hot Zone* (1989), provides a third perspective on the relationship between man, the environment, and specific viral diseases, such as HIV/AIDS and Ebola. The emergence of these diseases appears to be the result of man's ruining the tropical biosphere (Preston, 405). On this point, Preston and Naess occupy common ground. Since rain forests are reservoirs of viruses, when man strips the ecosystem through mining and deforestation, he is exposed to new diseases that might spread throughout the population (Preston, 406). Preston points to how badly man has treated nature and the degree to which the resulting danger has been underestimated. He imagines, in an ironic reversal, that the Earth is responding immunologically to the human species, the analogy being that either HIV/AIDS or Ebola is a kind of antibody to the human parasite or antigen; in these reductive terms, man-the-protein is open to the possibility of extinction; on this point, Lederberg and Preston would agree. Personifying nature (and depersonalizing man), Preston speculates that the biosphere may be reacting to an overpopulated, intrusive species. Mankind (in purely biological terms) is compared to an amplified virus, each person to a virion; deforesting humanity plunders woodlands and unknowingly becoming prey to the predatory microbe. The rain forest, Preston warns, can defend itself, and the Earth may be attempting "to rid itself of an infection by the human parasite" (Preston, 407).

Preston inverts Lederberg's anthropocentric view. For Preston, man can be thought of as a self-reflective parasite himself and the Earth as the host. The trope in which man is either parasite or a host is not new. William H. McNeill (1976), for example, calls those who raid an agricultural community, macro-parasites; and the agriculturalists against whom they transgress are hosts. Through trial and error, and to survive these forays, agriculturalists increased the crop production, in this way surviving such "predation" to maintain themselves. Such surpluses, he writes, "may be viewed as the antibodies appropriate to human macro-parasitism" (48). Just as governments improve immunity to foreign macro-parasitism by stimulating surplus production of sufficient food and raw materials, immunity to disease arises through the stimulation of antibodies and of other immunological defenses (48).

Case's antagonist, a sadist and megalomaniac, subscribes to a familiar doctrine that personifies and sacralizes the Earth as the source of life, a throwback to innumerable forms of natural religion. The Earth is the conventional maternal entity at the heart of their "religion"; and human behavior, in what amounts to biological matricide, is killing the planet and its children (all species). Man, Solange charges, has damaged the atmosphere, poisoned the groundwater, fouled the soil, and despoiled the forests (Case, 282). Few would argue with Solange's basic ecological assumptions, in view of waste dumping, the destruction of wetlands, municipal, agricultural and industrial pollution, flood control and damming, dredging, overfishing, expansion into rain forests, ranching, overhunting, over-logging, oil and mineral pollution, radioactive waste, acid precipitation, toxic chemicals, greenhouse gases and global warming, the depletion of atmospheric ozone, piles of plastic, and, as of December 2013, a population nearing 7.2 billion people (Campbell, Reece, et al., 1162–1165, 1168–1171, 1190–1191, 1237–1242; *Worldometers*). But no one would accept his solution to these problems: to unleash a hypervirulent flu virus into the population. Solange's rationale for initiating a near-extinction event, to damage the industrial West (Case, 327), is to support "Mother Nature" against a species (homo sapiens sapiens) that has caused a global crisis: "If one can create a vaccine against influenza, and that's natural, why is it unnatural to create a superflu" [?]. Doing so is a necessity, in view of the damage the Earth has incurred. Solange compares the human species not to a virus, but rather to a cancer cell, "metastasizing out of control" (Case, 327). As Walter Laqueur observes, "extreme environmentalists, particularly the so-called restoration ecologists, believe that environmental disasters will destroy civilization as we know it ... and regard the vast majority of human beings as expendable"; and the idea of using a lethal virus like smallpox is in their playbook ("Postmodern Terrorism").

Case's cult leader promulgates an eclectic variant of Deep Ecology. This system has four elements: (1) it is *axiological*, professing the ethical equity of all living things, as noted above; (2) it is *philosophical*, subscribing to the principle of "ecological holism": "that the biosphere does not consist of discrete entities but rather [of] internally related individuals that make up an ontologically unbroken whole," which is also noted above (Keller, 206–207). Deep Ecology (3) is *theological*, appropriating aspects of Judeo-Christian millenarianism: in ecological terms, using revolutionary action to preserve biodiversity; and, of course, (4) it is *biological*. I will expand on (3) and 4) below.

Solange's Deep Ecology doctrine is (3) *theological* and eschatological in worldview, and it relates directly to the Revelation to John. Ernest Tuveson explains that Millenarianism, in the Christian understanding of the term, finds its authorization in the Revelation to John, 20: 1–5, describing the cosmic warfare between the divine and the Satanic powers (*History of Ideas*, Vol. III: 223–235; and Cohn, 21). The war will culminate when the evil powers dwelling in Babylon are driven out. An angel will descend from Heaven to imprison the evil cohort, symbolized as a dragon, for one thousand years (hence: millennialism). Revelation 10: 7 reads: "And war broke out in heaven; Michael and his angels fought against the dragon. The dragon and his angels fought back, but they were defeated, and there was no longer any place for them in heaven. The great dragon was thrown down, that ancient serpent, who is called the Devil and Satan, the deceiver of the whole world—he was thrown down to the earth, and his angels were thrown down with him" (Rev. 10:7, 436). The Satanic powers will then be released upon the Earth after this interval of time, and Satan will gather his forces from all the nations of the Earth for Armageddon, a final battle. Once Satan is defeated, he will be cast into a lake of fire (Rev. 20:16, 446). A universal judgment will follow and then an eternal heavenly state. The New Heaven and the New Earth will be the culmination of God's triumph over evil (Rev. 21:1–27, 446–448). Solange professes a doctrine in which humanity is an evil force violating the sanctity of Nature. This is not a form of Pantheism equating God with the forces of nature but is more in the tradition of atheistic naturalism: the source of life is imminent and organic, but not intelligent.

The personages in the narrative of Revelation, chapters 20–21, are redefined in the millenarian terms of Deep Ecology. In Case's fiction, Luc Solange, the Angel of Light, is the messianic revolutionary who will free the natural world from its human oppressors and inaugurate an era of biological interconnectedness in which mankind, no longer at the apex either of the Great Chain of Being or of the food chain, lives in harmony with natural laws. Humanity, in this apocalyptic (Greek, *apokalypsis*: revelation) drama, is equated to the Satanic powers; and human extinction, through pandemic influenza, corresponds to the immersion of evil beings in a lake of fire (i.e., high fever and asphyxiating edema). The persona of Solange is, therefore, a fusion of the avenging angel who imprisons mankind and of the ecological messiah who subverts global anthropocentrism.

Finally, Deep Ecology is (4) *biological*, founded as it is on the concept of the *biosphere*: "The entire portion of Earth inhabited by life; the sum of all the planet's eco-systems" (Campbell, Reece et al. [Glossary, 5]). On this fundamental tenet, Deep Ecologists have little in common with the Judeo-

Christian tradition. After the cosmic conflict, the victory of good over evil in a culminating battle, and after the radical transfiguration of humanity in Creation, as opposed to a new heaven and a new earth in which "God is among mortals" (Rev. 21:1–3, 446), they envisage a pristine Earth and a re-naturalized humanity. With the revitalized Eden devoid of a divine Creator, man is left to adore the ecological order. As a Deep Ecologist, Solange builds his religion upon the foundations of chemical biology: on the regional exchange, distribution, and influence of energy and materials in each region, and on how this process sustains life (Campbell and Reece, 1149).

Case's ascription of Revelation, chapters 20–22, to The Temple of Light is consistent with the historical tradition of *millenarian* (violent overthrow) thought; and, ideologically, with descriptions of cultic terrorism in Tucker's paper. The Scriptural allusion to the First Horseman in Revelation (6:1–8, 19), however, is misapplied. It is likely that the *Fourth* Horseman should have been invoked, and I would like to investigate this possibility briefly.

Of the Fourth Horseman, St. John of Patmos writes: "I looked and there was a pale green horse! Its rider's name was Death, and Hades followed with him; they were given authority over a fourth of the earth, to kill with sword, famine, and pestilence, and by the wild animals of the earth" (Rev. 6:8, 429). Furthermore, the fall of Babylon/Rome, representing the corrupt city, is forecast by an angel who declares, in verse 18:8, "her plagues will come in a single day—pestilence and mourning and famine—and she will be burned with fire; for mighty is the Lord God who judges her" (Rev. 18:8, 443). This eschatological vision, rather than being rarefied, is mundane: war brings famine and disease, breaks down civilization, and jeopardizes the survival of refugees. Thus, Solange who sees himself as minister of Deep Ecology is waging a covert war against industrial civilization. But, in one important respect, he has more in common with the Fourth, rather than with the First, Horseman. The First Horseman of Revelation appears in three passages: (1) "I looked, and there was a white horse! Its rider had a bow; a crown was given to him, and he came out conquering and to conquer" (Rev. 6:2; 429); (2) "Then I saw heaven opened, and there was a white horse! Its rider is called Faithful and True, and in righteousness he judges and makes war" (Rev. 19:11, 444); and (3) "And the armies of heaven, wearing fine linen, white and pure, were following him on white horses" (Rev. 19:14, 445). The rider in Revelation 6:2 is a secular militarist, whereas the rider on the white horse is widely interpreted to be Jesus Christ, followed by an angelic army returning to Earth to rout the beast and its cohorts (Rev. 19:11–16, 444–445 & notes); the Second Horseman on a red steed signifies war and bloodshed (Rev. 6:4, 429 & note); the Third Horseman on a black steed signifies famine; but the Fourth Horseman on a "pale green horse" kills with sword, famine, and pestilence (Rev. 6:7–8, 429). Solange's messianic aspirations tie him to the white horse, his terrorist aggression to the Second Horseman, but the Fourth Horseman (as Katherine Anne Porter well knew) is the spirit of bioterrorism, the bearer of pestilence.

Daniel Kalla, Pandemic: A Novel *(2005)*

The third novel in the Characterization group, Daniel Kalla's *Pandemic: A Novel*, reflects current events and biomedical realities: the terrorists are committed to a radical tradition that envisions the transformation of human society through the exercise of force; its leaders are established members of financial, military, and scientific communities; international cooperation is as essential to the conspiracy as it is to its overthrow; the lethality of a viral pathogen is artificially enhanced through crude experiments; counterterrorism scientists and law enforcement agencies overpower the attackers. This discussion has three foci: on the bioterrorists themselves; on the viral pathogens they use; and on the counterterrorist campaign.

The premise of the story is that Islamist terrorists, based in downtown Cairo, Egypt, and in Hargeysa, Somalia, plan to infect suicide combatants with genetically-engineered influenza viruses (not the exhumed H1N1 strain but a descendant) and to spread this lethal hybrid in European and North American cities. Their theocratic motive is to establish Shar'ia Law: "a legal framework to regulate public and private aspects of life based upon specific Islamic teachings" (Kalla, 23, 245–46; "Shar'ia," *Glossary*). Two viral strains will be employed as ordnance: one is a naturally-occurring H2N2 virus; the other is a more virulent mutant, one that the terrorists create through the serial passage of both H2N2 and H3N2 in pigs (recalling Richard Shope's experiments), conducive to the exchange of genetic information and to the possibility of increased virulence. Their mode of acquiring the original strain is to dispatch Malay agents to China, one of whom self-infects with the Gansu flu (the reputed Type A/H2N2), ingesting the bloody secretions of a Chinese flu sufferer and filling vials with the dying man's blood. The infected agent, functioning as a human incubator, then brings the pathogen to terrorist bases in Somalia. By acting as an *in vivo* and *in vitro* carrier (the H2N2 strain is carried in blood samples from the index case and in his own body), the agent has committed suicide. Once the H2N2 virus is inoculated into suicide terrorists, they are deployed to Western urban centers to start epidemics (Kalla, 24). In the initial phase of the plan, suicidal carriers of the Gansu virus contaminate a London hotel (Kalla, 113). The more lethal and transmissible variant, H3N2, will be deployed in a second wave of attacks. The Brotherhood of One Nation, the terrorist organization, takes credit for the initial attacks in London, Hong Kong, Vancouver, and Chicago, and they demand the withdrawal of U.S. and Allied forces from Muslim territories (Kalla, 201–202). The plot outline is actually quite authentic, but there are discrepancies.

The idea of a suicide carrier of infectious disease is a theoretical possibility (Söderblom). This tactic, as it appears in the novel, is part of a two-pronged strategy: one being short-term and geopolitical; the other being long-term and millenarian. Consistent with Tucker's research, this terrorist cell has a theocratic vision in the reinstatement of the Caliphate or successor to the Islamic Prophets, who will unify all of Islam, under Shar'ia or halakhic Law ("Caliphate," *Glossary*). The main bioterrorist cell in Egypt features a zealous and rich financier, a rogue militarist, and an unscrupulous virologists working in a makeshift lab. Since their purpose is to realize this theological vision through force, they are ideologically aligned with Al Qaeda ("Al Qaida's Ideology"). The plan fragments as the theocratic financier and his sociopathic leader clash; the latter, with the seed cultures of an H3N2 Subtype, then tries to culture the virus for use against New York City. The terrorist cells in Seattle and New York are eventually destroyed (Kallas, 383–387).

A minor discrepancy concerns the H2N2 Subtype and the phyletic history of influenza. The H2N2 virus used as the initial weapon was the cause of the 1957 "Asian" flu pandemic. According to experts, however, H2N2 became extinct in 1968 and was subsequently replaced by H3N2 (Taubenberger & Morens, "1918 Influenza," 15–16; Palese & Wang, 1; Mahy, 193). Kalla's recrudescent H2N2, in reality, is extinct. As in the fictions of Crane and Case in which live virus is retrieved from permafrost burial sites, Kalla's use of an extinct Subtype conveys the idea that, with notable exceptions, bioterrorism is cost-effective and not necessarily dependent on state-of-the-art technology.

At the vanguard of the counterterrorist forces are epidemiologists. The protagonist, Dr. Haldane, working from WHO headquarters in Geneva, tracks the first documented case of H2N2 to a farm, fifty miles north of Jianyuguan City, Gansu Province. Other cases reported north of the index case also suffer a mortality rate of 25 percent. This strain causes the cytokine overreaction: acute respiratory distress, organ failure, and toxic shock. Kalla's scientists use the acronym ARCS for Acute Respiratory Collapse Syndrome, a variant of ARDS (Acute Respiratory Distress Syndrome) (Kalla, 34–35). Yet the virus, given an air of mystery, seems to be as chimerical as the Andromeda Strain: the returning H2N2 does not conform to the Type A and B categories, but its lineage from the Spanish flu is not ruled out (Kalla, 34). While this investigation is going on, the reader is introduced to Dr. Moskor, developer of an antiviral drug that would prove an important addition to the Western arsenal (Kalla, 40–42).

Like field investigators today who routinely study patient clusters in Asia, Kalla's epidemiologists go to Jiayuguan City, to examine a town doctor who contracted the disease while caring for two patients (Kalla, 64–65). They find that Dr. Fung is suffering from ARCS, an inflammatory, hemorrhagic syndrome. The index case, a northern farmer with similar symptoms, expired in 24 hours (Kalla, 66). The attending physician, Dr. Wu, suspects that the current virus is much worse than SARS. Though reputedly not an avian virus, this pathogen is contagious from person to person. Having found that no medicines work, the hospital requires that all staff wear biohazard suits while in negative-pressurized, patient-care areas (Kalla 68). Unknown to the international investigators, for a considerable price Dr. Wu had allowed the Malays access to the index patient, from whom secretions and venous blood had been initially drawn (Kalla, 71–72). Wu's activities (he confesses and commits suicide) were prompted by greed (a motive Tucker notes); and his collusion with the Malays and the Islamic cell is disclosed as the counterterrorists build their case (Kalla, 228).

The identity of the recrudescent virus will be revealed once the WHO investigators and Chinese virologists have completed RNA sequencing. The Gansu pathogen, they theorize, is indeed a product of zoonosis. A natural reassortment of avian and of human genetic material, it is a novel virus evolving in the porcine system; therefore, poultry and pigs must be destroyed en masse, despite the economic impact on local farming (Kalla, 102). In other words, this virus, like 1918 H1N1, is the product of an antigenic shift. Like H1N1, H2N2 is the product of genetic interchange between avian and human influenzas in the mixing vessel of swine.

Although the clinical syndrome of the Gansu strain is far worse than SARS in that it causes multi-organ failure, severe pneumonia, and death in two days, this degree of debilitation ironically provides an epidemiological advantage. Since people are sickened severely and bed-ridden quickly, they cannot spread the infection publicly, as they might have otherwise if they carried a virus with a longer incubation period (Kalla, 126–127). Most important is that in its natural form, the new H2N2, though dangerous, is not very contagious (Kalla, 127).

The Gansu strain, as the WHO ultimately determines, is indeed an H2N2 Subtype of the 1957 Asian influenza virus (Kalla, 177–78). Despite the phyletic discrepancy, the idea that novel H2N2 and H3N2 can be recombined genetically is possible (Taubenberger & Morens, "1918 Influenza," 15–16).

If Kalla's premise is to revive the extinct virus, then that makes for some interesting biomedical fiction.

Coordination between counterterrorist agencies continues to yield positive results. Scientists at the Department of Homeland Security in Washington, learning of the London hotel infections, suspect it is the work of bioterrorists, since there is no apparent geographical or epidemiological connection between the Gansu and London outbreaks and since the London incident involves a more virulent agent, one striking healthy children and adults the hardest (Kalla, 156–158). Because time is of the essence, researchers consider using Dr. Moskor's promising, but untested, antiviral medicine (Kalla, 161–166). Another piece of the puzzle is found when, Dr. Gwen Savard, Haldane's co-worker, deduces from epidemiological and forensic evidence that, "Someone has weaponized the Gansu Flu" and is using human beings both as incubating vessels and as suicide vectors (Kalla, 195). The time had come for an all-out international response (Kalla, 197). Meanwhile, the London outbreak has worsened: 700 cases with 20 percent mortality and sporadic clusters are detected in Amsterdam, Brussels, and Hamburg (Kalla, 235).

The concerted effort of counterterrorist forces and intelligence operatives gradually foils the aggressors' strategy. The CIA discovers Dr. Wu's activities and traces the London event to Gansu (Kalla, 200–201). An Egyptian policeman, Sergeant Achmed Eleish, before terrorists can execute him, sends a cryptic e-mail message, identifying not only the suicide vector in Vancouver, but also the major operatives and their sites in Somalia: the financier and publishing magnate Hazzir Kabaal, and a disaffected soldier, Major Abdul Sabri, are identified (Kalla, 250, 253–254). Law enforcement agencies and intelligent services in Islamic countries, it is important to note, are partners with the West in the counterrorist investigation.

The Gansu Flu is medically contained in Asia, in Europe, and in North America (Kalla, 343). But the CDC confirms, at this juncture, that *two* types of Gansu Flu are co-circulating: a novel H2N2 which is highly-pathogenic but poorly transmissible; and an H3N2 Subtype, genetically engineered into a highly-pathogenic *and* transmissible form, exactly what the bioterrorists needed. The existence of a novel Gansu H3N2 Subtype, detected in the blood serum of a terrorist lab monkey in Somalia, proves that the terrorists were still at work (Kalla, 351–53). To complicate matters for the investigators Haldane, Savard, and McLeod, Dr. Moskor's antiviral has serious side-effects (a risk of hepatitis), so its use on a broader scale would likely meet FDA resistance (Kalla, 358). With respect to the H2N2 bioweapon, Kalla's fiction adumbrates Zimmerman and Koch's 2009 argument for the infeasibility of an influenza bioweapon. Although the initial phase of the Islamists' bioweapons project had fizzled out, Dr. Aziz, using 1930s methods, is still able to introduce influenza viruses into pigs in the hope of increasing the contagiousness of Gansu. Aziz exclaims: "along with the Gansu strain [H2N2], we inoculated our pigs with the more contagious but far less lethal forms of the common flu [H3N2]. We tried several recent flu strains without success. But when we introduced the Beijing Flu to the mix ... we have developed a more infective version of the Gansu flu" (Kalla, 297). Trial and error and conventional procedures yield "a more infective version of the Gansu Flu," one in which the 20 percent level of infectivity is tripled (Kalla, 395–397). Dr. Savard describes to her colleagues how, "One of the terrorists ... managed to introduce sections of the Beijing Flu's genetic code into the Gansu Flu. The end result is the much more contagious H3N2 strain of Gansu Flu" (Kalla, 356). This fantastic supergerm, the terrorists believe, will give them enough leverage to force the U.S. and Coalition forces to withdraw from Islamic territory and to desist from supporting Israel (Kalla, 297).

Even though they are armed with a lethal agent, the terrorist cell undergoes a climactic split along ideological and strategic lines. Kabaal rejects the drastic use of the supervirus since it will neither dislodge their enemy nor further their cause, while Sabri thoughtlessly calls for mass destruction as the means of garnering popular support in the Islamic world (Kalla, 313–314). Major Sabri then murders his moderate co-conspirator (Kalla, 315) and embarks as a lone wolf to enforce divine justice through martyrdom. His impossible plan is to cultivate the H3N2 Gansu under makeshift conditions and to release the virus in New York City. Predictably, Sabri is killed in a shootout with the investigators. His accomplices in Seattle and New York are apprehended, and the terrorist cells are destroyed (Kalla, 383–397).

Pandemic: A Novel is an informative work but one that may have exaggerated the terrorists' ability to manufacture and disperse a recombinant pathogen for use as a weapon of mass destruction. With government backing, such a sinister plan is conceivable; but the likelihood of its success is low. First of all, influenza is, by its nature, ill-suited for use as a bioweapon. Soviet scientists in the Vector program, according to the defectors Pasechnik and Alibek, were at work on chimera organisms, combining smallpox and Ebola viruses, to be loaded onto missiles aimed at European and American cities (Alibek, *Biohazard*, 137–145, 259–261); influenza, however, seems not to have been in the arsenal. Considering the time and technological expertise required to create an influenza construct, the Brotherhood's plot strains credibility. A suicidal carrier of a highly pathogenic but moderately contagious H2N2 influenza virus is within the realm of possibility. Even if mortality was low, such an event would instill fear and burden public health services. A terrorist attack is designed to create fear, to disrupt everyday life, and to achieve a geopolitical or philosophical aim. Dr. Tara O'Toole, in her "Smallpox: An Attack Scenario" (August 1999), states that an attack using the much more dangerous smallpox virus "would deliberately seek to sow public panic, disrupt official institutions, and shake public confidence in government." It is reasonable to assume that any biological attack would have these effects.

The novels of Crane, Case, and Kalla reflect modern history. A flagrant modern incarnation, as mentioned above, is the Soviet's mass production of warhead-deliverable, Category A pathogens, a program justified, in the Russian mind, by the perception of a shifting balance of power between East and West. This mentality prevailed in the early 1980s, according to the defecting scientist Ken Alibek: "Our soldiers [i.e., Soviet] were dying in Afghanistan at the hands of U.S.-backed guerrillas, and Washington was about to deploy a new generation of cruise missiles in Western Europe, capable of reaching Soviet soil in minutes. Intelligence reports claimed that Americans envisioned the death of at least sixty million Soviet citizens in the case of a nuclear war" (*Biohazard*, 89). In the 1980s, "germ warfare was on the fringes [of] American military strategy," but President Reagan's idea of a "Star Wars shield" against Soviet nuclear warheads was in the headlines (Miller et al., *Germs*, 90–91). The prospect that the U.S. was working on ways to neutralize Soviet nuclear capability with space technology, while at the same time doubling funds for biodefense annually, may have sent the wrong message to the Russians. Already bogged down in Afghanistan, they may have perceived that they were losing ground in conventional, in nuclear, *and* in biological capability (Miller, et al., *Germs*, 83). These signals may have prompted the Soviets to develop a covert, retaliatory capability in direct violation of the 1972 *Biological Weapons Convention*: the production of enormous amounts of lethal biological weapons that could be delivered via long-range missiles. Ten bio-warheads on each MIRV (Multiple Independently Targetable Reentry Vehicle) "could be filled with dry powder or with liquid smallpox" (Preston, *The Demon*, 91–92). The long-term effects of Soviet policy had not been calculated (Miller et al., 83, 91). Nor are the whereabouts of "the many tons of frozen smallpox or the biowarheads" known (Preston, *The Demon*, 94).

Since the use of the influenza virus as a biological weapon is unlikely, and since the retrieval of live viruses (as distinguished from viable RNA fragments) from interred corpses is impossible, the fiction of the Characterization Period is more imitative than it is predictive; nevertheless, the historical research involved in these novels is impressive. The Inglesby-Bartlett Anthrax scenario, in contrast to the novelistic fiction, is a learning tool having a higher degree of predictive value.

Part Three

The Novelistic Period (1997–2014)

7

Avian Influenza

Definitions and Background

In a series of informative reports and papers, to which this chapter is largely indebted, the CDC outlines the history and characteristics of pandemics, generally, and of avian influenza, specifically.[1] This chapter provides a historical framework for the fiction on avian influenza, discussed in chapter 8. Background information on avian influenza will help us to appreciate the scientific work and the fiction it inspired.

Avian viruses normally do not affect human beings, but under certain circumstances they can make human beings and certain animals sick. For example, people who live and work in virus-contaminated environments, such as poultry markets, can pick up the infection directly from organic material, through tactile contact or inhaled dust. Another less apparent but more dangerous process can take place on the genetic level. A host, such as a pig, can be infected with the avian virus through direct environmental contact, for example, on a farm where poultry and pigs are kept, or if pigs drink from a trough contaminated with avian waste. A pig could be infected with a human influenza Type A virus, one of three viral Types (Types A and B cause seasonal epidemics; C, only mild disease) (Webster & Walker, 123). If it were to then pick up an avian Type A strain as well, then the two viruses in the pig's system could interchange or reassort genetic material, producing a new and dangerous influenza Type A virus. Having most of the genes from a human virus and several from the avian virus, this mutant could have the capacity to spread from human to human in a sustained manner. Influenza Type A viruses, comprised of eight gene segments, have the capacity to transfer genetic material between species.

The human experience with avian flu, though chronologically brief, is nevertheless worrisome since the disease is so virulent. Avian Flu Scares, as distinguished from epidemics, happened in 1997 and in 1999. The 1997 event involved several hundred people who had contracted an H5N1 avian virus in Hong Kong. The 1997 Scare, to use the CDC descriptor, was the first instance of an Asian lineage of H5N1viruses causing human respiratory disease (Harder & Werner, "Transmission to Humans"). The 1997 virus had, in this instance, crossed the species barrier, moving directly from chickens to humans, but fortunately had not reached man via an intermediate porcine host, a route whereby it could have picked up genetic material for human transmissibility. Approximately 1.5 million chickens had to be destroyed to contain its spread and to preclude further mutations. The 1999 Scare was also traced to Hong Kong, but this time, to the Subtype, H9N2 strain, also a novel avian virus. Both the strains of 1997 and of 1999 persist today in birds.

The CDC lists four recent North American outbreaks with documented transmission to humans. An avian Type A/H7N2 appearing in November 2003 involved a medically compromised individual. A second outbreak occurred in February 2004, in Texas. A highly virulent H5N2 was detected in a flock of chickens in south-central Texas, the first U.S. outbreak since the 1980s. Also in February 2004, a poultry outbreak was attributed to an avian strain in British Columbia, Canada. Ten poultry workers became ill, none died, and no evidence was found of person-to-person transmission. Interrelated outbreaks were also recorded in Delawarean chicken farms and in live bird markets in New Jersey, on 4 February 2004. In March of 2004, the same strain—a mildly pathogenic H7N2—was detected in Maryland. At the time of this writing, the WHO, the CDC, associated international surveillance facilities, and cooperating governments are monitoring the evolution of a virulent H7N9 bird flu virus that has a human fatality rate of approximately 20 percent and, as of 25 April 2013, had spread from mainland China to Taiwan.

Research, 2003–2012

Three papers on the H5N1 epizootic in Asia, from 2003 to 2007, indicate that poultry in confined Asian markets or farms have been breeding grounds for H5N1 outbreaks and that people working with poultry or whose living conditions bring them into close proximity to infected birds, under certain conditions are susceptible to infection from the avian virus. In none of the reports surveyed below is it suggested that the virus was transmitted from person to person through airborne transmission, the way mild seasonal influenza efficiently spreads. In other words, avian virus had not, in the documented Asian cases, crossed the species barrier as a highly contagious organism. The circuit of infection extended from a poultry worker who picked up the disease tactilely to family members who, while providing crude domestic care, presumably picked up the virus from contaminated surfaces and bedding.

Ungchusak and colleagues reported that, in 2004, a highly pathogenic H5N1 avian influenza virus was responsible for widespread poultry disease in eight Asian countries. Incredibly, thirty-two of the forty-four persons or 76 percent of those who contracted the virus died. Most of them had had close contact with infected birds. But the most important finding, in this case, was that there was no evidence of "person-to-person transmission." Investigators closely studied the transmission route in the Thai family where the outbreak originated. Information pertaining to the circumstances and timing of exposures was gathered for each of the three family members; in addition, their relationship to other ill persons was tracked. Three procedures were conducted: sick patients were isolated, treated, and tested to determine the genetic character of the pathogen; those who were exposed to the infected persons were kept under surveillance and treated prophylactically; and poultry in the infected village was destroyed.

Investigators found that the female index patient had become sick three or four days after her last exposure to dying chickens that were in the household. Her mother, who had come from a distant city and who had no previous poultry exposure, died of the infection after having cared for her daughter for sixteen to eighteen hours. Five days after the mother became febrile an aunt who had also arrived to provide nursing care developed fever and, on the seventh day of her stay, developed pneumonia. Laboratory tests indicated that both the mother and the aunt were infected with H5N1 avian influenza Type A virus. No other transmission chains were identified. The eight viral segments of the pathogen, when compared to other H5N1 genetic sequences of recent Thai avian isolates closely matched one another. The investigators concluded that the disease in the mother and aunt came through person-to-person direct contact during nursing care for the critically ill index patient (Ungchusak et al., 2005). The virus, in other words, had not been communicated through aerosolized droplets.

The second paper surveyed here focuses on an incident in Indonesia. I. N. Kandun and others (2006) point out that an avian influenza Type A/H5N1 poultry epidemic, also affecting birds, had caused similar, human viral infections in ten countries. In July 2005, the first Indonesian case was identified. Data were gathered from three groups of Indonesians, each group having had at least two hospitalized patients suffering from H5N1 infection during the period of June to October 2005. Clinical and virological information showed that in all three groups, severe disease was present, with mortality resulting in four of the eight patients. In each of the three groups, patients with H5N1 infection belonged to the same family, and most lived in the same household. The source of the infection in the index case was not determined, but molecular sequence analysis showed the isolates were H5N1 viruses of avian origin. The infection, it appears, had spread through close contact within the family circle. As in the Thai outbreak, the circuit of contagion did not extend beyond the immediate locations.

A third paper evaluates an outbreak in China. In December 2007, according to H. Wang and colleagues (2008), two individuals living in Jiangsu Province, China, contracted a severe form of avian influenza, Type A/H5N1. Public health authorities analyzed clinical, viral, and epidemiological data. While tracking down and monitoring those with whom the index cases had come into contact, they were especially interested in anyone who developed respiratory symptoms, so as to eliminate the dangerous possibility of a virus communicable through respiration rather than through physical contact. Although the twenty-four-year-old index case died, his fifty-two-year-old father survived the infection because he had already received anti-viral medicine and post-vaccination plasma, drawn from a person who had taken part in an H5N1 vaccine trial. Nevertheless, the father who had substantial exposure to his son became ill, presumably through personal contact as he cared for the young man. Investigators determined that the index case had been exposed to the H5N1 virus at a poultry market six days before becoming symptomatic.

The next phase of the Wang investigation focused on all those who had come into contact with either father or son, to eliminate the possibility of respiratory contagion. Of the ninety-one persons in this category, all agreed to undergo serological tests. Seventy-eight received the anti-viral drug oseltamivir, only two developing mild illness. Significantly, the ninety-one close contacts tested negatively for H5N1 antibodies. As for the father and son, both were infected with a genetically-identical virus. Wang's team concluded that this outbreak was a limited one, involving "non-sustained person-to-person transmission of H5N1 virus that occurred through close contact in a common living environment."

The three papers outlined above suggest that human beings did not readily contract avian influenza virus during the Asian outbreaks. The gray area that epidemiologists are studying involves the possibility of "non-sustained," person-to-person transmission. The most important factor on the minds of Ungchusak, Kandun, Wang, and colleagues was whether the virus could be transmitted from one person to another via sneezes and coughs.

What would happen if a genetically-reassorted H5 avian virus were to acquire the capacity to spread between persons in a sustained manner via an aerosolized route? This question can only be explored under controlled laboratory conditions. Four papers reviewed below, published from 2006 to 2009, describe efforts to understand the pandemic potential of H5N1. Taronna R. Maines and her colleagues summarize the biomedical problem in 2006. Avian influenza Type A/H5N1 viruses spread globally in wild bird populations, and the occasional transmission of the pathogen to human beings is highly probable. Although human-to-human transmission has "rarely" been documented (the word "rarely" requires gloss), the question remains: how are scientists sure that the index cases did not transmit the flu by sneezing or coughing in the faces of those who cared for them? Did the sick person's secretions carry communicable virus, or did the care givers become infected in the same manner as did the index case: by breathing in fomites or contaminated fecal dust?

The pandemics of 1957 and of 1968, as Maines et al. (2006) point out, were the result of reassorted avian-human influenza viruses—that is, of mutations or gene exchange. The avian virus had, in those outbreaks, naturally acquired "human virus-like receptor binding properties," genetic qualities making it more readily transmissible to human cells. This revelation could account for the species jump from poultry to poulterer. Since the mechanisms controlling human internal proteins and efficient transmission of influenza virus in humans is not well understood, Maines' team conducted experiments to learn more about the transmission efficiency of H5N1. Using ferrets in their experiments, they employed a highly transmissible, human H3N2 virus, and they exposed it to the internal protein genes of an avian virus. The purpose was to induce genetic recombination to see if the avian virus acquired from the human H3N2 had the capability to spread between human beings. The mutant strain, as it turned out, replicated efficiently within individual ferrets but was inefficiently transmitted from ferret to ferret (so far, so good).

Maines' team took the next step: to engineer the 1997 H5N1 avian influenza strain to acquire human virus internal proteins. Here, the results were even more encouraging. Viral replication in infected ferrets actually declined (in comparison to the previous experiment); and, again, there was no evidence of efficient (or aerosolized) transmission from ferret to ferret. These tests showed that human H3N2 surface proteins alone "did not confer efficient transmissibility." Nor was the 1997 H5N1's experimental acquisition of human transmissibility proteins (through the second step in the experiment) sufficient to create a dangerous virus, one both highly contagious and deadly to man. This finding was verified by serial passages in the ferrets, a process that would induce more mutations. Maines et al. circumspectly concluded that H5N1 viruses might require further adaptation to become the source of a pandemic ("Lack of Transmission of H5N1"). Thankfully, the laboratory results were negative.

Using Asian avian strains (H5N1 isolates from 2003–2006) and the ferret model, Hui-Ling Yen and co-workers (2007) also tested transmissibility. They made experimental groupings, each of which consisted of one ferret inoculated with avian virus and two placed in close proximity to the infected animal. In this way, they simulated what had occurred on poultry farms. They were trying to find out if the infected animal could transmit the virus to the nearby ferrets through the air.

Using four strains of H5N1s, harvested from people who had already been exposed to the virus, presumably through close contact, Yen and co-workers also searched for molecular changes in the human convalescents' virus that might affect its pathogenicity and transmissibility in human beings. Two H5N1 strains from Vietnam (outbreaks in 2004 and in 2005, respectively), when isolated from these people, showed they were "avian-like"; and two ferrets had positive reactions to these strains. When inoculated into the ferrets, this virus caused neurological symptoms and death. But further results were equivocal. A 2003 avian strain from Hong Kong and a 2006 one from Turkey, for example, were also found to have "binding affinity" for avian and human cell receptors (the authors use the hyphenated adjective "human-like"); these avian-human viruses, in other words, could be attracted either to bird and or to human cells. Despite these genetic propensities, these reassortant strains when inoculated into ferrets caused only mild symptoms and no mortality. Both humans and ferrets were susceptible to these avian strains (as the molecular analyses confirmed), but the ensuing illness was mild, and there was no evidence of aerosol-droplet transmission either from human to human or from ferret to ferret. The hypothesized route of transmission, again, was close contact between a sick and a healthy organism.

An infected ferret in proximity to a healthy one could indeed communicate the disease. This was shown to be true in the Yen experiments, as healthy ferrets in close proximity to an animal infected with 2003 Hong Kong developed antibodies. The results, however, were encouraging. Animals with antibodies to the virus (proof of exposure to viral antigens) were neither sick nor did they spread the infection. But a positive finding appeared soon afterward when unexposed or *naïve* ferrets were housed with animals that had been inoculated with 2005 Vietnam. Over a six-to-eight-day period, several of the healthy animals showed not only antibodies to the virus, but also virus infection. These clinical manifestations were variable. Although the naive animals with 2005 Vietnam became severely ill, unexpectedly virus was barely detectable in nasal secretions. Because of limited virus shedding (secretions from the inoculated ferrets), no secondary transmission occurred between the infected contact ferret and nearby healthy animals (simulating poultry farm conditions). Yen's group concluded that, despite receptor-binding affinity (a molecular change in the avian hemagglutinin protein conferring affinity to human cells), H5N1 viral strains possessed "molecular determinants" that *limited* their spread among mammals; that transmission of the virus did not occur through the respiratory route; and that inefficient transmission produced variable disease ("Inefficient Transmission of H5N1").

Erin M. Sorrell and co-workers (2009) tested Eurasian avian H9N2 influenzas that possessed "human-like" receptor specificity, finding that they were *sometimes* transmissible to humans and pigs (italics added). Their research was also aimed at determining if an avian-human H9N2 reassortant could be transmitted between ferrets. The experiments raised a red flag: a laboratory-reassorted virus, one containing genetic proteins of an avian H9N2 *and* of a human H3N2, could be transmitted via respiratory droplets between ferrets, inducing an infection similar to human influenza infections. Sorrell and colleagues discovered that a reassortant virus expressing *only* the hemagglutinin and the neuraminidase of the ferret-adapted virus could acquire mammalian transmissibility. This meant that a circulating avian H9N2 virus, if acquiring through reassortment the internal genes of a human virus such as H3N2, could adapt to mammals and possibly be contagious through coughs and sneezes. Furthermore, they concluded that H1, H2, and H3 influenza Subtypes were not the only variants capable of aerosolized respiratory transmission. The question as to whether avian flu could adapt to the human population and cause a pandemic remains unanswered. These studies suggest that such an event, though unlikely, cannot be ruled out.

Sarah Jackson and co-workers (2009) co-infected ferrets with a Thai 2004 avian Type A/ H5N1 influenza virus and a human H3N2 virus. The two viruses exchanged genetic material in the ferrets, and the reassorting of genes between these two viral Subtypes probably occurred in the ferrets' upper-respiratory tracts. From these results, Jackson's group learned that "continued exposure of humans and animals to H5N1 alongside seasonal influenza viruses" increases the risk, and the inevitability, that H5 Subtype reassortant viruses might be generated and shed from the respiratory tract. The research of the Sorrell and Jackson investigators raises the theoretical possibility that avian influenza virus, through genetic reassortment, could acquire the capability to spread from person to person via aerosol droplet spray. Their experiments also showed that genetic reassortment between H5N1 and human H3N2 occurred in the upper airways of ferrets. They reasonably concluded from this discovery "that continued exposure of humans and animals to H5N1 alongside seasonal influenza viruses" risks the emergence of an H5 Subtype, a novel virus or reassortant that could be shed through airway secretions. The determining factor in the Jackson experiment was *long-term exposure of human to avian influenza* (italics added).

This historical and scientific survey suggests that ground zero of the next pandemic would be a poultry farm located near aquatic bird habitats; the critical time period would be flu season; and the most dangerous organism in the area would be a poulterer who, while nursing a mild case of seasonal flu, cannot afford to take a week off from work.

Investigators agree that close contact between poultry processors and infected fowl is likely to blame for recent avian-to-human influenza transmissions. Humans, therefore, are at highest risk when in close contact with infected poultry, with surfaces and objects contaminated with droppings, and during the slaughtering, de-feathering, and butchering process (Harder & Werner, "Transmission to Humans"). Viral-contaminated dust or dirt is termed *fomes* (singular)/*fomitēs* (plural). The Latin term fomites was adapted as a medical term in 1773 to mean "the morbid matter of disease" and is in the modern lexicon (*OED*, V: 394/Compact, I: 1043); the term derives from Latin and means, "chips of wood" [*Pocket Oxford Latin Dictionary*, 77]). Contagion through particulate matter carrying avian virus can occur tactilely during poultering and find its way into a person's system from hand-to-mouth movements. The next question is: can the inhalation of avian fomites in poultry dust kill a healthy person? The second hypothetical is as follows: If the poulterer was infected with human flu, and if he or she breathed in contaminated particles, what would be the chances of a novel recombination, one having the ability to be conveyed through aerosolized human secretions rather than through poultry dust? Or is such a possibility simply unpredictable?

These bird-to-human infections continue to occur. On 22 January 2012, a second man in southern China was reported as having died from H5N1 bird flu. Investigators were, at first, alarmed to learn that neither man had been exposed to poultry in an occupational or domestic setting, raising the anxious possibility that they had caught the virus through the airborne route. The alarm was cancelled when it was learned the decedents *had not* directly infected human contacts. Because avian flu has pandemic potential, and because the fatality rate is greater than 50 percent, any outbreak must be thoroughly evaluated (Wines, A6). A recent outbreak of H7N9 bird virus, late spring of 2013, has been under surveillance in China and Southeast Asia.

Questions regarding transmissibility and virulence remain central to influenza research today. In June 2012, scientists publicized research describing how laboratory-induced mutations could render the lethal H5N1 bird flu transmissible between mammals. The more controversial of the two papers, written by scientists at the Erasmus Medical Center, The Netherlands, identified five mutations that were needed to make avian flu spread more easily in a ferret model, approximating human susceptibility. In view of the fact that at the time, 622 people had contracted H5N1, all presumably through occupational and environmental contact, and that more than half have died, this experiment made some apprehensive. Fouchier and colleagues (Herfst et al.) justified their work on the grounds of public health: enhancing H5N1's transmissibility to human beings under controlled conditions was a method through which vaccines and antiviral medications might be developed. These experiments and the information derived from them would be pre-emptively useful if a mutant avian virus were to appear in the wild. But publicizing the procedures has made some people uncomfortable about terrorism or laboratory accidents.

In 2011, news of the Fouchier project led to a polarized debate. Critics were alarmed over the possibility of an accidental release of the virus, that it could fall into the hands of terrorists, or that amateur virologists could produce it. In a 22 December 2011, *New York Times'* interview, Fouchier counterargued that if the mutations enhancing transmissibility were known, then the appearance of a novel virus of this kind in outbreak-prone countries could be detected and aggressively treated (Carvajal, A28). Furthermore, having the mammalian-adapted virus in the lab would give scientists a head start in the formulation of effective vaccines and antiviral drugs. Fouchier and colleagues discounted the possibility that bioterrorists could make a novel strain because technical sophistication is difficult to acquire and because other, more dangerous, pathogens are easier to wield.

The risks inherent to avian virus investigations of this kind have fomented a bio-safety/bio-security debate. Valid questions have been asked: (1) should these experiments be conducted in the first place, given the possibility of an accidental laboratory release, which could be catastrophic; (2) and should the methods employed in creating an efficient avian virus be publicized, allowing terrorists or deranged persons to have access to this know-how? These are legitimate concerns. But do they outweigh the imperative of understanding and preparing for a novel avian pandemic? Expert opinions on both sides of the issue are sampled below.

Several prominent scientists favor H5N1 experimentation and unfettered public disclosure. In 2012, Dr. Peter Palese of Mount Sinai School of Medicine/NYU, a contributor to the genomic characterization of the 1918 H1N1 influenza virus, calls for unrestricted publication of the H5N1 transmission experiments ("Don't censor"). Publication of the H1N1 genome in 2005, he points out, led to several important discoveries, most notably H1N1's sensitivity to seasonal flu vaccine and to common antiviral medications; consequently, the dual use of H1N1, its "positive and negative applications," was no longer a serious concern (Fauci & Collins, "Benefits and Risks," 1523).

In regard to the H5N1experimentation, Palese rejects the advice of the National Science Advisory Board for Biosecurity that, "the mutations behind the virus's transmissibility" should not be publicly revealed. To redact their findings as a dual-use security measure, in Dr. Palese's view, would be contrary to the interests of science and public health. Nor should "approved experts" alone be privy to the results. Limiting availability by mandate will not work, he argues, given the amount of workers in the field and the likelihood of the information leaking out. Nor is it clear on what basis scientists will qualify for approval. Since knowing which mutations make the virus more virulent or transmissible would lead to the development of vaccines and antiviral drugs, the entire community, Palese maintains, should contribute in an atmosphere of open dialogue.

For Dr. David M. Morens et al., laboratory research is vital, since "little is known about determinants of human influenza pathogenicity and transmissibility" ("Engineering H5N1"). Surveying dual-use debates over the last two decades, they observe that the question of whether or not to publish sensitive material has always ended in favor of open access. This was true for research on smallpox, for that on SARS, for that on ferret-model transmissibility using H2N2 influenza virus (a novel virus in 1957, H2N2 became extinct after 1968 [Palese, "Virus Subtypes,"2]), for that on H9N2 avian virus, and for that on the reconstruction of the 1918 virus genome. The reconstruction of H1N1, as mentioned, has contributed to present knowledge about the emergence, transmissibility, and pathogenicity of influenza viruses. All of this work was conducted, Morens et al. assert, "with appropriate oversight, and without negative consequences."

Opponents of full disclosure are also persuasive. Thomas V. Inglesby, Anita Cicero, and Donald A. Henderson (leader of the WHO campaign to eradicate smallpox) are uneasy about the mutation experiments because avian viruses, though not yet airborne transmissible to humans, are more virulent than H1N1 ("The Risk"). They point out that the mortality rate for H5N1 (involving a very limited number of persons, compiled from 2004 to 2012), stands at 59 percent. According to one estimate, the H1N1 virus sickened 20 percent to 40 percent of the world population of 1.8 billion in 1918–1919: that is, between 360 and 720 million persons. If only 2 percent of those infected succumbed to the disease, then global mortality would range from 7.2 to 14 million ("Pandemic Flu History"). This means that 98 percent of those contracting influenza—between 352.8 to 705.6 million persons—recovered without the benefit of vaccines, antivirals, or antibiotics. Should H5N1 acquire transmissibility, similar to seasonal influenza, a global pandemic inestimably worse than that of 1918–1919 could ensue.

Arguing that the benefits of these experiments "do not outweigh the risks" touched upon above, Inglesby et al. enumerate four arguments in favor of censorship: (1) the risk of a deadly strain of avian flu accidentally escaping the laboratory, though low, is not zero. In 1977, a pre–1957 strain of H1N1, thought to be extinct, was accidentally released from a Russian laboratory and is now circulating in the human population. The possibility of a containment breach, involving a bioengineered, highly-pathogenic avian flu virus, cannot be ruled out, either; (2) research and development geared to vaccines and antivirals, they say, does not require the creation of a virulent and highly contagious H5N1 virus; (3) should a deadly strain of virus be created "in the hopes that the frightening results invigorate R & D for vaccine development?"; and (4) the possibility exists that the viral mutations could indeed be used for terrorist purposes. Engineering avian strains to make antivirals and vaccines, from the standpoint of Inglesby et al., is too risky.

Andrew T. Pavia tries to reconcile these antipodal views. Though he acknowledges that the possibility of accidental release of an engineered H5N1 is low and the use of H5N1 as a weapon improbable, he concurs with Palese, Morens, and others that full disclosure of the Fouchier and Kawaoka experiments will benefit the biomedical community. In his words, "Understanding which genes and which regions must change [in H5N1 RNA], and ultimately understanding the structural and phenotypic changes that allowed the creation of a readily transmissible H5N1 virus," can facilitate screening of H5N1 strains and other "novel influenza viruses for pandemic potential"; and disclosure will also provide ideas for developing targets for antiviral and vaccine therapies (464).

Though favoring disclosure, Pavia is mindful of the need for safeguards. Society can balance the risks and advantages of H5N1 research that is designated "dual use" (that is, as having health benefits but concomitant risks), he writes, if agencies review scientific work in advance, especially in terms of biosecurity, because it is unclear if sufficient oversight is nationally or internationally in place. Thus, on the danger of misuse, he sides with Inglesby et al.: preventing this eventuality overrides the right to free and open access if potentially dangerous scientific information is involved. This is not a self-contradiction on Pavia's part. Full disclosure is needed, but a review board or oversight committee comprised of an "independent, expert, accountable and transparent group of scientists" should also be convened. The advice and supervision such a committee would bring to the table, in Pavia's view, is a better alternative than government oversight.

The laboratory containment breach is not science fiction. Tony Della-Porta, a microbiologist, describes several incidents related to viral pathogens that have been attributed to poor containment measures, inadequate training, and occupational shortcomings ("Laboratory Accidents"). All of these problems combined in a Taiwanese incident in December 2003, involving a senior scientist at the Institute of Preventative Medicine, National University in Taipei. This scientist reputedly had experience in the use of the Biosafety Level–4 laboratory, the securest facility in which researchers don pressurized space suits. But noncompliance with protocols can deflate training and experience. According to the article, having spilled SARS in an isolator cabinet, he hastily tried to decontaminate it, using 70 percent ethanol rather than the prescribed decontaminant, vaporized hydrogen peroxide; and he did so without donning respiratory protection. As a result, he developed SARS and was critically ill for six days. The WHO investigators identified a number of problems in this case: the scientist had worked alone; his compliance with decontamination procedures was inadequate; he departed from standard safety requirements in not donning respiratory protection; and medical staff, aware that he routinely worked with SARS, had not routinely tested him for infection.

Lapses in judgment and human errors in the presence of virulent microorganisms, Della-Porta relates, can imperil persons both inside and outside of the laboratory. An occurrence in Beijing, China, in April 2004, exemplifies how a serious procedural failure led to dangerous results. At China's Center for Disease Control and Prevention, scientists planning to study inactivated SARS coronavirus antigen outside of isolation did not realize that their attempt to neutralize the virus had failed. As a result, because they unwittingly had exposed themselves to live virus, four staff members contracted the infection, and they transmitted it to seven others *outside* of the Center, one of whom died. In addition, it was later revealed that two staff members, exposed to SARS in February 2004, had not been routinely monitored through blood tests. Nor had the responsible medical practitioners checked for SARS exposure in the facility. Had they acted routinely in this way, as Della-Porta concludes, the faulty inactivation procedure in April would not have gone undetected.

In hindsight, and from the perspective of the nonscientist, the causes of these dangerous accidents seem to be rather obvious. Working alone on a virulent strain appears foolhardy. One does not need a manual to know that admitting inadequately trained or unsupervised workers to a lab experiment using lethal pathogens is asking for trouble. A biosafety lab having containment flaws, or one not designated for use with a specific microbe, should not be used. Not reporting a safety breach in a timely fashion, a serious omission, jeopardizes workers and the public. Being unfamiliar with or using the wrong method of decontamination is difficult to understand, as is the failure to don protective clothing or respiratory devices, especially if the agent attacks the respiratory system. Medical services that fail to monitor healthy researchers or followup on symptomatic ones, in effect, have deactivated an early-warning system, designed to protect the health of workers and their families. Wrong choices, fatigue, hastiness, muddled thinking, and negligence have caused containment breaches.

Prior to the publication of the controversial studies described above, thirty-nine prominent scientists, including members of Fouchier's team, agreed to observe a 60-day moratorium on the research. According to a joint *Letter*, the co-signatories recognized that "more research is needed to determine how influenza viruses in nature become human pandemic threats," so that they can be contained before being transmitted from person to person or countered if adaptation to humans were to occur. But the "perceived fear that the ferret-transmissible viruses may escape from the laboratories" has continued to generate public dialogue over benefits and risks. An international forum was to be planned through which the scientific community could arrive at a consensus regarding issues surrounding this research ("Pause on Avian Flu Transmission Research"; Saey, "Moratorium Ends").

When the moratorium expired in March 2012, however, the Fouchier and Kawaoka groups, working independently of each other, modified the Type A/H5N1 virus genetically, allowing it to acquire mutations during passage in ferrets. The genetically modified virus, ultimately, became "airborne-transmissible in ferrets" ("*Science* Publishes the Fouchier Ferret Study"). Altogether, the Dutch researchers had induced viral mutations as the organism was passed through ten generations of ferrets, using nasal secretions continuously transferred from one to another animal (McNeil, A7). Throughout this period, Fouchier et al. argued that the benefits of their work outweighed the potential risks, their primary goal being to raise awareness of the pandemic potential of H5N1 viruses occurring naturally. Because of this imminent danger, they affirmed that experimentation and surveillance could fend off or contain a pandemic (Butler, "Benefits of Mutant Flu Research"). In a paper describing similar experiments, Yoshihiro Kawaoka et al. produced "respiratory droplet transmission" in a reassortant avian-human virus. Using the ferret model, they, too, made the virus "transmissible among mammals" (Imai et al., "Experimental Adaptation").

In February 2013, The Department of Health and Human Services amended the National Institute of Health Guidelines for research involving Recombinant DNA Molecules ("Changes to the *NIH* Guidelines"). The detailed amendments appear to constitute a direct response to the debate over the experiments of Fouchier, Kawaoka, and their colleagues. The amendments reconcile polarized opinions over dual-use projects, such as those involving avian influenza strains, putting Pavia's ideas into practice. The Notice of Changes is explicit in regard to avian influenza: "Experiment with influenza viruses containing genes or segments from 1918–1919 H1N1 ... human H2N2 (1957–1968) and highly pathogenic avian influenza (HPAI) H5N1 virus strains ... including, but not limited to strains ... that are transmissible among mammals by respiratory droplets, as demonstrated in an appropriate animal model or clinically in humans ... shall be conducted at BL3 *enhanced* containment" (p. 12076; italics added). The BioSafety Level 3 protocol, according to the CDC, is to be used, "where work is performed with indigenous or exotic agents that may cause serious or potentially lethal disease through the inhalation route of exposure." Laboratory personnel must receive (1) specific training in handling pathogenic and potentially lethal agents, and must be (2) supervised by scientists competent in handling infectious agents and associated procedures. Furthermore, all procedures involving the manipulation of infectious materials (3) must be conducted within BSCs [Biosafety Cabinets] or other physical containment devices." ("Biosafety Level 3").

The NIH Recombinant DNA Advisory Committee (R.A.C.) found that existing laboratory safety and security measures in the standard Biosafety Level 3 (BL-3) facility *were inadequate* for experimentation on mammalian-transmissible, highly pathogenic H5N1 viruses (p. 12074). Thus, the R.A.C.'s amendments are explicitly aimed at lowering the possibility of a containment breach during experimentation with avian influenza virus. The Committee members made their recommendations, no doubt, mindful of the history and psychology of microbiological accidents. Each of the fourteen categories and subsets that the Committee articulates seems earmarked to minimize human error and to optimize biosafety. Thus, scientists must effectively decontaminate liquid effluents, animal tissues, carcasses, and bedding (e.g., by autoclaving) before the material is removed from the containment area. Anyone working with highly pathogenic H5N1 mammalian-transmissible strains must provide baseline serum samples before, and periodically during, the experimental period (recalling the February-April 2004 SARS breach in Taiwan). If research is conducted on mammalian-transmissible, highly-pathogenic H5N1 viruses, exhaust air "must be HEPA filtered," the ductwork must be sealed from the containment barrier to the filter"; and, should the air-handling system fail, its design must ensure that the airflow cannot reverse (perhaps, with the accidents at Birmingham and Sverdlovsk in mind). The HEPA filters, moreover, must be checked, and backup power must be available. Powered air-purifying respirators are mandatory for all workers in the containment zone. Street clothes must be replaced by protective clothing (wrap-back disposal gowns, olefin protective suit); everyone must wear double-disposable gloves, with protective sleeves over the gown when at work in a biosafety cabinet; double, disposable shoe coverings or a facsimile must be worn. Before exiting the laboratory, everyone is to receive a decontaminating shower. To lessen the chance of fomites infection, all personal equipment exposed to live virus has to be disinfected by spray or wiping, a far cry from conditions on a farm.

Along with essential material protocols, the R.A.C. comments on training and accountability. To ensure compliance with suiting up and decontamination, workers are mandated "to report any loss of containment or exposures." On the level of common sense is the regulation that at least two people must be in the laboratory during experimentation, especially if procedures involve animals, sharp instruments, or when "the generation of aerosols is reasonably anticipated" (pp. 12077–12078). Furthermore, the R.A.C. requires laboratory workers to sign what sounds like a legal document indicating that: (a) they understand these biosafety regulations and that they intend to abide by them; and (b) that they will "report any exposures or accidents, including those by other individuals in the lab." So that the excitement of discovery does not override biosafety, any research on *an antiviral resistant virus* must cease immediately (p. 12078). Any loss of containment, accidents, spills, or possible exposures must be reported to the public health authorities within 24 hours (p. 12079).

Perhaps with the Beijing and other accidents in mind, the R.A.C. requires: annual influenza vaccination for all workers unless medically contraindicated; virus-specific vaccination if a licensed highly-pathogenic H5N1 vaccine is available; and the collection of post-vaccination serum samples to identify an asymptomatic carrier. Along with these protocols, workers must be monitored for flu-like symptoms (p. 12079). Anyone who is symptomatic will receive medical evaluation and treatment, the decision to isolate that person depending on medical diagnosis (p. 12080). Presumably, this is to prevent a person already infected with a seasonal flu virus from coming in contact with an avian organism in the event of a breach. The Biosafety Level 3 enhancements for research on highly pathogenic H5N1 are reasonable responses to those who voiced concern about accidents.

No amendments can prevent noncompliance absolutely, even if the consequences are severe. Improvements can heighten awareness in the laboratory but not prevent criminality, irrationality, or negligence, the consequence of boring routine, fatigue, distraction, arthritis, overconfidence, a squirming lab animal, or the need to catch a flight. Biosecurity could be breached for profit; it could be the act of a deranged scientist; or it could be the fault of an established expert who loses sight of the danger. But even if containment were breached in any one of these scenarios, judging from the backup systems, the strengthening of oversight, and re-training that goes with it, it is unlikely (not impossible) that a public health emergency or global crisis would result from an avian flu accident.

The R.A.C. amendments regarding highly-pathogenic H5N1 research were intended to reduce the chance of an accident. If a fictionist wishes to achieve realism in a novel about a release of avian flu, he or she must be familiar with the professional debate which would frame the story and motivate the characters. If a credible story were created demonstrating a weakness in the system—for the sake of argument, one that the R.A.C. had *not*, or had only vaguely, addressed—or a situation involving a precipitating event, such as a natural disaster compromising the laboratory, then an imaginative writer could contribute to the public health effort, exposing an unseen factor or predicting an unanticipated danger. In this capacity, believable fiction could augment scientific papers, public reports, and "computer-based interactive simulations" of a pandemic influenza outbreak. Researchers at the Pennsylvania State University College of Medicine, in a recently conducted simulation of this kind, tested the response of hospital personnel in an avian influenza crisis (Leaming et al.) Conjectural historiography can reveal possibilities and conceivable events, but only if a logical thread connects medical science and history to the fiction.

It is of some comfort that person-to-person transmission of Type A/H5N1 avian influenza has very rarely occurred. When it has, it has been attributed to fomites, has been limited to close physical contact between an infected individual and family members or caretakers, and has been confined to what epidemiologists call a *family cluster*.

8

Novel Virus and the Approval of *Q-Pan*

Richard Preston, The Cobra Event *(1998)*

Early in 1998, President Bill Clinton, who was already concerned about biosecurity, read Richard Preston's *The Cobra Event* (1997), a bioterrorist novel in which a mad scientist plans mass homicide by unleashing a chimeric pathogen on New York City; the construct, "engineered with skill and subtlety," is a genetic recombinant of smallpox, a nerve-destroying insect virus, and a common cold virus, the latter ensuring transmissibility (Preston, 278). Preston understood that movies and popular literature can effectively educate the public about the bioterrorist reality and that public awareness, in turn, "can help shape a constructive response from governments and scientists around the world far more effectively than the lone warnings of a few experts" ("The Reality behind *The Cobra Event*," 421). Preston's novel accurately portrays bioterrorist history and capabilities, and its setting in lower Manhattan is prescient and disturbing, especially the scene in the Second Avenue tunnel as viral glass housing the microbe is made airborne through detonation, "filling the tunnel with a gray haze that was alive and aching to find blood" (Preston, *The Cobra Event*, 408).

The novel impressed President Bill Clinton to the extent that he instructed his military advisers, in 1998, to determine if the story was plausible, and if what they learned from it could be applied to bio-security. Deputy Secretary of Defense, John Hamre, reported to the President that Preston's "scenario was theoretically plausible." President Clinton explains, in his autobiography, *My Life*, how the molecular biologist Craig Venter confirmed that terrorists could find ways to develop synthetic genes, to reengineer existing viruses or to combine pathogens to make deadly weapons (Clinton, 788–790;

Miller et al., 225–226). President Clinton then urged cabinet members and Speaker of the House Newt Gingrich to read Preston's novel because it reflected current political history (Tucker, "Scourge," 192). The World Trade Center bombing, in 1993, had already heightened awareness about attacks on the homeland, and the Russian scientist Ken Alibek, a defector, would later shock the intelligence community with descriptions, in "Behind the Mask: Biological Warfare" (1998) and in the book *Biohazard* (1999), of the huge stores of bio-engineered anthrax, smallpox, Ebola, and other microbes that the former Soviet Union had manufactured on an industrial scale for bio-warfare purposes. They had engaged in these programs in direct violation of the 1972 *Biological Weapons Convention.* All of this information was instrumental in the broadening of U.S. programs for defense against biological attack.

In March of 1998, members of the Clinton Administration met at Blair House to participate in a "table top exercise," a scenario designed to examine ways of dealing with terrorist attacks employing biological, chemical, and radiological weapons (Clinton, 789). The smallpox simulation revealed defensive weaknesses: it took too much time to get the outbreak under control; too many lives were lost in the interim; the supplies of vaccine and medicines were inadequate; quarantine laws were obsolete; public health systems were ill-equipped for the emergency; and state emergency plans were not suitable. Conferral with scientific advisers, including Nobel Laureate Dr. Joshua Lederberg, and with those responsible for emergency management, confirmed that the country was not ready for a biological attack. As a result, two billion dollars was requested to improve public health capabilities from 1998 to 2006. A series of scenario exercises have contributed to the reinforcement of national defense. They include Tara O'Toole's "Smallpox: An Attack Scenario" (August 1999); the *Dark Winter Bioterrorism Exercise* (22–23 June 2001); the *Atlantic Storm,* smallpox exercise (January 2005); and the *Black Ice Bioterrorism International Coordination Exercise* (2006). Antibiotic, antiviral, and vaccine production has been stepped up; and numerous counterterrorist initiatives, developed.

Preston's fiction was a catalyst for the improvement of national defense against biological terrorism. It was an important contribution to a greater narrative consisting primarily of scenarios, of government and military assessments, and of medical evaluations. In synthesizing historical, scientific, and contemporary events, Preston's novel publicized a real danger which, in turn, led officials to conduct a computer-simulated scenario disclosing severe inadequacies. Consistent with biomedical science and with the psychology of terrorism, Preston's cautionary tale had become a national defense asset. Both the government and the popular writer had consulted the experts, notably Dr.

Lederberg. Thus, Preston, the scientific community, and government leaders were able to pool their ideas and capabilities to enhance biosafety and national security.

Imaginative representations of biomedical crises are more than archival, therapeutic, and public health resources. An outgrowth of contemporary history, these productions can influence political behavior, shape defensive strategies, and anticipate catastrophic events. The remainder of this chapter looks at a film and three novels on influenza and influenza-like outbreaks that dramatize the consequences of unpreparedness and that, in the struggle with emergent diseases, imagination is our greatest asset.

Contagion *(2011)*

If conjectural historiography and realistic fiction can reveal possibilities and conceivable events, can productions in non-print media inform the public, disclose risks, and predict possible dangers, as well? Movies certainly have this potential. Patricia Wald writes at great length about the 1995 film *Outbreak*, in which a hemorrhagic-fever outbreak renders a small California town and its population expendable if the disease is to be controlled, and if its nefarious origin is to be covered up (29).

WHO consultants and medical experts, Drs. W. Ian Lipkin and Lawrence Brilliant, reviewed the biomedical content of the 2011 thriller, *Contagion*, directed by Steven Soderbergh (*contagionmovie*). A virulent influenza-like virus, causing neurological disease, suddenly emerges, leading the WHO, the CDC, and Homeland Security to the discovery that the virus had originally spread tactilely but then underwent an antigenic shift, making it airborne and transmissible between human beings, avian flu's worst-case scenario. MEV-1 (Meningoencephalitis Virus One) turns out to be a genetic reassortant, comprising bat, human and swine influenza virus genes. The pig's virus, presumably, endowed the hybrid with the capacity for sustained human-to-human infection.

The virus in *Contagion* has a real analogue. A zoonotic organism, *Nipah virus* is transmissible from animals to humans, causing both brain inflammation and respiratory disease, and by virtue of the latter is an analogue to avian flu. Nipah virus, upon which MEV-1 may have been modeled, is not really an exotic choice, although at first glance it may seem to have been. A newly-discovered entity, in 1999 the virus was identified in Malaysia. Most of those who contracted the disease got it from direct contact with pigs; and (here is where it gets interesting) it may have been spread from pigs to humans "via respiratory droplets" ("Nipah virus," WHO); so it has that in common with H1N1, although it is believed that swine caught it from human beings, and that the novel virus of 1918 was avian-like. Outbreaks of Nipah virus in Bangladesh and India, from 2001 to 2008, were attributed to contact with contaminated human secretions (the "dead-end" theory). The case-fatality rate, however, ranges from 40 to 75 percent; and there is no vaccine (in the movie, one is developed over time). Its natural hosts are fruit bats immune to the virus. The infection strikes pigs, horses, goats, sheep, cats, and dogs; but in piglets, mortality is low. In the film, an infected bat drops a half-chewed contaminated banana into a piglet trough; the piglet consumes the banana, and there starts the recombinant process. The piglet, in turn, is slaughtered and served at a high-end restaurant, infecting the index case, and leading to the deaths of 100,000,000.

The central premise of the movie is reasonable. Direct transmission of Nipah virus from bats to humans can indeed happen through the consumption of contaminated fruit or animal flesh. Human-to-human transmission in the case of Nipah is similar to what is found in H5N1 clusters: dead-end infections caused by direct contact with sick individuals. The scientific advisers to the film, in all probability, sought a recombinant analogue to avian flu: a Bat-Human-Swine influenza virus. The swine, susceptible to both the human and bat viruses, become the vessel within which these viruses exchange genetic material, producing a hybrid that is lethal to humans and extremely contagious. In the movie, the virus undergoes a mutation to reach this hybridic form, turning from dead-end (as we have seen in Asian family clusters) to sustained transmission.

On 14 May 2013, *The New York Times* reported that a second case of novel coronavirus had been found, suggesting human-to-human transmission; the details of the case, however, are unclear (Erlanger: A9). The French theorized that the virus was zoonotic, that is, it had jumped *from bats to humans*; and they consider the possibility that the virus had spread from the second case to a patient in a nearby bed. If "close contact" is thought to have spread the disease from patient to patient in a shared hospital room, does that mean this particular SARS virus was airborne and inhaled? All those who were in contact with the index case, including health care professionals caring for him, tested negatively; so this hospital or nosocomial infection appears to be a mystery, although an outbreak in Toronto, ten years earlier, caused similar hospital infections. Bat-to-human-to-human contagion, once again, poses a conundrum. As of 16 December 2013, the mainstream media has said nothing further about it. The central virological premise of the film *Contagion*, however, is in the mainstream.

This brings us to influenza fiction that is prospective. Writers envisioning an imminent pandemic are interested in the idea of a novel H5N1 avian flu virus. According to the WHO, a loud alarm was raised on 30 April 2005 when, in the vicinity of Qinghai Lake, central China, 6,345 mixed species waterfowl died off en masse. The cause was a highly pathogenic avian influenza virus. Other locations reported avian outbreaks. In June 2005, poultry markets in Xinjiang and in other provinces began to experience a mass dying-off of poultry due to the infection. On 6 July 2005, the virus responsible for the Qinghai Lake occurrence was officially identified as a novel H5N1 variant, a strain lethal to birds that could experimentally infect mice ("H5N1 Avian Influenza: Timeline").

Surveillance and biomedical experimentation on the novel strain has continued without interruption worldwide. On 25 April 2013, *The New York Times* reported on a new strain of avian influenza that, since February 2013, had infected more than one hundred people on mainland China and had reached Taiwan. The 53-year-old Taiwanese victim, presumably, picked up the virus while travelling to the Chinese city of Suzhou. Tests on 24 April revealed that he had contracted the H7N9 bird flu virus. As of April 23, Chinese officials had recorded 22 deaths out of 108 cases, a fatality rate of 19 percent. Since the emergence of H5N1 in 2003, nearly 60 percent of the more than 600 persons infected have died (Feng & Grady).

This information serves as background to the avian influenza fiction of Craig DiLouie (2008), D. W. Hardin (2009), and Steven Konkoly (2010). My main concern is how these stories represent the biomedical history surveyed in the previous chapter, and, as dramatic scenarios, if the stories are instructive and in some degree prescient.[1]

Craig DiLouie, The Thin White Line *(2008)*

Craig DiLouie's 2008 novel is a work of speculative fiction. A "near-future scenario," the story describes the impact of an avian influenza pandemic on Ontario, Canada; however, "its effects," according to one critic, "are modeled explicitly on the 1918–1919 pandemic (an H1N1 virus)" (Belling, 61). The connection between the two pathogens suggests that the author, a journalist, views the past pandemic and its imagined recrudescence on a phylogenetic continuum: both H1N1 and H5N1 belong to the family *Orthomyxoviridae*, and he may be implying that the avian form is as much a threat to an unprepared human population today as was H1N1 in 1918.

DiLouie's predictions, interspersed among imaginative eyewitness reports, are also based on careful research of government response plans, biomedical sources, and historical records of influenza. The epidemiological locus of the pandemic is a lake in Guangdong province, China, known for its abundant waterfowl species. DiLouie situates his scenario in the current history of H5N1. In 1997, the year that the Taubenberger team published the first 1918 sequencing paper, H5N1 broke out in Hong Kong. Chickens picked up the infection from waterfowl droppings, and human beings who had been in close contact with infected birds contracted the infection. Migrating birds continued to spread the virus to Southeast Asia, reaching Thailand. DiLouie's premise is consistent with epidemiological history and with the 2004 findings of Ungchusak et al., reviewed in chapter 7 (DiLouie, 5). In 2004, a mother and aunt caught the virus through personal nursing care, reputedly not through aerosolized person-to-person transmission. DiLouie is correct to cite this as, "the first case of human-to-human transmission of the virus. At this point, however, transmission required very close contact" (DiLouie, 5). Migratory aquatic birds, such as cormorants, spread the virus westward "into Europe, the Middle East, and Africa" (DiLouie, 5).

The narrative extrapolation begins at this point. As in *Contagion*, a transmissible strain develops, and the mortality rate begins to rise. The WHO knows that the virus "could evolve into a form that would be easily transmissible between the people." Scientists predicted that, within the coming decade, a pandemic could arise (DiLouie, 6). Economic recession, destabilized nations, and war are the consequence of this pandemic, an interesting inversion of the 1918–1919 pandemic that, some argue, had been caused by the circumstances of World War I. In the novel, only the first wave is recorded, but the virus would remain in circulation thereafter, "mutating, changing, adapting" (DiLouie, 179). A second wave, DiLouie writes, is nervously awaited in the next flu season.

Although it sounds like mankind's survival is given up to chance, DiLouie—whose scope is geographically limited to the Province of Ontario—considers several factors that could be improved to enhance pandemic preparedness, which is the aim of this perceptive scenario. One major question is whether the health care system will be able to respond to the catastrophe with sufficient resources (DiLouie, 185). Adequate hospital care, especially in ICUs, the availability of ventilators, government intervention, social-distancing measures to limit contagion, media programs emphasizing hygiene, pharmaceutical and vaccine supplies in national stockpiles, adequate means of distributing supplies, are all cited as essential to the Canadian national plan to withstand a severe pandemic in the future (DiLouie, 188–194). DiLouie compiles statistics (presented in four tables) to estimate Canada's ability to defend against the worst situation.

The Thin White Line is a literary hybrid form, having characteristics of conventional fiction (first and third person narrators, imagined eye witness reports, and a beginning, middle, and end) and the elements of a scenario, including simulated social, public health, and government reactions. Extrapolated statistics are markedly scenaristic. In the appendix, the author charts exponential increases in numbers of clinically ill and hospital admissions over a four-week period, considers acute-care bed capacity versus how many require such beds, how many require ICU beds versus ICU capacity, how many ventilators are available versus how many need them, and the mortality rate of clinically ill versus how many die in the hospital (DiLouie, 187). He recalculates the numbers over a ten-week period: if hospital capacity were increased due to social distancing, admissions would be reduced (DiLouie, 192); in turn, morbidity could be lowered, hospital capacity increased, and the availability of antiviral drugs to treat the majority of clinically ill cases made greater (DiLouie, 194). DiLouie's simple model, though it shows gradual improvement in the health care system with each intervention, also reveals the high probability that an influenza pandemic "would overwhelm Canada's health systems and result in mass casualties"; it exhibits social disruption, and severe economic shocks would be felt, "even with additional capacity, antiviral drug and social distancing interventions" (193).

D.W. Hardin, Hidden and Imminent Dangers *(2009)*

D. W. Hardin's novel describes an epidemic arising not in the Far East but in the state of Kentucky, on a poultry farm. This is not far-fetched, for science writers have argued for the North American or European, rather than for the Far Eastern, origin of the 1918 influenza virus (Barry, *Influenza*, 91–97). Another irony is that an antigenic shift happens in this narrative not in pigs, as in Kalla's novel, but in the body of a Kentucky farm worker. An *antigenic drift*, we recall, is a mutation occurring during viral replication when the microbe is under selective pressure in response to the host's immune system; mutant viruses, which can then evade the immune system of the host, have acquired selective advantages, to become the "dominant variant" in the host population (Harder & Werner). An *antigenic shift*, on the other hand, is a sudden recombination of H and N Subtypes "within a single replication cycle," as exemplified by the novel viruses of 1957 (H2N2) and 1968 (H3N2), to which human populations had no immunity (Harder & Werner).

Billy Keeling, the index case in Hardin's fiction, is a young man at work in the family's poultry farm. He discovers a mass dying-off of chickens, a red flag he ignores and simply clears away. After his exposure to the carcasses and to the waste products of the chickens, he begins to show symptoms of a respiratory ailment: fever, malaise, and coughing (Hardin, 81). Billy is hospitalized and declines rapidly. His mother tells health authorities that Billy had been ill, on and off, for eight days. At the onset, he had been acutely ill for three days, feels better, but is still febrile. Does that mean he has entered the intermediate phase in the disease, between the initial virus infection and the bacterial sequel?

At this juncture in the illness, and reminiscent of H1N1's co-pathogenicity sequel, severe symptoms return. Doctors at University Community Hospital in Louisville diagnose it correctly as flu (Hardin, 93). When his condition became critical, with hemorrhaging and blood-filled lungs, a doctor suspects the worse: "he may have a form of avian influenza. The H5N1 virus could have mutated, making the leap to a human. Worse yet, if he had a human flu, the genetic material could have been exchanged between the two viruses, creating a highly infectious mutant H5N1. Under the right conditions, it could be spread through respiratory droplets or even contact" (Hardin, 94–95).

As Billy Keeling nears death with a cerebral hemorrhage, doctors assert that it takes "only one viral mutation to start an epidemic" (Hardin, 105). If a novel virus were indeed confirmed, intercontinental air travel would make confining its spread nearly impossible (Hardin, 105). Clearly, the author, a medical professional himself, has researched the literature. One doctor in the story reiterates the biomedical findings that I surveyed earlier: that "Studies of avian influenza show it is not easily transmissible from one human to another. Most cases of avian flu have been confined to small populations such as the family unit" (Hardin, 131). This demonstrates the author's familiarity with ideas central to the work of Ungchusak, Kandun, Wang, Maines, and others.

When the pathogen is confirmed as H5N1, and after Billy Keeling dies, the question then arises as to whether the strain is transmissible to humans and, specifically, whether his parents were infected (Hardin, 142, 167). Is the infection confined to the Keeling "family cluster"? Avian virus acquired through unprotected exposure to poultry and/or to the infected index case had been established in the Asian studies. The infectious disease specialist in the novel, Mercato Marcus, M.D., is well aware of these facts. She is alarmed by the clinical picture, believing it to be a new strain, a reassortant virus. The warning sign is that "it appears to be highly contagious, infecting the upper respiratory tract first. That's unlike other cases of avian flu I've studied. It reminds me of the 1918 flu" (Hardin, 172). High pathogenicity and a proclivity for the upper-respiratory tract suggest that, through mutagenesis, the hemagglutinin protein could bind to mammalian sialic-acid receptors on human cell surfaces.

The outbreak becomes an epidemic. The Louisville Children's Hospital reports that they are overwhelmed by the influx of sick children presenting with flu-like symptoms and, worse, with hemorrhaging (Hardin, 181). A CDC investigator, Dr. Zinsky, confirms Mercato's worst fears: "It's obvious the H5N1 virus has had an antigenic shift and is extremely contagious. I suspect some kind of genetic recombination with another Type A virus allowing it to attack the upper respiratory system and then spread through the body" (Hardin, 182). And this suspicion proves to be true: "the virus has genetically mutated to become highly contagious in regard to humans—very similar to the Spanish flu. There has been one survivor of this nova [*sic* novel] virus, so there is hope" (Hardin, 198). The survivor is Mrs. Keeling; however, Herbert Keeling, Billy's father, had contracted the infection through aerosolized droplets (Billy's coughing) and becomes a secondary fatality (Hardin 81). Mrs. Keeling's resistance suggests that she has antibodies to the disease or that its spread was limited to direct physical contact, but the latter hypothesis proves a dead end, as the disease begins to spread from person to person.

Scientists in the fiction try to determine how an avian strain could acquire airborne transmissibility in mammals. They conjecture that chickens at the farm must have been infected with avian flu from an outside carrier, probably a bird, and that Billy Keeling had carried a Type A human flu when he came into contact with the avian strain (Hardin, 340). This brings us back to T. R. Maines et al. (2006) and to their creation of an avian-H5N1/human-H3N2 reassortant that proved to be innocuous in experiments. In the novel, Hardin's researchers find that the quality of contagiousness intrinsic to the H3N2 virus had transferred to the avian virus (similar to Kalla's premise). This theoretically improbable occurrence, in Hardin's imagined world, is the source of imminent danger. The secretary of state informs his audience of a worst-case scenario: "Now we have a person infected with two different types of flu at the same time. The avian flu probably wasn't all that contagious at the time, but the human type A was a contagious flu that attacked the upper respiratory tract. The odds of what happened next are exponentially high! There was a genetic transfer between the two flus" (Hardin, 341). Whereas, in the 1918 pandemic, pigs are theorized as having been the intermediate or mixing vessel within which avian H5N1 acquired the capacity for airborne infection in humans, in Hardin's story a human being becomes the reassortant vessel: avian Type A flu, human Type A flu, and "the hybrid flu" were all isolated from Billy's specimens (Hardin, 352); and he served as "the incubating vessel" (Hardin, 353). Epidemiologists suspect that infected migrating birds had contaminated the farm "with their droppings," and that the virus subsequently made its way into the poultry and, ultimately, into the human population (Hardin, 379).

In several areas, the novel is not believable. The emergency vaccine program, for one, stems the American pandemic in an incredible 30 days. In the area of fatality statistics, moreover, the author may have exaggerated. These figures are so elevated that it is difficult to conceive of global commerce, government, health systems, and industrial civilizations not collapsing under the weight of numbers. Such a massive dying-off, in reality, would probably damage underdeveloped countries to the degree that starvation and secondary diseases of all kinds would engulf the survivors. In terms of the survival of the human species, what does this aspect of the story imply?

Let us take a close look at the numbers. To grasp what this could mean, we can begin by comparing Hardin's figures with death tolls in 1918–1919. The U.S. population in 1918 was 103.2 million, of which 675,000 or 0.7 percent died of influenza (worldwide mortality was about 2 percent). In the novel, the imagined death toll in the U.S. (2009 population: 307 million) is 70.6 million or 23 percent of the population (Hardin, 384). The global mortality figures in the novel are more difficult to envisage. Whereas somewhere between of 50 to 100 million deaths have been attributed to the Great Pandemic, 1918 to 1920 (Johnson & Mueller), Hardin's fictive estimate is 40–50 percent. Since the world population in 2009 (the narrative year) was 6.8 billion, the H5N1 mortality range in the novel is between 2.7 to 3.4 *billion* deaths (*Population Reference Bureau*). What are the implications of Hardin's estimates for narrative credibility? Given his figures, is *Hidden and Imminent Dangers* an extinction scenario?

The epidemiological ramifications of Hardin's statistics make recovery doubtful. He imagines that 50 percent of China's population is dead. According to the census of 2009 (if we use the narrative time-frame), this would mean 665,500,000 deaths on the mainland in one month and a swamped the health care system (*International Data Base*; Hardin, 385). The implications of so many deaths, in so short a time, for sanitation and the ecology are difficult to assess. The problem of secondary disease, however, will unavoidably affect segments of the surviving 50 percent who are displaced or who lack essential services. John T. Watson et al. argue that risk factors for secondary outbreaks in a natural disaster (nothing on the order of the pandemic) would include the lack of safe water and adequate sanitation facilities (exacerbated by the loss of power needed to run water treatment plants), communicable disease outbreaks in dense populations, displacement from homes, and the unavailability of health care services ("Epidemics after Natural Disasters"). Outbreaks of hepatitis A, B (bloodborne), and E, meningitis, diarrheal disease, leptospirosis (from rodent-contaminated food and water) are just some of the biological dangers. These threats are magnified in the pandemic-ravaged, densely-populated cities of China (Watson et al. "Epidemics"). In other countries in the narrative, the results are just as bad. Insurgents are reported to have carried the virus to Iran where influenza claimed 50 percent of the population (36,600,000 deaths). Consequently, Iran is reduced to fractious, decentralized governance and is considered to be a lesser threat to the West than before the pandemic (Hardin, 356, 384). In Pakistan and North Korea, the pandemic would most certainly have destroyed at least half of the population, leaving nuclear, chemical, and biological weapons in unknown hands and turning Shenyang, PRC, into the largest refugee camp and cholera mass grave in world history. I think that the excessive fatality figures in the novel inadvertently suggest the possibility of human extinction.

David M. Raup, in *Extinction: Bad Genes or Bad Luck?* (1991), comments on the extinctive possibilities of a disease targeting a single species: "The HIV virus causing AIDS in humans comes close to being species specific. Such viruses are common and have the potential to annihilate a species—several close calls have been recorded in animals" (116). Although pandemic disease targeting a single species has an extinctive potential, extinction ultimately depends on the size of a population and on its ability to rebound reproductively. Scientists call this the *minimum viable population* or MVP (Raup, 124–126). In a conjectural world in which 50–60 percent of the human species survives, it is *unlikely* that a pandemic could threaten extinction. But secondary effects must also be factored in, and these consequences could significantly affect the MVP. Survivors, for example, would have to contend with outbreaks, such as cholera and typhoid, which arise from insanitation and from the inability to bury billions of corpses; starvation would ensue; economies and social infrastructure would be damaged almost beyond repair; and human migrations, especially from underdeveloped countries, would begin on a massive scale. Joshua Lederberg points out that, while micro-organisms can sustain "vast fluctuations of population size" because they reproduce exponentially, "a fluctuation of 1 percent in our population size is a major catastrophe" ("Emerging Infections"). What then can be said for a fluctuation of 50 percent? The mood of the American government in the story, once the pandemic is over, is unreasonably optimistic, as if what had transpired was an epidemic rather than a megadeath event. As the president and his cabinet set forth emergency legislation regarding fuel and energy reserves, there is no indication that the short-term, international implications of the disaster are appreciated (Hardin, 383–384).

The aftermath of Hardin's book has much in common with George R. Stewart's *Earth Abides* (1949), where civilization must reconstitute itself after a pandemic. The pathogen, in Stewart's novel, is also familiar: it is suspected either of having sprung from an animal reservoir; of being "a new microorganism, most likely a virus, produced by mutation"; or of having escaped or having been intentionally released "from some laboratory of bacteriological warfare" (Stewart 14). Survivors in *Earth Abides* suffer from "Secondary Kill," a widespread, post-traumatic stress reaction: "Of those that the Great Disaster had spared, many would fall victim to some trouble from which civilization had previously protected them," namely alcohol poisoning, murder, suicide, mental illness, and accident (Stewart, 37). Stewart's protagonist, Isherwood, realizes that, "biologically speaking, there was a critical point in the numbers of any species—if the numbers were reduced below this point, the species could not recover" (Stewart, 37).

Biostatistics aside, Hardin's novel is potentially valuable as a scenario exploring the possibility of avian-human viral reassortment and its worst effects. *Hidden and Imminent Dangers* augments virology research on influenza in an important way: it educates the general reader and underscores the need for surveillance, global cooperation, and ongoing research in regard to pandemic influenza. Its message of preparedness aligns it with the scientific papers, discussions, and interviews on this subject, and the novel complements the factual compendia of the CDC reports. It could just as well have been retitled, *Overt and Immediate Dangers*. I think that, if Hardin had a sequel in mind, he could imagine what life in a post-pandemic world as humanity grappled with the consequences of a contagious and lethal virus. Just as secondary infections were responsible for most of the fatalities in 1918–1919, the *consequences* of an H5N1 pandemic, rather than the outbreak itself, could inhibit recovery and population growth to the degree that human extinction might become a possibility.

Steven Konkoly, The Jakarta Pandemic *(2010/2012)*

The Jakarta Pandemic is a scientifically accurate story on avian influenza and a commentary on social psychology. The avian influenza pandemic that sweeps the globe in the novel is a Type A/H16N1. Before 2004, influenza Type A avian viruses were known to carry 15 antigenic Subtypes of hemagglutinin (H) and 9 of neuraminidase (N). A March 2005 article in *The Journal of Virology* reports on 2004 research identifying the H16 antigenic Subtype.

The H16 Subtype had been circulating in Sweden among black-headed gulls. Sophisticated testing did not show that H16 reacted to H1, although it was found to be a genetic relative of H15 (HA), which is carried by shorebirds. The biochemical composition of its binding sites which allow it to adhere to healthy cells was "distinct" from viral Subtypes circulating in ducks and geese (Fouchier et al., "Characterization of a Novel Influenza A Virus Hemagglutinin Subtype"). An expert in the field of avian virus Subtypes, Dr. Hiroshi Koba, had been collecting HA Subtypes since 1978 ("Hunt for Duck Feces"). In March 2009, he completed his collection and, with the assistance of Dr. Yoshihiro Sakoda, developed a virus database. The elusive piece to the virological puzzle was H16N1, a virus he found to be relatively common in ducks. He was able to incubate H16N1, the last remaining Subtype in his collection, to derive genetic information that could help in the production of vaccines. H16 research has been going on over the last decade.

Extensive media and informational pages were expurgated from Konkoly's 2010 edition of his novel but made public online and in a 2012 re-release of the book, with the expurgated text or "Lost Scenes" in an appendix. Konkoly faced the dilemma of the pandemic fictionist: too much biomedical and geopolitical material bogs the narrative down; too little robs it of authenticity. From the present reader's perspective, the expurgated material was quite well done and grounded the story. In fact, I prefer the whole text to the 2010 redaction, primarily because the civil strife and the survivalist motif of the original text, though important to the reality of pandemic emergency, tended to crowd out the biological and geopolitical aspects of the story, which are causally related to each other.

Konkoly's viral menace, as the CDC is made to confirm, is an H16 variant, a strain classified as H16N1, Dr. Koba's microbe. This virus is the source of a growing pandemic in Asia (Konkoly, 37). It is a highly pathogenic and contagious virus, causing flu-like symptoms, the most serious being respiratory distress. I note that fictional virology and factual science diverge a bit at this point. In a 3 November 2013 fictional media-excerpt, a reporter states this is a novel virus and that previously only fifteen Subtypes had been discovered in either humans or animals; in light of the work of Fouchier (2004) and Kida (2009), this is obviously incorrect. The idea that, in 2009, very little was known about H16 Subtypes, however, is true. Moreover, Jakarta which has been a hotbed for avian flu infection since 2004 is a good choice for "the epicenter of the H16 virus" (Konkoly, 59).

Other aspects of the plot are believable: infected patients' air travel routes have been traced back via Hong Kong International Airport to Jakarta (Konkoly, 59); the H16N1 virus is highly contagious from person to person; the case-fatality rate is high, with ARDS deaths accounting for 20 percent of the fatalities (Konkoly, 109–110); and quarantine and social distancing are critical mitigation strategies (Konkoly, 110).

The most terrifying aspect of the novel is told in the section *Survival* (the narrative chronology, 30 November to 15 December 2013, recapitulating the second wave of 1918). The protagonist Alex Fletcher must defend against the flu and its infrastructural effects (e.g., the widespread power failures throughout New England [Konkoly, 307]), while trying to protect his family from looters who invade the suburban community of 33 households on Durham Road. The flu recesses to the background, as Fletcher and a neighbor engage the criminals in nerve-wracking backyard fire-fights (Konkoly, 362).

To dismiss this part of the book as stock disaster-novel footage misses an important point. Criminality is not uncommon after hurricanes, earthquakes, floods, and pandemics. People brandish guns in gas lines and rob generators during blackouts. The United States government in its "Law Enforcement Pandemic Influenza Planning Checklist," which is a guide for local, state, and federal government, points out that local and State law enforcement, in conjunction with the National Guard, are to coordinate their resources in the pre-pandemic phase in the interests of public safety. Although most of their work will lie in the realm of public health, traffic control, and securing vaccination sites and hospitals, they also have plans to deal with public disturbances and unrest: the "management of panic and/or public fear, crowd/riot control, enforcement of public health orders." Their preparatory measures are intended for "community vulnerabilities"—a euphemism for vulnerable populations, such as the elderly. Law enforcement is clear on "crimes of opportunities" and "fraudulent schemes." Under bad conditions, states need to use the National Guard "to perform law enforcement and security functions," and they would have the authority of federalized military forces.

Controlling a disease, and not the criminals, appears to be the first order of business in government planning documents. Both state and federal officials have this dominant concern ("Interim Pre-pandemic Planning Guidance"; "Law Enforcement"). This includes hospital preparedness, vaccine research and supply, social-distancing measures, evaluations of the immediate impact of the outbreak on labor, schools, families, food supplies, energy resources, and so on. How to deal with marauding gangs is not explicitly outlined in the public domain, though no doubt it is spelled out in tactical briefings for state and local police. If contingencies are not in place, the secondary effects of a pandemic, like that in Konkoly's novel, are bound to occur. Konkoly gives us a ground-level view of creeping civil deterioration, and, from this perspective, his novel has something in common with Thomas Mullen's and, to a lesser extent, with James Rada's, in terms of how people behave in crises.

The police force in eastern Maine is clearly stressed to the point of collapse in Konkoly's fiction. No pre-pandemic plan seems to have been formulated. The National Guard has not been deployed. Police who call on Alex Fletcher's home to investigate calls about a rifle shot (Fletcher was responsible) uncharacteristically wear full body armor (Konkoly, 233); the police department is at less than half strength; only two cars are on patrol at any time; and the shifts are round the clock (Konkoly, 235). Break-ins, vandalism, and minor fights are happening in Maine. But Boston, the epicenter of arson and "limited riots," teeters on "the brink of a complete breakdown" (Konkoly, 237). People are fleeing northward to Maine in search of food and vacant houses. Police blockades can neither stem the flow of migrants nor evict the squatters. Reports from York County are that "nighttime battles" are taking place in neighborhoods (Konkoly, 237–238). Much of this activity has not involved break-ins; but indiscriminate shootings are reported (Konkoly, 238). Fletcher reads an online news article (he still has power) about volunteers blocking northbound travelers, not for the purpose of quarantine, but to stop looting (Konkoly, 240). By 28 November, less than one month since the pandemic began, newspapers are warning of "the sudden decline of civil order within the major Boston metropolitan area." At this belated point in time, while similar events are taking place in other coastal cities, the National Guard is finally called up. Fletcher reflects on this lack of preparedness: "Sounds like they needed to put the Guard into action a few weeks ago" (Konkoly, 243). The media assessment is that civil disorder can be traced to a "complete breakdown of the food and essentials supply chain in the northeast, compounded by an overwhelmed healthcare system that has far exceeded its capacity to handle the flu pandemic" (Konkoly, 243–244).

The Jakarta Pandemic exploits a gap in Maine's influenza preparation protocol, as far I can see from public documents. Konkoly is focused squarely on the social effects of an influenza pandemic. The "Maine CDC 2009 H1N1 Influenza Pandemic After-Action Summary" (December 2010) is rightly concerned with surveillance, mitigation, vaccination, communication, and recovery. But nowhere in this 23-page document is there any reference to public safety or where to find information in that regard. The implication seems to be that, if preparedness works to mitigate the disease and promote recovery, then criminality would gradually decline. Konkoly's fiction imagines what could happen if a comprehensive plan were not in place. Thus, it is a social scenario.

Although the specific duties of law enforcement in regard to criminal conduct during a health emergency are, arguably, secondary to mitigation strategies in public health, they are no doubt discussed in closed-door briefings.

Most police agencies in the country have emergency communication systems or reverse 911 phone alerts to keep citizens informed. The situation that Konkoly imagines suggests how rapidly society can come apart during a pandemic if a comprehensive pre-pandemic plan is not ready or if it does not hold up against an outbreak that is more severe than predicted ("Interim Pre-pandemic Planning Guidance"). The Jakarta outbreak that impacts northeastern Maine has traveled more than 9,700 miles northwest of Indonesia. But in the modern world, geographical distance offers no immunity, only a brief window of time.

Human fallibility, technical failure, accidents, the unpredictability of natural selection, and unforeseen factors provoke debate, justify moratoria, and are often catalysts in pandemic fiction. Highly Pathogenic Avian Influenza (HPAI) viruses, such as H5N1or H7N9, are preoccupying scientists today and have gotten the attention of talented fictionists, such as Craig Di Louie, D. W. Hardin, and Steven Konkoly, who have imagined the public health and social impact of naturally-occurring pandemics.[1]

Biomedical scientists, equipped with astonishing technology and with the advantage of global networks and immediate communication links, do not underestimate the danger of avian viruses, which are unpredictable, unstable, and ubiquitous. The writers reviewed in this chapter advertise these ideas: even in the industrialized world, the morbidity rate will far exceed the capabilities of public health care, that is, at the outset of the pandemic (DiLouie); the emergence of a novel Type A influenza virus is neither fantastic nor statistically improbable; nor is its immediate detection guaranteed (Hardin); and Western society, however rich and resilient, is fragile if unprepared in time of pestilence (Konkoly).

Postscript (November 2013–January 2014)

The good news is that, on 22 November 2013, the FDA approved the use of *Q-Pan*, the first vaccine manufactured "to protect against H5N1 influenza" (Lurie; "Influenza A [H5N1]"). However, on Friday, 17 January 2014, another and more virulent avian flu strain is reported to be causing concern. Chinese health authorities have detected an increasing number of H7N9 bird flu cases, suggesting that the disease may be spreading on mainland China, where 14 cases were confirmed in the week of 12–17 January 2014. Other factors are complicating the problem. One is that the disease is worsening precisely when "the world's largest annual human migration begins ahead of Chinese New Year" (i.e., Friday, 31 January 2014). The potential will be there for great numbers of exposed persons to carry the virus far and wide. Second, H7N9 has a greater capacity to grow in human lung tissue than any other avian strain, as laboratory tests at Hong Kong University recently demonstrated. Health authorities, as expected, are watching "for signs of greater human-to-human transmission" (Bradsher, A10). The narrative continues.[2]

Chapter Notes

Introduction

1. The worldwide death toll in 1918–1919 due to influenza is grossly inexact, estimates ranging from a low of 20 to a high of more than 100 million. Johnson and Mueller point out that morbidity and mortality statistics are likely understated because of nonregistration, missing records, misdiagnoses, nonmedical certifications, and variances between locations. A 1920 calculation put the global death rate at 21.5 million. In 1991, this estimate was revised upward into the range of 24.7–39.3 million. These investigators suggest, initially, that mortality "was of the order of 50 million"; however, upon further reflection, they consider this figure "perhaps as much as 100 percent understated." They settle on a range of 50 to 100 million flu-related deaths from 1918 to 1920 ("Updating the Accounts").

2. Major historical works of World War I excluding, or passingly referring to, the pandemic are chronologically listed here: B. H. Liddell Hart, *The Real War: 1914–1918* (Boston: Little, Brown, 1930; Cyril Falls, *The Great War, 1914–1918* (New York: G. P. Putnam's Sons, 1959), 347; Barbara Tuchman, *The Guns of August*, foreword by Robert K. Massie, preface by B. Tuchman (1962, New York: Presidio Press/Random House, 2004); Frank Freidel, *Over There: The Story of America's First Great Overseas Crusade* (Short Hills, NJ: Burford Books, 1964); Cyril Falls, *Armageddon: 1918* (Philadelphia: J. B. Lippincott, 1964), 132; Marc Ferro, *The Great War: 1914–1918*, translated by Nicole Stone (1969; New York: Routledge & Kegan Paul, 1973); David M. Kennedy, *Over Here: The First World War and American Society* (1980; New York: Oxford Univ. Press, 2004); James L. Stokebury, *A Short History of World War I* (New York: HarperCollins, 1981), 278; Gordon Brook-Shepherd, *November 1918* (Boston: Little, Brown, 1981); J. M. Winter, *The Experience of World War I* (New York: Oxford Univ. Press, 1989); *The Oxford History of the 20th Century*, edited by Michael Howard and William Roger Louis (New York: Oxford Univ. Press, 1998); Stuart Robson, *The First World War*, Seminar Studies in History, gen. eds., Clive Emsley and George Martel (London: Longmans, 1998); David Rosner, "Twentieth-Century Medicine," 483–507, in *The Columbia History of the Twentieth Century*, edited by Richard W. Bulliet (New York: Columbia Univ. Press, 1998), 492; John Mosier, *The Myth of the Great War: A New Military History of World War I* (New York: HarperCollins, 2001); Susan R. Grayzel, *Women and the First World War*, Seminar Studies in History (Harlow, UK: Pearson Education, 2002); Neil H. Heyman, *Daily Life during World War I.* Daily Life through History Series (Westport, CT: Greenwood Press, 2002); Michael Howard, *The First World War* (New York: Oxford Univ. Press, 2002); Simon Adams, *World War I* (New York: Darling Kindersley, 2007); G. J. Meyer, *A World Undone: The Story of the Great War, 1914 to 1918* (New York: Random House, 2007); Peter Graves and Peter Englund, *The Beauty and the Sorrow: An Intimate History of the First World War* (London: Profile Books, 2011), 465, 478, 482, 483–484, 499; and Adam Hochschild, *To End All Wars: A Story of Loyalty and Rebellion, 1914–1918* (Boston: Houghton Mifflin Harcourt, 2011); Louisa Thomas, *Conscience: Two Soldiers, Two Pacifists, One Family—A Test of Will and Faith in World War I* (New York: Penguin, 2011).

3. For a comprehensive history of the influenza genome project, see the papers of Taubenberger, Morens, and co-workers cited in the Bibliography. John M. Barry incisively describes the mechanism of viral infection. A spherical particle, its outer envelope houses its genome or genetic composition. About 1/10,000th of a millimeter in diameter, its genetic material is an eight-segmented single strand of RNA (ribonucleic acid). Its surface is studded with protein stems or spikes called hemagglutinin (H; hema+glutinin: sticks to blood cells); a second kind of protuberance (a stalk with a box-shaped head) is the enzyme neuraminidase. As the virus approaches a healthy cell, H-spikes contact the cell's outer membrane, binding biochemically to sialic acid receptors on its surface. Once H-spikes have attached to, or become adsorbed onto the cell, the virus enters by enclosing itself in a bubble, made from the cell surface, a cloaking maneuver preventing the immune system from detecting the invader. As the virus's outer form dissolves, its genes penetrate the cell nucleus, replacing the cell's genetic components with its own. Mass production of the virus ensues. The neuraminidase, with its box-like head on a stalk, breaks up the sialic acid on the cell's surface, preventing the acid from trapping emergent influenza viruses. In this way, a swarm of 100,000 to 1 million new viruses exit the dying cell, unhindered by the sticky outer membrane, through which the viral progeny bud (*Influenza*, 103–104).

4. The Recovery writers practiced a form of *pathography*, as this modality was defined in 1853. A neologism combining the Greek prefix *pathos* (suffering, experience, and emotion) and the suffix *graphicos* (formed by writing, drawing, or engraving), pathography's English usage dates back to 1853; its first reported usage, cited as Dunglison's in his *Medical Lexicon*, is simply, "the ... description of disease" (*OED*, 12: 553/Compact, II: 2098). The neurologist Paul Julius Mobius (1853–1907) appropriated the term *pathographische* to describe psychoanalytical case studies but has incorrectly been credited with coining the word, although his use of it in psychoanalysis might have been original (Roback; Hilken et al., 11–26). Its meaning in English usage, however, has become nebulous. The 1971 edition of *The Merriam-Webster Dictionary*, for example, omits *pathography* altogether, whereas the 2004 edition defines it, narrowly, as "*biography* focusing on a person's flaws or misfortunes" (italics added; 528), thus, excluding autobiographical writing, currently its popular meaning. In an effort to redefine pathography, medical and literary professionals have created a list of cognate phrases, each with a particular emphasis. These include Narrative Medicine (Rita Charon [2001]), Illness and Life Writing (Kay Cook), the Case History (Margaret Homberger), Disability and Life Writing (G. Thomas Couser), Insanity and Life Writing (G. Thomas Couser), and Trauma and Life Writing (Leigh Gilmore).

The scholars and medical practitioners, to whom I refer below, have shaped the modern understanding of pathography and its related forms. In 1993, Anne H. Hawkins described how, through pathography, the seriously ill writer can find coherence in a life which illness had made chaotic ("Pathography," 2–3). Pathography, as an autobiographical form, communicates the person's sense of isolation, pain, and disorientation, and the text then becomes the focus of reflection and understanding. As a medium through which the patient can move through "the disordering process" of illness to a state in which new meaning is found, pathography connects "the suffering self and the outside world by an overt act of communication"; moreover, the need to tell others allows the teller to move from alienation to relationship ("Pathography," 2–3, 25).

Kathryn M. Hunter (1991, 2006) conceives of the patient and the physician as participants in an ongoing dialogue. The narrative structure of medical knowledge is fundamentally a literary activity and the means through which clinician and patient routinely communicate. Their dialogue has a common goal: the patient's well-being. She likens the physician's diagnosis (a composite of clinical, laboratory, and diagnostic evidence) to "a plot summary of a socially constructed pathophysiological sequence of events" (*How Doctors Think*, 13). Medicine, in her view, is essentially "an interpretive activity ... that begins with the understanding of the patient and ends in therapeutic action on the patient's behalf." If the physician-patient record is understood as a narrative activity, patient care will gain priority over diagnostics (*Doctors' Stories*, xxi). Hunter also emphasizes the idea that two texts are essential to the dialogue: the patient's consultative story and "the medical account constructed by the physician from selected, augmented parts of the patient's story and from the signs of illness in the body" (*How Doctors Think*, 13); thus, the physician, whom Hunter compares to a critic or editor, analyzes "the original motivating account" that the patient brings, and then constructs a medical narrative from it on the basis of the story and the bodily illness (*How Doctors Think*, 13).

Rita Charon (2001) believes that the physician needs to acquire "narrative competence": "the ability to acknowledge, absorb, interpret, and act on the stories and plights of others." On this point, she agrees with Hunter that the physician is critic or editor who sorts through data to arrive at a clear-cut diagnosis. Charon's concept of "Narrative Medicine" involves close readings of personal literature. The practice of "Narrative Medicine" is central to medical dialogues between physician and patient, physician and colleagues, and physicians and society. Like Hunter, Charon believes that this kind of interconnectivity benefits the practice of medicine. Through narrative medicine, physicians develop a better understanding of patients' condition, deepen their own experiences as physicians, and promote public discourse on health care matters. Empathic medicine, according to Charon, is a process initiated and supported by the material text ("Narrative Medicine").

The illness narrative or patient account has emerged as an interdisciplinary approach to medicine, generating studies and databases of diverse works, including poetry, drama, fiction, historiography, and literary criticism. The Medical Humanities Program, directed by Dr. Felice Aull and sponsored by the New York University School of Medicine, has created the *Medicine Database: Illness Narrative/Pathography*, featuring a list of nearly 300 titles and an annotated bibliography, including a wide variety of works pertaining to the understanding of disease. The Program in Narrative Medicine, sponsored by the Columbia University, College of Physicians and Surgeons, aims to help medical professionals and academics in other fields to explore the intersection between "narrative and medicine." At the University of California, the Program in Narrative Medicine's mission statement describes its scope as "profoundly multidisciplinary," involving medicine and literature. Further, from 1998 to the present, *JAMA* has published more than 300 psychological narratives and analyses under the series title, "A Piece of My Mind."

Other major contributors to the development and use of pathography in its modern form include G. Thomas Couser, "The Body and Life Writing," *Encyclopedia of Life Writing*, Vol. 1, A-K, 121–123; and his *Recovering Bodies: Illness, Disability, and Life Writing* (Madison: University of Wisconsin Press, 1997). See also Arthur W. Frank, *The Wounded Storyteller: Body, Illness, and Ethics* (Chicago: University of Chicago Press, 1995); Arthur Kleinman, *The Illness Narratives: Suffering, Healing, and the Human Condition* (New York: Basic Books, 1988); and Susan Sontag, *Illness as Metaphor and AIDS and Its Metaphors* (New York: Farrar Straus Giroux, 1978).

5. (1) The virus classification system utlizes lettered categories, code, and definitionss: thus, influenza viruses belong to the family *Orthomyxoviridae.* This family comprises four genera: Types A, B, C, and the tickborne *Thogotovirus.* Types A and B cause disease in humans, and avian lineages cause pandemics (Webster & Walker, 123); (2) an incisive, linear classification system identifies a virus sample in terms of its location, date of retrieval, and Subtype; for example, the phrase "A/Sydney/5/97 (H3N2) Subtype" transcribes to: a Type A influenza virus, of the Subtype H3 (hemagglutinin 3) and N2 (neuraminidase enzyme 2), first discovered in Sydney, Australia, in 1997; and the "5" signifies the specific isolate (N. Johnson, *Dark Epilogue*, 10–12); and (3) an influenza virus can undergo two kinds of genetic mutation. One, according to the CDC, is *antigenic drift*: the production of new virus strains the immune system does not recognize ("How the Flu Virus Can Change"; Webster & Walker, 122–124); if this happens, antibodies acquired from exposure to older strains cannot defend against the "newer" virus, resulting in reinfection. Because of this phenomenon, one or two of the three virus strains in influenza vaccines may be annually updated to keep up with changes in circulating viruses. A new virus combining avian lethality, immunological stealth, and human-to-human transmissibility would be the consequence of an *antigenic shift*. A *shift* can produce either an entirely new influenza A Subtype or one resulting from the genetic reassortment of human and animal viruses; in the event of a *shift*, human beings will have no immunity to a novel virus ("How the Flu Virus Can Change"). For an influenza pandemic to occur, then, three factors must coincide: a

novel virus having the capacity for "sustained transmission from human-to-human" must appear; the population, in such a case, would have very low or no immunity; and a localized outbreak would spread widely, in large part because of modern travel ("Avian Influenza" Fact Sheet, *World Health Organization*).

Chapter 1

1. Ironically, Koch's postulates would eventually be used to diagnose influenza. In 1937, using Koch's method, the American virologist Thomas Milton Rivers (1888–1962) outlined criteria, any one of which if satisfied could establish viral pathogenicity. Rivers proposed six criteria based on Koch's thinking: (1) the virus is isolable from blood and tissue; (2) it is histologically classifiable; (3) antibodies to the suspected virus increased in specific tissue samples; (4) in control populations, there was a low incidence, or a complete absence, of the virus; and (5) the isolated virus or its associated pathology directly related to phases of clinical disease (Rivers [1937]; Robinson [1958]). Koch's method, however, was of no use in 1892, since the existence of the influenza virus would be gradually established over decades.

2. Co-pathogen(ic) refers to the activity of concurrent disease-causing microbes; comorbid(ity), to the concurrent diseases caused by at least two pathogens.

3. Michael Bresalier has recently observed that approaching influenza etiology bacterially was not an absolute dead end. Work on Pfeiffer's microbe, in his view, contributed to the development of bacteriology: the knowledge accumulated in this field would interact with epidemiology and ultimately support definitions of influenzal disease based largely on clinical symptoms. Pfeiffer's hypothesis that a bacillus caused influenza, though incorrect, would have the unanticipated effect of helping to align clinical, epidemiological, and laboratory efforts in the study of influenza. ([2012], 481–510).

4. The actual number, according to a later report by the epidemiologist Dr. George A. Soper, was 9,717 patients, diagnosed over a period of 36 days (12 September to 18 October 1918) ("The Influenza Pneumonia"). On average and over a 16-hour shift, each physician, with no medical treatment to offer beyond palliation, was responsible for more than 150 patients, many of whom were in critical condition. If we compare Grist's numbers to those of Major Soper who relied on War Department statistics for Camp Devens, the caseload figures appear to need adjustment. If as Grist claims, there were 250 doctors on the compound, and if Soper's total of 9,717 influenza cases is correct, then each physician was responsible for about 40 cases. A discrepancy such as this really was meaningless: whether each physician's caseload was 40 or 140, it was apparent that the medical staff could do very little.

5. See also: S. Burt Wolbach, "Comments on the Pathology and Bacteriology of Fatal Influenza Cases, as Observed at Camp Devens, Mass.," *Johns Hopkins Hospital Bulletin* XXX, no. 338 (1919): 104–109; O. J. Walker, "Pathology of Influenza-Pneumonia," *The Journal of Laboratory & Clinical Medicine* 5 (1919):154; E. R. LeCount, "Disseminated Necrosis of the Pulmonary Capillaries in Influenza Pneumonia," *JAMA* 72 (1919): 1519–1520; M. C. Winternitz, I. M. Mason, F. P. McNamara, *The Pathology of Influenza* (New Haven: Yale Univ. Press, 1920); E. L. Opie, F. G. Blake, J. C. Small, and T. M. Rivers, *Epidemic Respiratory Diseases: The Pneumonias and Other Infections of the Respiratory Tract Accompanying Influenza and Measles* (St. Louis: C. V. Mosby, 1921); W. G. McCallum, "Pathological Anatomy of Pneumonia Associated with Influenza," *Johns Hopkins Hospital Reports* 20 (1921): 149; Mervyn H. Gordon, "The Bacteriology of Influenza. I.," Article: Nineteenth Annual Meeting of the British Medical Association, *British Medical Journal* 2 (19 August 1922): 289; reprinted in *International Medical and Surgical Survey*, edited by Henry O. Reik and F. J. Stockman, vol. 4, no. 4 (New York: American Institute of Medicine, October 1922), Section 5d-273, p. 831; and Jeffery K. Taubenberger and David M. Morens, "The Pathology of Influenza Virus Infections," *Annual Review of Pathology* 3 (2008): 499–522.

Chapter 2

1. Letter 582: To Mary Austin (18 March 1922); Letter 675: To Dorothy Canfield Fisher (2 March 1922); and Letter 681: to Lorna Birtwell (12 March 1933), in *A Calendar of the Letters of Willa Cather*, edited by

Janis P. Stout (Lincoln, NE: The Univ. of Nebraska Press, 2000), 88–89, 101

Chapter 3

1. The federal government authorizes isolation and quarantine for influenza cases, as well as for eight other communicable diseases. The last time a federal quarantine was invoked was during the 1918–1919 pandemic ("Isolation and Quarantine"). Today, the President of the United States has the power to authorize large-scale isolation, which, according to the CDC, is defined as separating persons sick with a communicable disease from those who are healthy. Quarantine, according to the CDC, is employed to restrict the movement of healthy or of asymptomatic persons, suspected of having been exposed to a listed communicable disease. Cordoning off a town to prevent the ingress of possible germ carriers is *not* quarantine in the CDC sense, although the term has long been used synonymously with the isolation of individuals or of vessels suspected of harboring a communicable disease. The underlying purpose of both practices is to limit contagion.

The Commerce Clause of the U.S. Constitution gives the government authority to invoke these measures ("Legal Authorities for Isolation and Quarantine"). The "Quarantine and Inspection" section, Part G, paragraphs 264–272, of the *Public Health Service Act* (The U.S. Department of Health and Human Services/U.S. Food & Drug Administration), describes the government's responsibility, and constitutional right, to prevent the entrance of communicable disease into the country and its transmission between states. The CDC is delegated to detain, medically examine, and release whoever is suspected of having a disease specified on the list. Individual states and tribal jurisdictions have the right to assert these restrictions and detain persons or bar their ingress, but the supreme authority in this regard rests with the federal government.

2. Ibid.

Chapter 4

1. I am indebted to three primary texts here to summarize the exhumation and sequencing of the 1918 influenza virus: Taubenberger, "Genetic Characterization of the 1918 'Spanish' Influenza Virus," pp. 39–47; Taubenberger et al., "Historical Context"; and commentary by Jeffery K. Taubenberger, Johan V. Hultin, and David M. Morens, in the post-production script, "We Heard the Bells: The Influenza of 1918," writer/producer, Lisa Laden, 4 December 2009, *Centers for Medicare & Medicaid Services/ U.S. Department of Health and Human Services.*

2. Ibid.

3. Ibid.

4. The primary Characterization papers consulted here are: Taubenberger, et al., "Initial Genetic Characterization of the 1918 'Spanish' Influenza Virus," 1793–1796; Taubenberger et al., "Integrating Historical, Clinical, and Molecular Genetic Data," 1829–1839; Reid and Taubenberger, "The Origin of the 1918 Pandemic Influenza Virus," 2285–2292; Taubenberger et al., "Characterization of the 1918 Influenza Virus Polymerase Genes," 889–893; Tumpey et al., Characterization of the Reconstructed 1918 Spanish Influenza Virus" (Abstract); Taubenberger and Morens, "1918 Influenza," 15–22, esp. 15; D. M. Morens et al., "The Persistent Legacy," 225–229.

5. Ibid.

6. Ibid.

7. Ibid.

8. Ibid.

9. Ibid.

Chapter 7

1. The ten CDC articles, which I paraphrase in this chapter, were accessed at http://www.cdc.gov: "Pandemic Influenza/ Pandemics: How They Start, How They Spread, and Their Potential Impact"; "Pandemic Influenza/Pandemics and Pandemic Scares in the 20th Century: Historical Overview"; "Influenza: Familiar, but Not Friendly"; "Pandemic Influenza/Ongoing Influenza Defense Tactics"; "Preparing for the Next Pandemic," *CDC-National Vaccine Program Office* / Retrieved 14 October 2003; Avian Influenza (Flu)/Influenza Viruses"; "Transmission of Avian Influenza A Viruses between Animals and People"/ Retrieved 9 January 2012; "How the Flu Virus Can Change: 'Drift' and 'Shift,'" *CDC-Seasonal Influenza (Flu)* / Retrieved 20 March 2013; "Highly Pathogenic Avian Influenza A (H5N1) in People"; "Public Health Threat of

Highly Pathogenic Avian Influenza A (H5N1) Virus"; and "Emergence of Avian Influenza A (H7N9) Virus Causing Severe Human Illness—China, February-April 2013," *CDC-Morbidity and Mortality Weekly Report* 62 (1 May 2013):1–6; Retrieved 4 May 2013.

Chapter 8

1. The accidental release of a novel virus and its consequences has not been fully explored. One well-known fictional precursor of this theme is Stephen King's *The Stand* (1978, 1990), in which an antigenic shift is induced in a Type A influenza virus. The superflu which escapes a CDC lab (of all places) has been bioengineered to shift selectively, eluding antibodies, resisting vaccines, and having a mortality rate of 99.4 percent (King, 28–31, 151, 171, 1136). King, in effect, is imagining an extinctive event.

2. Donald G. McNeil, Jr., "Cases of New Deadly Bird Flu [H7N9] Surge in China, Experts Say." *The New York Times/International* (5 February 2014): A8.

Bibliography

Adams, Simon. *World War I.* New York: Darling Kindersley, 2007.

"Additional H7N9 Cases Reported in China; CDC Receives H7N9 Virus Isolate." *Centers for Disease Control and Prevention.* 12 April 2013; http://www.cdc.gov/ Retrieved 5 April 2013.

"Al Qaida's Ideology." *Security Service Mi5*; http://www.clarionproject.org/ Retrieved 13 December 2013.

Alibek, Ken. "Behind the Mask: Biological Warfare." *Institute for the Study of Conflict, Ideology, and Policy/Perspective* IX, no. 1 (September-October 1998); http://www.bu.edu/ Retrieved 28 July 2013.

_____, with Stephen Handelman. *Biohazard.* New York: Random House, 1999.

American Psychiatric Association. *DSM-III R; Diagnostic and Statistical Manual of Mental Disorders.* 3rd ed., rev. Washington, D.C.: American Psychiatric Association, 1987.

"Amerithrax or Anthrax Investigations." *Famous Cases & Criminals. The Federal Bureau of Investigation.* 2011; http://www.fbi.gov/ Retrieved 17 December 2013.

"Amerithrax Documents: Exhibits A. to M." *United States Department of Justice.* 19 February 2010; http://www.justice.gov/ Retrieved 17 December 2013.

Anderson, Jeffrey. *Sleeper Cell: A Novel.* New York: Berkley Books, 2005.

Andrewes, Christopher. *In Pursuit of the Common Cold.* London: William Heinemann Medical, 1973.

_____. P. P. Laidlaw, and Wilson Smith. "Influenza: Observations on the Recovery of Virus from Man and On the Antibody Content of Human Sera." *The British Journal of Experimental Pathology* 16, no. 6 (December 1935): 566–582; www.ncbi.nlm.nih.org/ Retrieved 16 August 2012.

Armstrong, James F. "Philadelphia, Nurses, and the Spanish Influenza Pandemic of 1918." *The Navy Department Library*; http://www.history.navy.mil/ Retrieved 23 September 2013.

Atkinson, Kate. *Life after Life: A Novel.* New York: Little, Brown, 2013.

Atlantic Storm Interactive. UPMC Center for Health Security. 2011; http://www.atlantic.storm.org/ Retrieved 9 December 2013.

"Avian Influenza." *World Health Organization/Fact Sheet.* April 2011; www.who.int / Retrieved 9 January 2012.

"Avian Influenza (Flu)/Influenza Viruses." *The Centers for Disease Control and Prevention*; www.cdc.gov/ Retrieved 9 January 2012.

Barry, John M. *The Great Influenza: The Epic Story of the Deadliest Plague in History.* New York and London: Viking Penguin, 2004.

_____. "The Site of Origin of the 1918 Influenza Pandemic and Its Public Health Implications." *Journal of Translational Medicine/BioMed Central* 2 (20 January 2004): 3; http://www.translational-medicine.com/ Retrieved 29 January 2012.

_____. Cecile Viboud, and Lone Simonsen. "Cross-Protection between Successive Waves of the 1918–1919 Influenza Pandemic: Epidemiological Evidence from U.S. Army Camps and from Britain." *Journal of Infectious Diseases* 198, no. 10 (15 November 2008): 1427–1434; http://www.ncbi.nlm.nih.gov/ Retrieved 22 October 2013.

Bartlett, John G. "Applying Lessons Learned from Anthrax Case History to Other Scenarios." *Centers for Disease Control and Prevention/Emerging Infectious Diseases* (1999); http://www.cdc.gov/ Retrieved 13 November 2003.

Basler, C.F., et al. "Sequence of the 1918 Pandemic Influenza Virus Nonstructural Gene [NS] Segment and Characterization of Recombinant Viruses Bearing the 1918 NS Genes." *Proceedings of the National Academy of the Sciences [of the United States of America]* 98 (2001): 2746–2751.

Beijerinck, M. W. A *Contagium Vivum Fluidum* as the Cause of the Mosaic Disease of Tobacco Leaves (1898)." *Milestones in Microbiology: 1546 to 1940.* Translated and edited by Thomas D. Brock. 1961. Washington, D.C.: ASM Press, 1999. 153–156.

Bell, Quentin. *Virginia Woolf: A Biography.* New York: Harcourt, Brace, Jovanovich, 1972.

Bellevue Literary Press; http://www.blp.books.org.

Belling, Catherine. "Overwhelming the Medium: Fiction and the Trauma of Pandemic Influenza in 1918." *Literature and Medicine* 28, no. 1 (Spring 2009): 55–81.

Benson, Jackson J. *Wallace Stegner: His Life and Work.* Lincoln, NE: The Univ. of Nebraska Press, 2010.

"Berkefeld Filter." www.http://lexic.us/ Retrieved 11 November 2013.

"Berkefeld Filter"; www.http://thesciencedictionary.org/ Retrieved 11 November 2013.

Beveridge, W. I. B. *Influenza: The Last Great Plague: An Unfinished Story of Discovery.* New York: Prodist, 1977.

"Biosafety Level 3." *Biosafety in Microbiological and Biomedical Laboratories*; www.cdc.gov/ Retrieved 16 April 2013.

"Biotechnology Activities, Office of." Notice of Changes to *NIH Guidelines*. Department of Health and Human Services / National Institutes of Health. *Federal Register* 78, no. 35 (21 February 2013): 12074–12082; pkisupport@gpo.gov/ Retrieved 11 April 2013.

"Bioterrorism Agents/Diseases." *Centers for Disease Control and Preparedness/Emergency Preparedness and Response*; www.bt.cdc.gov/ Retrieved 4 July 2011.

"Biowarfare, History of." *NOVA Online*; http://www.pbs.org/ Retrieved 16 November 2002.

"Biowarfare and Bioterrorism, History of." *Epidemiology and Surveillance.* Arizona Department of Health Services; http://www.hs.state.az.us / Retrieved 16 November 2002.

Birken, Gary. *Plague: A Novel of Bioterrorism.* New York: Berkley Books, 2002.

Black Ice: Bioterrorism International Coordination Exercise (2006 After-Action Report); http://merln.ndu.edu/ Retrieved 15 July 2013.

Bloy, Marjie. "Florence Nightingale (1820–1910)." *The Victorian Web: Literature, History, & Culture in the Age of Victoria*; http://www.victorianweb/history/crimea /Retrieved 13 November 2013.

Bono, Michael Joseph. "Micoplasmal Pneumonia." *Medscape.* Edited by Robert E. O'Connor; www.medscape.com/ Retrieved 17 June 2013.

Bostridge, Mark. *Florence Nightingale: The Making of an Icon.* New York: Farrar, Strauss, and Giroux, 2008.

Bradford, John Rose, E. F. Bashford, and J. A. Wilson. "Preliminary Report on the Presence of a 'Filter Passing' Virus in Certain Diseases." *The British Medical Journal* 1 (1 February 1919):127–128; http://www.ncbi.nlm.nih.gov/ Retrieved 20 January 2013.

Bradsher, Keith. "Rise in Bird Flu Cases in China Stokes Worry before Peak Travel Time." *The New York Times/International.* 18 January 2014, A10.

Bresalier, Michael. "Fighting Flu: Military Pathology, Vaccines, and the Conflicted

Identity of the 1918–1919 Pandemic." *Journal of the History of Medicine & Allied Sciences* 68, no. 1 (2013): 87–128.

_____. " 'A Most Protean Disease': Aligning Medical Knowledge of Modern Influenza, 1890–1914." *Medical History* 56, no. 4(October 2012): 481–510; http://www.ncbi.nlm.nih.gov/ Retrieved 5 June 2013.

_____. "Uses of a Pandemic: Forging the Identities of Influenza and Virus Research in Interwar Britain." *Social History of Medicine* (15 December 2011); www.escholar.manchester.ac.uk / Retrieved 7 July 2012.

Bristow, Nancy K. *American Pandemic: The Lost Worlds of the 1918 Influenza Pandemic.* New York: Oxford Univ. Press, 2012.

_____. "'It's as Bad as Anything Can Be': Patients, Identity, and Influenza Pandemic." *Public Health Reports/Community Response* 125, supp. 3 (2010); www.ncbi.nlm.nih.gov/ Retrieved 1 January 2013.

_____. "'You Can't Do Anything for Influenza': Doctors, Nurses and the Power of Gender during the Influenza Pandemic in the United States." *The Spanish Influenza Pandemic of 1918–1919: New Perspectives.* Edited by David Killingray, Howard Phillips, John S. Oxford, and Terry Ranger. Introduction by Howard Phillips and David Killingray. *Studies in the Social History of Medicine.* New York: Routledge, 2003. 58–70.

Broad, William J., and Scott Shane. "Scientists' Analysis Disputes F.B.I. Closing of Anthrax Case." *The New York Times/National.* 10 October 2011, A1, A13.

Brook-Shepherd, Gordon. *November 1918.* Boston: Little, Brown, 1981.

Brundage, John F. "Interactions between influenza and Bacterial Respiratory Pathogens: Implications for Pandemic Preparedness." *The Lancet/Infectious Diseases* 6 (2006): 303–312.

_____, and G. Dennis Shanks. "Deaths from Bacterial Pneumonia during 1918–1919 Influenza Pandemic." *Emerging Infectious Diseases* 14, no. 8 (August 2008): 1193–1199; http://www.ncbi.nlm.nih.gov/ Retrieved 16 December 2012.

Bulloch, William. *The History of Bacteriology.* New York: Dover Publications, 1938.

Burdick, Eugene, and Harvey Wheeler. *Fail-Safe.* 1962. Hopewell, NJ: The Ecco Press, 1999.

Burkhardt, Barbara. "Interview with William Maxwell." In *William Maxwell: A Literary Life.* By Barbara Burkhardt. Urbana: The Univ. of Chicago Press, 2005. 19–22.

Burnet, F. M. "Influenza Virus on the Developing Egg: I. Changes Associated with the Development of an Egg-Passage Strain of Virus." *British Journal of Experimental Pathology* 17, no. 4 (2 June 1936): 282–294; http://www.ncbi.nlm.nih.gov/ Retrieved 7 January 2012.

Butler, Declan. "Researchers Defend Benefits of Mutant Flu Research." *Nature/News & Comment: Q&A.* 26 January 2012; http://www.nature.com/ Retrieved 28 March 2012.

Byerly, Carol R. *Fever of War: The Influenza Pandemic in the U.S. Army during World War I.* New York: New York Univ. Press, 2005.

_____. "The U.S. Military and the Influenza Pandemic of 1918–1919." *Public Health Reports* 125, supp. 3 (2010): 82–91; http://www.ncbi.nlm.nih.gov/ Retrieved 23 September 2012.

Byrne, Joseph P. "Flu Pandemics Past and Present: *Cordon Sanitaire.*" ABC-CLIO Schools; http://www.historyandtheheadlines.abc-clio.com/ Retrieved 28 May 2012.

_____. "Flu Pandemics Past and Present: Influenza Pandemic, 1889–1890." ABC-CLIO Schools; http://www.historyandtheheadlines.abc-clio.com/ Retrieved 22 July 2012.

_____. "Flu Pandemics Past and Present: Influenza Pandemic, 1918–1919." ABC-CLIO Schools; http://www.historyandtheheadlines.abc-clio,com / Retrieved 26 May 2012.

Calderon, Fernando. "The Influence of Influenza on Menstruation, Pregnancy and Puerperium." *The Journal of the American Medical Association* 73, no. 13 (27 September 1919): 982–983; www.Google.com/ Retrieved 26 July 2012.

"Caliphate." *Glossary of Islamic Terms. The Clarion Project*; *http://www.clarionproject.org/* Retrieved 13 December 2013.

Campbell, Neil A., Jane B. Reece et al. *Biology*. Edited by Beth Wilber. 8th ed. San Francisco: Pearson/Benjamin Cummings, 2008.

Camus, Albert. *The Plague*. Translated by Stuart Gilbert. New York: The Modern Library, 1947.

Caperton, William B. "Personal Account by Rear Admiral William B. Caperton of the 1918 Influenza on Armored Cruiser No. 4, USS *Pittsburgh*, at Rio de Janeiro, Brazil." *The Navy Department Library/Naval Historical Center*; http://www.history.navy.mil / Retrieved 8 August 2011.

Carus, W. Seth. "Bioterrorism and Biocrimes: The Illicit Use of Biological Agents since 1900." *Center for Counterproliferation Research/National Defense University*. August 1998; www.ndu.edu/ Retrieved 12 June 2012.

Carvajal, Doreen. "Scientist in Bird Flu Study Says He is Not Convinced Censorship is Safeguard." *The New York Times/National*. 22 December 2011, A26.

Case, John. *The First Horseman*. New York: Ballantine Books, 1998.

Cather, Willa S. *A Calendar of the Letters of Willa Cather*. Edited by Janis P. Stout. Lincoln, NE: The Univ. of Nebraska Press, 2002.

_____. *One of Ours*. Lexington, KY: Cassia Press, 1922.

Cello, J., A. V. Paul, and Paul G. Thomas. "Dangerous for Ferrets: Lethal for Humans?" *BioMedCentral Biology/Comment* 10, no. 10 (2012); http://wwwbiomedcentral.com/ Retrieved 2 April 2012.

Centers for Disease Control and Prevention. "How the Flu Virus Can Change: 'Drift' and 'Shift.'" Seasonal Influenza (Flu); http://www.cdc.gov/ Retrieved 12 November 2013.

_____. *Influenza Playbook* (CDC); http://cdc.gov./story / Retrieved 18 September 2013.

"Chamberland, Charles." *Repères chronologiques*; http://pasteur.fr/infosci/archives/ Retrieved 11 November 2013.

Charon, Rita. *Honoring the Stories of Illness*. New York: Oxford Univ. Press, 2006.

_____. "Medical Interpretation: Implications of Literary Theory of Narrative for Clinical Work." *Journal of Narrative and Life History* 3, no. 1 (1993): 79–97.

_____. "Medicine, the Novel, and the Passage of Time." *Annals of Internal Medicine* 132 (2000): 63–68.

_____. "Narrative Medicine: Form, Function, and Ethics." *Annals of Internal Medicine* 134 (2001): 83–87.

_____. "Narrative Medicine: A Model for Empathy, Reflection, Profession, and Trust." *The Journal of the American Medical Association* 286, no. 15 (17 October 2001):1897–1902; www.jama.jamanetwork.com/ Retrieved 11 July 2012.

_____. "The Narrative Road to Empathy." *Empathy and the Practice of Medicine: Beyond Pills and the Scalpel*. Edited by H. Spiro, M.G.M. Curnen, E. Peschel, and D. St. James. New Haven, CT: Yale Univ. Press, 1993. 147–159.

_____, J. T. Banks, J. Connelly et al. "Literature and Medicine: Contributions to Clinical Practice." *Annals of Internal Medicine* 122 (1995): 599–606.

"Chinese Media Report Fourth Bird-flu Death." *CNN* Staff. 4 April 2013; http://www.cnn.com/ Retrieved 4 April 2013.

Christian, Henry A. "Incorrectness of the Diagnosis of Death from Influenza." *The Journal of the American Medical Association* 71, no. 19 (19 November 1918): 1565–1566; http://jama.ama-assn.org/ Retrieved 1 January 2012.

Clark, Liat. "Study: Engineered Airborne Hybrid Flu Contagious between Animals." *Scientific Method/Science & Exploration*. 5 May 2013; www.arstechnica.com/ Retrieved 19 May 2013.

Clinton, Bill. *My Life*. New York: Alfred A. Knopf, 2004.

Clodfelter, Michael, ed. *Warfare and Armed Conflicts—A Statistical Reference to Casualty and Other Figures, 1500–2000*. Jefferson, NC: McFarland, 2002.

Coffman, Edward M. *The War to End All Wars: The American Military Experience in World War I.* 1968. Lexington, KY: The Univ. of Kentucky Press, 1998.

Cohen, Stanley N., Annie C. Y. Chang, Herbert Boyer, and Robert B. Helling. "Construction of Biologically Functional Bacterial Plasmids in Vitro" [Abstract]. *Proceedings of the National Academy of Science. USA* 70 (1973): 3240–3244.

Cohn, Norman. *The Pursuit of the Millennium: Revolutionary Millenarians and Mystical Anarchists in the Middle Ages.* Rev. and expanded ed. New York: Oxford Univ. Press, 1977.

Collier, Richard. *The Plague of the Spanish Lady: The Influenza Pandemic of 1918–1919.* New York: Atheneum, 1974.

Conner, Lewis A. "The Symptomology and Complications of Influenza." *The Journal of the American Medical Association* 73, no. 5 (2 August 1919): 321–325; www.Google.com/ Retrieved 25 July 2012.

Contagion. Perf. Marion Cotillard, Matt Damon, and Laurence Fishburne. Dir. Steven Soderbergh. Participant Media, Imagination Abu Ghabi, Double Feature Films, 9 September 2011.

_____. *Internet Movie Database.* http://www.imdb.com.

_____. Official Website; http://www.contagionmovie.com.

"Contagion/*Contagium*." *Pocket Oxford Latin Dictionary.* Edited by James Morwood. New York: Oxford Univ. Press, 2005.

Convention on the Prohibition of the Development, Production and Stockpiling of Bacteriological (Biological) and Toxin Weapons and on Their Destruction [Biological Weapons Convention]. Signed at London, Moscow and Washington on 10 April 1972. Entered into force on 26 March 1975; http://www.opbw.org/ Retrieved 16 August 2011.

Cook, Kay. "Illness and Life Writing." *Encyclopedia of Life Writing: Autobiographical and Biographical Forms.* Edited by Margaretta Jolly. 2 vols. London: Fitzroy Dearborn, 2001. Vol. 1, A-K, 457–458.

Cook, Robin. *Vector.* 1999. New York: Berkley Books, 2000.

Cooper Cole, C. E. "Preliminary Report on the Influenza Pandemic at Bramshott in September-October 1918." Introductory note by R. D. Rudolf. *The British Medical Journal* 2 (23 November 1918): 566–568; *The Canadian Medical Association Journal* 9, no. 1 (January 1919): 41–48; http://www.ncbi.nlm.nih.gov/ Retrieved 28 December 2011.

Cornwell, Patricia. *Unnatural Exposure.* New York: Berkley Books, 1997.

Couser, G. Thomas. "The Body and Life Writing." *Encyclopedia of Life Writing: Autobiographical and Biographical Forms.* Vol. 1, A-K, 121–123.

_____. "Disability and Life Writing." *Encyclopedia of Life Writing: Autobiographical and Biographical Forms.* Vol. 1, A-K, 277–279.

_____. *Recovering Bodies: Illness, Disability, and Life Writing.* Madison: The Univ. of Wisconsin Press, 1997.

Crane, Leonard. "The 1918 Spanish Flu Pandemic and the Emerging Swine Flu Pandemic"; http://www.ninthday.com/ Retrieved 7 September 2012.

_____. *Ninth Day of Creation.* Los Angeles: Connection Books, 1998.

Cromwell, Judith Lissauer. *Florence Nightingale, Feminist.* Jefferson, NC: McFarland, 2013.

Crosby, Alfred W. *America's Forgotten Pandemic: The Influenza of 1918.* 2nd ed. 1976. New York: Cambridge Univ. Press, 2003.

_____. Review of *American Pandemic: The Lost Worlds of the 1918 Influenza Epidemic.* By Nancy K. Bristow. Oxford: Oxford Univ. Press, 2012. *Journal of the History of Medicine and Allied Sciences* 68, no. 1 (January 2013): 150–152; *www.jhmas.oxfordjournals.org/* Retrieved 2 January 2013.

Dark Winter: Bioterrorism Exercise Script, Andrews Air Force Base (June 22–23, 2001); http://www.upmchealthsecurity.org/ Retrieved 15 June 2013.

Davies, Peter. *The Devil's Flu: The World's Deadliest Influenza Epidemic and the Scientific Hunt for the Virus That Caused It.* New York: An Owl Book/Henry Holt, 2000.

DeKruif, Paul. *Microbe Hunters*. Introduction by F. Gonzalez-Crussi. 1926. San Diego: Harcourt Brace, 1996.

"Delirium: Symptoms." The Mayo Clinic; www.http://mayoclinic.com/ Retrieved 10 May 2013.

Della-Porta, Tony. "Laboratory Accidents and Breaches in Biosafety—They Do Occur!" *Microbiology Australia/In Focus* (May 2008): 62–65.

DeQuincey, Thomas. *Confessions of an English Opium Eater and Other Writings*. Edited with a foreword by Aileen Ward. 1822. New York: Signet Classic/New American Library, 1966.

DiLouie, Craig. *The Thin White Line: A History of the 2012 Avian Flu Pandemic in Canada*. Calgary, Alberta, Canada: Future Shock Books, 2008.

Dochez, A. R., K. C. Mills, and Yale Kneeland, Jr. "Disease of the Upper Respiratory Tract: Problems Connected with the Etiology and Prophylaxis." *The Journal of the American Medical Association* 101, no. 19 (4 November 1933): 1441–1444; http://jama.jamanetwork.com/ Retrieved 3 June 2012.

_____. "Studies of the Etiology of Influenza." *Proceedings of the Society for Experimental Biology and Medicine*. New York, NY 30, no. 8 (May 1933): 1017–1022; *http://ebm.rsmjournals.com/* Retrieved 3 June 2012.

_____. "Studies on the Virus of Influenza" [Abstract]. *The Journal of Experimental Medicine* 63, no. 4 (1 April 1936): 581–598; http://jem.rupress.org/ Retrieved 23 February 2012.

Dochez, A. R., G. S. Shibley, and K. C. Mills. "Studies in the Common Cold. IV. Experimental Transmission of the Common Cold to Anthropoid Apes and Human Beings By Means of a Filterable Agent." *The Journal of Experimental Medicine* 52 (1930): 701–716.

Doherty, Peter C., and Paul G. Thomas. "Dangerous for Ferrets: Lethal for Humans?" Comment: *BioMed Central/Journal of Biology* 10, no. 10 (2012); http://www.biomedcentral.com/ Retrieved 2 April 2013.

Doležal, Joshua. "'Waste in a Great Enterprise': Influenza, Modernism, and *One of Ours*." *Literature and Medicine* 28, no. 1 (Spring 2009): 82–101; http://muse.jhu.edu/ Retrieved 19 June 2013.

Donald, David Herbert. *Look Homeward: A Life of Thomas Wolfe*. Boston: Little, Brown, 1987.

Donnelly, Pat. "Myla Goldberg Found Inspiration in the 1918 Flu Epidemic." *The Montreal Gazette*. 10 December 2005, H1.

Dudley, Sheldon P. "The Biology of Epidemic Influenza, Illustrated by Naval Experience." *Proceedings of the Royal Society of Medicine* 14 (1921) (War Section): 37–50; http://www.ncbi.nlm.nih.gov/ Retrieved 16 December 2012.

Duncan, Kirsty. *Hunting the 1918 Flu: One Scientist's Search for a Killer Virus*. Toronto: The University of Toronto Press, 2003.

_____. "Biosafety at the Top of the World: Unearthing the Secrets of Spanish Flu." 2007; www.phaenex.uwindsor.ca/ Retrieved 11 December 2011.

Eagan, Sean P. "From Spikes to Bombs: The Rise of Eco-Terrorism." *Studies in Conflict & Terrorism* 19 (1996): 1–18; www.tandfonline.com/ Retrieved 24 September 2012.

"Emergence of Avian Influenza A (H7N9) Virus Causing Severe Human Illness—China, February-April 2013." *Centers for Disease Control and Prevention /Morbidity and Mortality Weekly Report* 62 (1 May 2013): 1–6; http://www.cdc.gov/ Retrieved 4 May 2013.

Engelberg, Stephen, et al. "New Evidence Adds Doubt to FBI's Case Against Anthrax Suspect." *Propublica: Journalism in the Public Interest*. 10 October 2011; http://www.propublica.org/ Retrieved 22 December 2013.

Erkoreka, Anton. "Origins of the Spanish Influenza Pandemic (1918–1920) and Its Relation to the First World War." *Journal of Molecular and Genetic Medicine: An International Journal of Biomedical Research* 3, no. 2 (December 2009): 190–194; www.ncbi.nlm.nih.gov/ Retrieved 29 July 2012.

Erlanger, Steven. "France Confirms 2nd

Case of Virus Linked to SARS." *The New York Times/ International.* 14 May 2013, A9.

"The Etiology of Influenza." The Work of the Central Council of the British Medical Association. *The British Medical Journal* 2, no. 3019 (2 November 1918): 493–498; http://www.ncbi.nlm.nih.gov/ Retrieved 23 October 2013.

Eyler, John M. "The Fog of Research: Influenza Vaccine Trials during the 1918–1919 Pandemic" [Abstract]. *Journal of the History of Medicine and Allied Sciences* 64, no. 4 (2009): 401–428; http://jhmas.oxfordjournals.org/ Retrieved 14 June 2012.

_____. *Sir Arthur Newsholme and State Medicine, 1885–1935.* Cambridge Studies in the History of Medicine. 1997. Cambridge, UK: Cambridge Univ. Press, 2002.

_____. "The State of Science, Microbiology, and Vaccines circa 1918." *Public Health Reports: The Science of Influenza* 125, sup. 3 (2010): 27–36; www.ncbi.nlm.nih.gov/ Retrieved 6 April 2012.

Falls, Cyril. *Armageddon: 1918.* Philadelphia: J. B. Lippincott, 1964.

_____. *The Great War: 1914–1918.* New York: G. P. Putnam's Sons, 1959.

Fauci, Anthony S., and Francis S. Collins. "Benefits and Risks of Influenza Research: Lessons Learned." *Science Magazine / H5N1 Policy Forum* 336 (22 June 2012): 1522–1523; www.sciencemag.org/ Retrieved 2 April 2013.

Feng, Bree, and Denise Grady. "As Bird Flu Spreads to Taiwan, Governments Act to Prepare." *The New York Times.* 25 April 2013; www.nytimes.com/ Retrieved 20 June 2013.

Ferro, Marc. *The Great War: 1914–1918.* Translated by Nicole Stone. 1969. New York: Routledge & Kegan Paul, 1973.

Fisher, Jane A. *Envisioning Disease, Gender, and War: Women's Narratives of the 1918 Influenza Pandemic.* Balingstoke, UK: Palgrave Macmillan, 2012.

Foote, Horton. *Courtship, Valentine's Day, 1918: Three Plays from the Orphans' Home Cycle.* Introduction by Reynolds Price. New York: Grove Press, 1986.

Fouchier, Ron A. M., et al. "Characterization of a Novel Influenza A Virus Hemagglutinin Subtype (H16) Obtained from Black-Headed Gulls" [Abstract]. *Journal of Virology* 79, no. 5 (March 2005): 2814–2822; http://www.ncbi.nlm.nih.org/ Retrieved 11 November 2013.

Fox, Herbert. "Vaccines in Influenza." *The Journal of the American Medical Association* 71, no. 20 (16 November 1918): 1682; http://jama.ama-assn.org/ Retrieved 1 January 2012.

Francis, Thomas, Jr., and T. P. Magill. "The Antibody Response of Human Subjects Vaccinated with the Virus of Human Influenza. *The Journal of Experimental Medicine* 63, no. 1 (28 October 1936): 251–259; www.jem.rupress.org/ Retrieved 18 February 2012.

_____, and Richard E. Shope. "Neutralization Tests with Sera of Convalescent or Immunized Animals and the Viruses of Swine and Human Influenza" [Abstract]. *The Journal of Experimental Medicine* 63, no. 5 (1 May 1936): 645; www.jem.rupress.org/ Retrieved 23 February 2012.

Frank, Arthur W. *The Wounded Storyteller: Body, Illness, and Ethics.* Chicago: The Univ. of Chicago Press, 1995.

Freidel, Frank. *Over There: The Story of America's First Great Overseas Crusade.* Short Hills, NJ: Burford Books, 1964.

Frost, W. H. "The Epidemiology of Influenza." *The Journal of the American Medical Association* 73, no. 5 (2 August 1919): 313–318; www.Google.com/ Retrieved 25 July 2012.

Garrett, Laurie. *The Coming Plague: Newly Emerging Diseases in a World Out of Balance.* New York: Penguin, 1994.

Gensheimer, Kathleen F., Martin I. Meltzer, Alicia S. Postema, and Raymond A. Strikas. "Influenza Pandemic Preparedness." *Commentary/Emerging Infectious Diseases. Centers for Disease Control and Prevention* 9, no. 12 (December 2003); http://wwwnc.cdc.gov/ Retrieved 26 March 2012.

Gibson, H. Graeme, F. B. Bowman, and J. I. Connor. "A Filtrable Virus as the

Cause of the Early Stage of the Present Epidemic of Influenza." *The British Medical Journal* 2, no. 3024 (14 December 1918): 645–646; http://www.ncbi.nlm.nih.gov/ Retrieved 21 October 2013.

Gilbert, Martin. *The First World War: A Complete History*. New York: Henry Holt, 1994.

Gilmore, Leigh. "Trauma and Life Writing." *Encyclopedia of Life Writing*. Vol. 2, L-Z, 885–887.

Gladwell, Malcolm. "A Reporter at Large: The Dead Zone." *The New Yorker*. 29 September 1997, 52–64; http://www.gladwell.com/ Retrieved 18 May 2011.

"The Global Initiative on Sharing All Influenza Data"; http://www.gisaid.org.

Gold, Hal. *Unit 731 Testimony: Japan's Wartime Human Experimentation Program*. Boston: Tuttle Publishing, 1966.

Goldberg, Myla. *Wickett's Remedy*. New York: Doubleday, 2005.

"Goldberger, Joseph [1874–1929]." *The Great Pandemic: The United States in 1918–1919*; http://1918.pandemicflu.gov/ Retrieved 7 April 2012.

Goldleaf, Steven. *John O'Hara: A Study of the Short Fiction*. Twayne's Studies in Short Fiction, No. 76. Gen. eds., Gary Scharnhorst and Eric Haralson. New York: Twayne Publishers, 1999.

Goodpasture, Ernest W. "Bronchopneumonia Due to Hemolytic Streptococci Following Influenza." *The Journal of the American Medical Association* 72, no. 10 (January-June 1919): 724–726. Edited by George H. Simmons. Chicago: The American Medical Association, 1919; http://books.google.com/ Retrieved 28 May 2012.

Gordon, Mervyn H. "The Bacteriology of Influenza. I." *The British Medical Journal* 2 (19 August 1922): 289. Reprinted in *International Medical and Surgical Survey*. Edited by Henry O. Reik and F. J. Stockman. Vol. 4, no. 4. New York: The American Institute of Medicine, October 1922. Section 5d-273; p. 831.

Grady, Denise. "Bird Flu Studies to Be Published Despite Concern." *The New York Times*. 18 February 2012, A1, A3.

_____. "Genetically Altered Bird Flu Virus Not as Dangerous as Believed, Its Maker Asserts." *The New York Times*. 29 February 2012; www.nytimes.com/ 20 June 2012.

_____. "Scientists to Pause Research on Deadly Strain of Bird Flu." *The New York Times*. 20 January 2012; www.nytimes.com/ Retrieved 20 June 2013.

_____, and Donald G. McNeil, Jr. "Debate Persists on Deadly Flu Made Airborne." *The New York Times*. 27 December 2011, A1, A11.

Graves, Peter, and Peter Englund. *The Beauty and the Sorrow: An Intimate History of the First World War*. London: Profile Books, 2011.

Grayzel, Susan R. *Women and the First World War*. Seminar Studies in History. Harlow, UK: Pearson Education, 2002.

Grist, Roy. "A Letter from Camp Devens." *Influenza 1918: WGBH American Experience*; http://www.pbs.org/ Retrieved 23 September 2012.

Harder, Tim C., and Ortrud Werner. "Introduction: Avian Influenza." *Influenza Report*. Edited by Bernd Sebastian Kamps, Christian Hoffmann, and Wolfgang Preiser. 2006–2009; http://www.influenzareport.com/ Retrieved 28 April 2013.

Hardin, D. W. *Hidden and Imminent Dangers*. Seattle: Create Space, 2009.

Harmon, William, and Hugh Holman. *A Handbook to Literature*. 10th ed. Upper Saddle River, NJ: Pearson Prentice Hall, 2006.

Harris, Richard C. "Getting Claude 'Over There': Sources for Book Four of Cather's *One of Ours*." *Journal of Narrative Theory* 35, no. 2 (Summer 2005): 248–256; http://muse.jhu.edu/ Retrieved 18 December 2011.

Harris, Sheldon H. *Factories of Death: Japanese Biological Warfare, 1932–1945, and the American Cover-Up*. Rev. ed.. New York: Routledge, 2002.

Harrison, Charlotte. "Sepsis: Calming the Cytokine Storm." *Nature Reviews: Drug Discovery* 9 (May 2010): 330–331; www.Nature.com/ Retrieved 17 January 2013.

Hawkins, Anne Hunsaker. "Pathography:

patient narratives of illness." *Western Journal of Medicine* 17, no. 2 (August 1999): 127–129; www.ncbi.nlm.nih.gov/ Retrieved 12 January 2012.

_____. *Reconstructing Illness: Studies in Pathography*. West Lafayette, IN: Purdue Univ.Press, 1993.

Hays, J. N. *The Burdens of Disease: Epidemics and Human Response in Western History*. New Brunswick, New Jersey, and London: Rutgers University Press, 1998.

Henderson, D. A. "Bioterrorism as a Public Health Threat." *Emerging Infectious Diseases/Special Issue* 4, no. 3 (July-September 1998): 488–492; http://www.ncbi.nlm.nih.gov/ Retrieved 17 December 2013.

_____. *Smallpox: The Death of a Disease*. Foreword by Richard Preston. Amherst, NY: Prometheus Books, 2009.

Herfst, Sander, et al. "Airborne Transmission of Influenza A/H5N1 Virus Between Ferrets." *Science Magazine*, Vol. 336, no. 6088 (22 June 2012): 1534–1541; www.sciencemag.org/ Retrieved 7 December 2012.

Hilkin, Susanne, Matthias Bormuth, und Michael Schmidt-Degenhard. *Kunst und Krankheit: Studiern zur Pathographie*. Edieren bei Matthias Bormuth, Klaus Podoll, und Carsten Spitzer. Göttingen: Wallstein Verlag, 2007. 11–26.

Hochschild, Adam. *To End All Wars: A Story of Loyalty and Rebellion, 1914–1918*. Boston: Houghton Mifflin/Harcourt, 2011.

Holman, Hugh, William Harmon et al. *A Handbook to Literature*. 10th ed. Upper Saddle River, NJ: Pearson/Prentice Hall, 2006.

Homberger, Margaret. "Case Histories." *Encyclopedia of Life Writing*. Vol. I, A-K, 186–187.

Homer. *The Iliad*. Translated with an introduction by Richmond Lattimore. 1951. Chicago: The Univ. of Chicago Press, 1967.

Honigsbaum, Mark. *Living with Enza: The Forgotten Story of Britain and the Great Flu Pandemic of 1918*. Basingstoke, UK: Palgrave MacMillan, 2009.

Hovanec, Caroline. "Of Bodies, Families, and Communities: Refiguring the 1918 Influenza Pandemic." *Literature and Medicine* 29, no. 1 (Spring 2011): 161–181.

"How the Flu Virus Can Change: 'Drift' and 'Shift.'" *Centers for Disease Control and Prevention/ Seasonal Influenza (Flu)*. 8 February 2011; http://www.cdc.gov/ Retrieved 20 March 2013.

Howard, Michael. *The First World War*. New York: Oxford Univ. Press, 2002.

_____, and William Roger Louis, eds. *The Oxford History of the 20th Century*. New York: Oxford Univ. Press, 1998.

Hoyle, L. "The Structure of the Influenza Virus: The Relation between Biological Activity and Chemical Structure of Virus Fractions." *Journal of Hygiene* (London) 50, no. 2 (June 1952): 229–245.

Hugh-Jones, Martin E., Barbara Hatch Rosenberg, and Stuart Jacobsen. "The 2001 Attack Anthrax." *Journal of Bioterrorism & Biodefense/Review Article*. 2011; http://dx.doi.org/10.4172/2157-2526.S3-001/ Retrieved 9 September 2013.

"Hunt for Duck Feces." 18 March 2009; http://www.flutrackers.com/ Retrieved 11 November 2013.

Hunter, Kathryn M. *Doctors' Stories: The Narrative Structure of Medical Knowledge*. Princeton: Princeton Univ. Press, 1991.

_____. *How Doctors Think: Clinical Judgment and the Practice of Medicine*. New York: Oxford Univ. Press, 2006.

Husband, Joseph. *A Year in the Navy*. Boston: Houghton-Mifflin Company, 1919.

"Illness Narrative/Pathography." *Literature, Arts, Medicine Database, 1993–2012*. New York Univ.; http://litmed.med.nyu.edu/ Retrieved 18 May 2012.

Imai, Masaki, et al. "Experimental Adaptation of an Influenza H5 HA Confers Respiratory Droplet Transmission to a Reassortant H5 HA/H1N1 Virus in Ferrets." *Nature Magazine*. 2 May 2012;

www.nature.com/ Retrieved 17 January 2012.

"Influenza A (H5N1) Virus Monovalent, Adjuvanted VRBPAC Briefing Document." *Food & Drug Administration*; http://www.fda.gov/ Retrieved 19 December 2013.

Influenza Committee of the Advisory Board to the D[irectorate].G[eneral]. M[edical].S[ervice]., in France. "A Report on the Influenza Epidemic in the British Armies in France, 1918." *The British Medical Journal* 2, no. 3019 (9 November 1918): 505–509; http://www.ncbi.nlm.nih.gov/ Retrieved 21 October 2013.

"Influenza Epidemic Hits Camp Devens." *The New York Times*. 14 September 1918; www.query.nytimes.com/ Retrieved 21 June 2013.

"Influenza: Familiar, but not Friendly." *The Centers for Disease Control and Prevention/Pandemic Influenza*. 20 March 2002; http://www.cdc.gov/ Retrieved 14 October 2003.

"The Influenza Outbreak" [Editorial]. *The Journal of the American Medical Association* 71, no. 14 (5 October 1918): 1138; http://jama.ama-assn.org/ Retrieved 1 January 2012.

"Influenza Pandemics: How They Start, How They Spread, and Their Potential Impact." *Centers for Disease Control and Prevention/Pandemic Influenza*. 25 June 2001; http://www.cdc.gov/ Retrieved 14 October 2003.

Inglesby, Thomas V. "Anthrax: A Possible Case History." *Emerging Infectious Diseases/ Centers for Disease Control and Prevention* 5, no. 4 (1999); http://www.cdc.gov/ Retrieved 13 November 2003.

_____, Anita Cicero, and Donald A. Henderson. "The Risk of Engineering a HighlyTransmissibleH5N1 Virus." *Biosecurity and Bioterrorism* 10, no. 1 (1 November 2012): 151–152; http://www.upmc-biosecurity.org/ Retrieved 4 April 2013.

_____, Donald A. Henderson, John G. Bartlett et al. "Anthrax as a Biological Weapon: Medical and Public Health Management." *Journal of the American Medical Association* 281, no. 18 (12 May 1999): 1735–1745.

_____, Tara O'Toole, and Donald A. Henderson. "Preventing the Use of Biological Weapons: Improving Response Should Prevention Fail." *Clinical Infectious Diseases* 30 (2000): 926–929; http://cid.oxfordjournals.org/ Retrieved 23 April 2012.

"Interim Pre-pandemic Planning Guidance: Community Strategy for Pandemic Influenza Mitigation in the United States—Early Targeting, Layered Use of Nonpharaceutical Interventions." *The Centers for Disease Control and Prevention*; http://www.flu.gov/planning-preparedness/ Retrieved 2 December 2013.

International Committee on Taxonomy of Viruses. Virology Division-IUMS; http://www.ictvonline.org/ Retrieved 2 December 2013.

International Data Base. *United States Census*; http://www.census.gov/ Retrieved 6 November 2013.

"Isolation and Quarantine, Legal Authorities for." *Centers for Disease Control and Prevention*. 10 January 2012; http://www.cdc/ Retrieved 12 May 2012.

Ivins, Bruce E., et al. "Comparative Efficacy of Experimental Anthrax Vaccine Candidates Against Inhalation Anthrax in Rhesus Macaques." *Vaccine* 16, no. 11/12 (1998): 1141–1148; http://www.ncbi.nlm.nih.org/ Retrieved 14 August 2013.

_____. "Comparison of the Efficacy of Purified Protective Antigen and MDPH to Protect Non-human Primates from Inhalation Anthrax." *Proceedings of the International Workshop on Anthrax*. 19–21 September 1995. Winchester U.K. *Salisbury Medical Bulletin*. Special Supplement 87 (1996): 130.

_____. "Defining a Serological Correlate of Protection in Rabbits for a Recombinant Anthrax Vaccine." *Vaccine* 22, no. 34 (2 January 2004): 422–430; http://www.ncbi.nlm.nih.gov/ Retrieved 14 August 2013.

_____. "Efficacy of a Human Anthrax Vaccine in Guinea Pigs, Rabbits, and Rhesus Macaques Against Challenge by *Bacillus anthracis* of Diverse Geographical Origin." *Vaccine* 19 (2001): 3241–3247; http://www.vaccine.mil/ Retrieved 14 August 2013.

_____. "Efficacy of a Standard Human Anthrax Vaccine Against *Bacillus anthracis* Aerosol Spore Challenge in Rhesus Monkeys." *Proceedings of the International Workshop in Anthrax*. 19–21 September 1995. Winchester, U.K. *Salisbury Medical Bulletin*. Special Supplement 87 (1996): 125–126.

_____. "Efficacy of a Standard Human Anthrax Vaccine Against *Bacillus anthracis* Spore Challenge in Guinea Pigs." *Vaccine* 12, no. 10 (August 1994): 872–874; http://ncbi.nlm.nih.org/ Retrieved 14 August 2013.

_____. "Immunization Against Anthrax with Aromatic Compound-Dependent (Aro-) mutants of *Bacillus anthracis* and with Recombinant Strains of *Bacillus subtilis* that Produce Anthrax Protective Antigen." *Infection and Immunity* 58, no. 2 (February 1990): 303–308; http://www.ncbi.nlm.nih.gov/ Retrieved 14 August 2012.

_____. "In Vitro Correlate of Immunity in an Animal Model of Inhalational Anthrax." *Journal of Applied Microbiology* 87 (1999): 304.

_____. "In Vitro Correlate of Immunity in a Rabbit Model of Inhalational Anthrax." *Vaccine* 19, no. 32 (14 September 2001): 4768–4773; http://www.ncbi.nlm.nih.gov/ Retrieved 14 August 2013.

_____. "Passive Protection by Polyclonal Antibodies Against *Bacillus anthracis* Infection in Guinea Pigs." *Infection and Immunity* 65, no. 12 (December 1997):5171–5175; http://iai.asm.org/ Retrieved 14 August 2013.

_____. "Postexposure Prophylaxis Against Experimental Inhalation Anthrax." *Journal of Infectious Diseases* 167, no. 5 (1993): 1239–1242; http://jid.oxfordjournals.org/ Retrieved 14 August 2013.

Iwanowski, D. M. "On the Mosaic Disease of the Tobacco Plant." *Great Experiments in Biology*. Translated by Mordecai L. Gabriel. Edited by Mordecai L. Gabriel and Seymour Fogel. The Prentice-Hall Animal Science Series. Edited by H. Burr Steinbach. Englewood Cliffs, NJ: Prentice-Hall, 1955. 124–126.

Jackson, Sarah, et al. "Reassortment between Avian H5N1 and Human H3N2 Influenza Viruses in Ferrets: Public Health Risk Assessment." *Journal of Virology* 83, no. 16 (August 2009): 8131–8140; www.jvi.asm.org/ Retrieved 10 December 2012.

James, Reina. *This Time of Dying*. New York: St. Martin's Press, 2006.

Johnson, Niall P. *Britain and the 1918–1919 Influenza Pandemic: A Dark Epilogue*. Routledge Studies in the Social History of Medicine. New York: Routledge, 2006.

_____. "The Overshadowed Killer: Influenza in Britain in 1918–1919." *The Spanish Influenza Pandemic of 1918–1919: New Perspectives*, 132–155.

_____, and J. Mueller. "Updating the Accounts: Global Mortality of the 1918–1920 'Spanish' Influenza Pandemic." *Bulletin of the History of Medicine* 76, no. 1 (Spring 2002): 105–115; http://www.ncbi.nih.nlm.org/ Retrieved 29 July 2012.

Jordan, Edwin O. "Bacteriology of Influenza." *Journal of Infectious Diseases* [Chicago] 73, no. 2 (2 August 1919): 147–148; www.Google.com/ Retrieved 25 July 2012.

_____. *Epidemic Influenza: A Survey*. Chicago: The American Medical Association, 1927.

Kahn, Herman. *On Thermonuclear War*. 2nd ed. Princeton: Princeton Univ. Press, 1961.

Kalla, Daniel. *Pandemic: A Novel*. New York: A Tom Doherty Associates Book, 2005.

Kandun, I. N., et al., "Probable Person-to-Person Transmission of Avian Influenza (H5N1). *The New England Journal of Medicine* 355 (2005): 2186.

_____. "Three Indonesian Clusters of H5N1 Virus Infection in 2005" [Abstract]. *The New England Journal of Medicine* 355, no. 21 (23 November 2006): 2186–2194; www.ncbi.nlm.nih.gov/ Retrieved 10 December 2012.

Kausche, G. A., E. Pfankuch, and H. Ruska. "Die Sichtbarmaching von pflanzlichen Virus im Ubermikroskop." *Naturwissenschaften* 27 (1939): 292–299.

Keegan, J. J. "The Prevailing Pandemic of Influenza." *The Journal of the American Medical Association* 71, no. 13 (28 September 1918): 1051–1055; http://jama.ama-assn.org/ Retrieved 1 January 2012.

Keller, David R. "Deep Ecology." *Encyclopedia of Environmental Ethics and Philosophy*. Edited by J. Baird Callicott and Robert Frodeman. New York: Macmillan/Thomas Gale, 2008. 206–211; www.uky.edu/ Retrieved 17 September 2012.

Kelso, J. K., G. J. Milne, and H. Kelly. "Simulation Suggests that Rapid Activation of Social Distancing Can Arrest Epidemic Eevelopment Due to a Novel Strain of Influenza" [Abstract]. *BioMed Central/Public Health* 9 (29 April 2009): 117; http://www.ncbi.nlm.nih.gov/ Retrieved 26 May 2012.

Kendal, A.P., et al. "Antigenic Similarity of Influenza A (H1N1) Viruses from Epidemics in 1977–1978 to 'Scandanavian' Strains Isolated in Epidemics of 1950–1951." *Journal of Virology* 89 (1978): 632–636.

Kennedy, David M. *Over Here: The First World War and American Society*. 1980. New York: Oxford Univ. Press, 2004.

Kent, Susan K. *The Influenza Pandemic of 1918–1919*. Bedford Cultural Editions. New York: Bedford/St. Martin's Press, 2012.

Kilbourne, Edwin D. "Influenza Pandemics of the 20th Century." *Emerging Infectious Diseases. Centers for Disease Control and Prevention* 12, no. 1 (January 2006): 9–14; http://www.ncbi.nlm.nih.gov/ Retrieved 28 April 2013.

_____. "Introduction: A Virologist's Perspective on the 1918–1919 Pandemic." *The Spanish Influenza Pandemic of 1918–1919: New Perspectives*. Edited by David Killingray, Howard Phillips, John S. Oxford, and Terry Ranger. Introduction by Howard Phillips and David Killingray. Studies in the Social History of Medicine. New York: Routledge, 2003. 29–38.

King, Stephen. *The Stand*. 1978. New York: Doubleday, 1990.

Kirshner, Howard S. "Confusional States and Acute Memory Disorders." Edited by Michael Hoffmann. *Medscape Reference: Drugs, Diseases & Procedures*. 2 March 2010; http://emedicine.medscape.com/ Retrieved 7 August 2011.

Kitasato, Shibasaburo. "The Influenza Bacillus: II.—On the Influenza Bacillus and the Mode of Cultivating It." *The British Medical Journal* 1, no. 1620 (16 January 1892): 128; www.ncbi.nlm.nih.gov/ Retrieved 13 June 2012.

Klein, H. A. "The Treatment of 'Spanish Influenza.'" *The Journal of the American Medical Association* 71, no. 18 (2 November 1918): 1510; http://jama.ama-assn.org/ Retrieved 1 January 2012.

Kleinman, Arthur. *The Illness Narratives: Suffering, Healing, and the Human Condition*. New York: Basic Books, 1988.

Kobasa, Darwyn, et al. "Atypical Host Innate Immune Responses May Contribute to Lethality." *Nature: International Weekly Journal of Science* 445 (18 January 2007): 319–323.

Koch, Amanda M., and Burke K. Zimmerman. "Do Recent Scientific and Technological Advances Lower the Threshold for the Proliferation of Biological Weapons?" *The Nuclear Threat Initiative/Global Security Newswire*. 16 July 2009; www.nti.org/ Retrieved 4 September 2012.

Koch, Robert. "On Bacteriological Research" (1890). *Essays of Robert Koch*. 179–186.

_____."The Etiology of Tuberculosis [Koch's postulates] (1884)." *Milestones in Microbiology: 1546 to 1940*. Translated and edited by Thomas D. Brock. Historical introduction by Thomas D. Brock. Washington, D.C.: American Society for Microbiology, 1999. 116–118.

_____. "[Excerpts from] The Etiology of Tuberculosis" (1882). *Essays of Robert Koch*. Translated by K. Codell Carter. Contributions in Medical Studies, Number 20. New York: Greenwood Press, 1987. 129–150.

Koen, J. S. "A Practical Method for Field

Diagnoses of Swine Diseases." *The American Journal of Veterinary Medicine.* Edited by D. M. Campbell. Vol. 14. Chicago: The American Veterinary Publishing Company, September 1919. www.books.Google.com/ Retrieved 16 August 2012.

Koenig, Robert. *The Fourth Horseman: One Man's Mission to Wage the Great War in America.* New York: Public Affairs, 2006.

Kohn, George Childs, ed. *Encyclopedia of Plague and Pestilence from Ancient Times to the Present.* Foreword by Mary-Louise Scully. Rev ed. 1995. New York: Checkmark Books, 2001.

Kolata, Gina. *Flu: The Story of the Great Influenza Pandemic of 1918 and the Search for the Virus That Caused It.* New York: Simon & Schuster, 1999.

_____. "Lethal Virus Comes Out of Hiding." *The New York Times/Science.* 24 February 1998; http://www.nytimes.com/ Retrieved 8 March 2012.

Konkoly, Steven. *The Jakarta Pandemic: A Novel.* Charleston, SC: Booksurge, 2010.

Kuhn, Thomas S. *The Structure of Scientific Revolutions. International Encyclopedia of Unified Science: Foundations of the Unity of Science.* Vols. I-II of the *Encyclopedia.* Edited by Otto Neurath et al. Chicago: The University of Chicago Press, 1962.

Laden, Lisa. "We Heard the Bells: The Influenza of 1918" [Post-Production Audio Script]. *Centers for Medicaire & Medicaid Services/U. S. Department of Health and Human Services*; http://www.flu.gov/ Retrieved 7 May 2012.

Laidlaw, P. P. "Epidemic Influenza: A Virus Disease." *The Lancet* 225, no. 5828 (11 May 1935): 1118–1124.

Laqueur, Walter. "Postmodern Terrorism: New Rules for a New Game." *Foreign Affairs.* September/October 1996; http://www.foreignaffairs.com/ Retrieved 29 December 2013.

"Law Enforcement Pandemic Influenza Planning Checklist." *The Centers for Disease Control and Prevention*; http://www.flu.gov/ Retrieved 2 December 2013.

Leaming, James M., Spencer Adoff, and Thomas E. Terndrup. "Computer Simulation as a Tool to Enable Decision-Making in a Pandemic Influenza Response Scenario." *Western Journal of Emergency Medicine.* 2013; http://www.escholarship.org/ Retrieved 3 May 2013.

LeCount, E. R. "Disseminated Necrosis of the Pulmonary Capillaries in Influenza Pneumonia." *The Journal of the American Medical Association* 72 (1919): 1519–1520.

Lederberg, Joshua. "Biological Warfare and the Extinction of Man." *Stanford M. D.* 8, no. 4 (Fall 1969): 15–17. *The Joshua Lederberg Papers. Profiles in Science/National Library of Science*; http://profiles.nlm.nih.gov/ Retrieved 22 August 2012.

_____. "The Control of Chemical and Biological Weapons." *The Stanford Journal of International Studies* VII (Spring 1972): 22–44; http://profiles.nlm.nih.gov/ Retrieved 14 November 2011.

_____. "Emerging Infections: An Evolutionary Perspective." *Emerging Infectious Diseases. The Centers for Disease Control and Prevention* 4, no. 3 (July-September 1998); http://www.cdc.gov/ Retrieved 20 June 2003.

_____. "Infectious Disease and Biological Weapons: Prophylaxis and Mitigation." *Commentaries/Editorial. The Journal of the American Medical Association* 278, no. 5 (6 August 1997): 435–436.

_____. "Infectious Disease as an Evolutionary Paradigm." *Emerging Infectious Diseases/The Journal of the American Medical Association* 3, no. 4 (October–December 1997): 417–423.

_____. "Infectious History." The American Association for the Advancement of Science. 2000; http://www.univie.ac.at/ Retrieved 20 June 2003.

_____. "Pandemic as a Natural Evolutionary Phenomenon." *Social Research* 55, no. 3 (Autumn 1988): 343–349. *The Joshua Lederberg Papers. Profiles in Science/National Library of Science*; http://profiles.nlm.nih.gov/ Retrieved 23 August 2012.

Ledingham, J. C. G. "A Paper on Tissue Changes in Virus Diseases." *The British*

Medical Journal. 26 November 1932; www.ncbi.nlm.nih.gov/ Retrieved 16 August 2012.

Lee, Hermione. "Prone to Fancy" [Virginia Woolf's *On Being Ill*]." *The Guardian.* 2012; http://www.guardian.co.uk/ Retrieved 6 March 2012.

"Legacy of the Pandemic." *The Great Pandemic: The United States in 1918–1919*; www.flu.gov/ Retrieved 2 January 2013.

Lewis, Paul A., and R. E. Shope. "Swine Influenza: II. A Hemophilic Bacillus from the Respiratory Tract of Infected Swine. *The Journal of Experimental Medicine* 54, no. 3 (1 September 1931): 361–371; www.jem.rupress.org/ Retrieved 23 February 2012.

Lezzoni, Lynette. *Influenza, 1918: The Worst Pandemic in American History.* Foreword by David McCullough. New York: TV Books, 1999.

Liddell Hart, B. H. *The Real War: 1914–1918.* Boston: Little, Brown, 1930.

Lindemann, Marilee, ed. *The Cambridge Companion to Willa Cather.* Cambridge: Cambridge Univ. Press, 2005. 146–158.

Lipowski, Z. J. "Delirium (Acute Confusional States)" [Abstract]. *The Journal of the American Medical Association* 258, no. 13 (1987): 1789–1792; http://jama.ama-assn.org/ Retrieved 6 September 2011.

Literature, Arts, and Medicine Database. New York University School of Medicine; www.litmed.nyu.edu.

Literature: An Introduction to Reading and Writing. Edited by Edgar V. Roberts, and Robert M. Zweig. 10th ed. Upper Saddle River, NJ: Longman/Pearson, 2012.

Literature and Medicine; http://www.press.jhu.edu.

Litzinger, Mary. "The 1918–1919 Influenza Pandemic as Covered in *The Journal of Immunology* from 1919 to 1921." *Newsletter* (July/August 2012): 12–13; http://www.aai.org/ Retrieved 1 November 2013.

Loeffler, Friedrich, and P. Frosch. "Report of the Commission for Research on the Foot-and-mouth Disease" (1898). Translated by Thomas D. Brock. *Milestones in Microbiology.* 149–52.

Longcope, Wakefield. "Survey of the Epidemic of Influenza in the American Expeditionary Forces." *The Journal of the American Medical Association* 73, no. 3 (19 July 1919): 189–191; www.Google.com/ Retrieved 25 July 2012.

Lopez, Enrique Hank. *Conversations with Katherine Anne Porter: Refugee from Indiana Creek.* Boston: Little, Brown, 1981.

Lurie, Nicole. "FDA Approval of Avian Flu Vaccine Moves Preparedness Forward." *U.S. Department of Health & Human Services/News.* 22 November 2013; http://www.hhs.gov/ Retrieved 19 December 2013.

Lutz, Ralph Haswell. *The German Revolution, 1918–1919.* New York: Cambridge Univ. Press, 1967.

MacDonald, Peter, and J. C. Lyth. "Incubation Period of Influenza." *The British Medical Journal* 2, no. 3018 (2 November 1918); www.ncbi.nlm.nih.gov/ Retrieved 20 June 2013.

MacShane, Frank. *The Life of John O'Hara.* New York: E. P. Dutton, 1980.

Madjid, Mohammad, Scott Lillibridge, Parsa Mirhaji, and Ward Cascells. "Influenza as a Bioweapon." *Journal of the Royal Society of Medicine* 96, no. 7 (July 2003): 345–346; http://jrsm.rsmjournals.com/ Retrieved 3 September 2012.

Magill, T. P., and Thomas Francis, Jr. "The Action of Immune Sera on Human Influenza Virus in Vitro." *The Journal of Experimental Medicine* 65, no. 6 (1 June 1937): 861–872; http://jem.rupress.org/ Retrieved 23 February 2012.

_____. "Studies with Human Influenza Virus Cultivated in Artificial Medium." *The Journal of Experimental Medicine* 63, no. 6 (1 June 1936): 803–811; http://jem.rupress.org/ Retrieved 23 February 2012.

Mahy, Brian W.J. *The Dictionary of Virology.* 4th ed. Burlington, Massuchusetts, and London: Academic Press, 2009.

"Maine CDC 2009 H1N1 Influenza Pandemic After-Action Summary." *Maine Center for Disease Control and Preven-*

tion: An Office of the Department of Health and Human Services. December 2010; www.maine.gov/ Retrieved 26 June 2012.

Maines, Taronna R., et al. "Lack of Transmission of H5N1 Avian-human Reassortant Influenza Viruses in a Ferret Model" [Abstract]. *Proceedings of the National Academy of Sciences of the United States of America* 103, no. 32 (8 August 2006): 12121–12126; www.pnas.org/ Retrieved 10 December 2012.

Markel, Howard, et al. "Nonpharmaceutical Influenza Mitigation Strategies, U.S. Communities, 1918–1919 Pandemic." *Emerging Infectious Diseases/The Centers for Disease Control and Prevention* 12, no. 12 (December 2006): 1961–1964; http://www.ncbi.nlm.nih.gov/ Retrieved 26 May 2012.

_____. "Nonpharmaceutical Interventions Implemented by U.S. Cities during the 1918–1919 Influenza Pandemic." *The Journal of the American Medical Association* 298, no. 6 (8 August 2007): 644–654; http://www.ncbi.nlm.nih.gov/ Retrieved 26 May 2012.

Marr, John S., and John Baldwin. *The Eleventh Plague*. New York: HarperPaperbacks, 1998.

Mason, Kenneth C. "*The Big Rock Candy Mountain*: The Consequences of a Delusory American Dream." *Great Plains Quarterly* 6 (Winter 1986): 34–43; http://digitalcommons.unl.edu/ Retrieved 20 June 2013.

Mathers, George. "Etiology of the Epidemic Acute Respiratory Infections Commonly Called Influenza." *The Journal of the American Medical Association* 48, no. 9 (1917): 678–680. Reprinted in *Proceedings of the Institute of Medicine of Chicago*. Vols. 1–2; 7 November 1916, 85–92. Chicago: The American Medical Association, 1917; www.google.com/ Retrieved 20 June 2013.

Maugham, W. Somerset. *The Painted Veil*. 1925. New York: Vintage Books, 2004.

Maxwell, William. *They Came Like Swallows*. 1937. New York: Vintage Books, 1964.

McCallum, W. G. "Pathological Anatomy of Pneumonia Associated with Influenza." *The Johns Hopkins Hospital Report* 20 (1921): 149.

McCarthy, Mary. *Memories of a Catholic Girlhood*. 1957. San Diego: A Harvest Book/ Harcourt, 1974.

McCoy, G. W. "Status of Prophylactic Vaccination Against Influenza." *The Journal of the American Medical Association* 73, no. 6 (9 August 1919): 401–405; www.Google.com/ Retrieved 25 July 2012.

McGuire, L. W., and W. R. Redden. "Treatment of Influenza Pneumonia by the Use of Convalescent Human Serum: Preliminary Report." *The Journal of the American Medical Association* 71, no. 16 (1918): 1311–1312; http://jama.ama-assn.org/ Retrieved 1 January 2012.

McLeod, Melissa A., et al. "Protective Effect of Maritime Quarantine in South Pacific Jurisdictions, 1918–1919 Influenza Pandemic" [Abstract]. *Dispatch/The Centers for Disease Control and Prevention* 14, no. 3 (March 2008); http://wwwnc.cdc.gov/ Retrieved 12 May 2012.

McNeil, Donald G., Jr., "Bird Flu Paper Is Published after Debate." *The New York Times/International*. 22 June 2012, A7.

_____. "New Tools to Hunt Viruses." *The New York Times/Science Times*. 28 May 2013, D1, D3.

_____. "Scientist Plays Down Danger of Flu Strain." *The New York Times/National*. 26 January 2012, A16.

_____. "Cases of Deadly Bird Flu [H7N9] Surge in China, Experts Say." *The New York Times/International*. 5 February 2014: A8.

McNeill, William H. *Plagues and Peoples*. Garden City, NY: Anchor Books, 1976.

The Merriam-Webster Dictionary. Editor in chief, Frederick C. Mish. Springfield, MA: Merriam-Webster, 2004.

Meselson, Matthew, et al. "The Sverdlovsk Anthrax Outbreak of 1979." *Science* 266 (1994): 1202–1208; http://www.athrax.osd.mil/ Retrieved 22 July 2013.

Meyer, G. J. *A World Undone: The Story of the Great War, 1914 to 1918*. New York: Random House, 2007.

Miller, Judith, Stephen Engelberg, and

William Broad. *Germs: Biological Weapons and America's Secret War*. New York: Simon & Schuster, 2001.

Miller, Judith. "Mr. Bio-Defense, William C. Patrick, III: a Tribute." *City Journal*. 5 October 2010; http://www.city-journal.org/ Retrieved 12 December 2013.

Morens, David M., Kanta Subbarao, and Jeffery K. Taubenberger. "Engineering H5N1 Avian Influenza Viruses to Study Human Adaptation." *Nature Magazine/Perspectives* 486 (21 June 2012): 335–340; http://www.nature.com/ Retrieved 5 May 2013.

_____, Jeffery K. Taubenberger, and Anthony S. Fauci. "The Persistent Legacy of the 1918 Influenza Virus." *The New England Journal of Medicine/Perspective* 361 (16 July 2009): 225–229; http://www.nejm.org/ Retrieved 8 December 2011.

_____. "Predominant Role of Bacterial Pneumonia as a Cause of Death in Pandemic Influenza: Implications for Pandemic Influenza Preparedness" [Abstract]. *Journal of Infectious Diseases* 198, no. 7 (1 October 2008): 962–970; http://www.ncbi.nlm.nih.gov/ Retrieved 2 June 2011.

Mosier, John. *The Myth of the Great War: A New Military History of World War I*. New York: HarperCollins, 2001.

Mullen, Thomas. "Author's Note." *The Last Town on Earth*. 389–392.

_____. "A Conversation with Thomas Mullen." Held by the *Readers' Circle*." *The Last Town on Earth*. 397–402.

_____. "An Interview with Thomas Mullen." Conducted by Nicola. *Edible Geography*. 6 October 2009; http://www.ediblegeography.com/ Retrieved 29 May 2012.

_____. *The Last Town on Earth: A Novel*. New York: Ballantine Books, 2007.

Murphy, Frederick A. "The Foundations of Medical and Veterinary Virology." *Discoverers and Discoveries, Inventors and Inventions, Developers and Technologies. The American Society for Microbiology*; http://forms.asm.org/ Retrieved 26 November 2012.

Naess, Arne. "The Shallow and the Deep, Long-Range Ecology Movement. A Summary." Introductory lecture at the 3rd World Future Research Conference, Bucharest, 3–10 September 1972. *Inquiry* 16 (1973): 95–100; www.ecology.eth.ch.edu/ Retrieved 17 September 2012.

Narrative Medicine [*Program*], Columbia University, College of Physicians and Surgeons; www.narrative.medicine.org.

National Strategy for Pandemic Influenza Implementation Plan / Homeland Security Council. May 2006; http://www.flu.gov/ Retrieved 17 May 2013.

Newman, George. *Chief Medical Officer's Introduction. Report on the Pandemic of Influenza, 1918*. (October 1920): iv-xxiii; http://influenza.sph.unimelb.edu.au/ Retrieved 23 April 2012.

Newsholme, Arthur. "Discussion of Influenza." *Proceedings of the Royal Society of Medicine/General Reports* 129 (1919): 1–18/ Delivered 13 November 1918; http://www.ncbi.nlm.nih.gov/ Retrieved 22 October 2013.

_____. "Introductory Remarks on Epidemic Catarrhs and Influenza." *The Lancet* 192, no. 4969 (13 November 1918): 689–693; www.thefreelibrary.com/ Retrieved 5 June 2013.

_____. *Public Health and Insurance*. Baltimore: The Johns Hopkins University Press, 1920.

_____. "Some Considerations on Tuberculosis." National Tuberculosis Association. National Transactions of the Sixteenth Annual Meeting, St. Louis, MO, 22, 23, and 24 April 1920. New York: National Tuberculosis Association, 1921. 483–489.

Nicolle, Charles, and Charles LeBailly. "Certain Experimental Ideas about the Infectious Agent of Influenza." *Comptes Rendus de l'Academie des Sciences* 167 (1918): 607–610.

Nicolson, Juliet. *The Great Silence, 1918–1920: Living in the Shadow of the Great War*. London: John Murray; New York: Grove, 2009.

"Nipah Virus." *World Health Organization/Media Centre*. Fact Sheet No. 262; July 2009; http://www.who.int/ Retrieved 7 May 2013.

Nishiura, Hiroshi, Nick Wilson, and Michael G. Baker. "Quarantine for Pandemic Influenza Control at the Borders of Small Island Nations." *BioMed Central/Infectious Diseases* 9 (2009):27; http://www.ncbi.nlm.nih.gov/ Retrieved 26 May 2012.

Nowell, Elizabeth. *Thomas Wolfe: A Biography*. Garden City, NY: Doubleday, 1960.

O'Brien, Sharon. "Willa Cather in the Country of the Ill." *The Cambridge Companion to Willa Cather*. Edited by Marilee Lindemann. Cambridge: Cambridge Univ. Press, 2005. 146–158.

"Observations on the Present Epidemic of So-Called Influenza in Europe" [Editorial]. *The Journal of the American Medical Association* 71, no. 19 (9 November 1918): 1580; http://jamanetwork.com/ Retrieved 19 November 2013.

O'Hara, John. "The Doctor's Son." *The Doctor's Son and Other Stories*. New York: Avon Books, 1935. 5–32.

Olitsky, Peter K., and Frederick L. Gates. "Experimental Study of the Nasopharyngeal Secretions from Influenza Patients." *The Journal of the American Medical Association* 74, no. 22 (1920): 1497–1499; http://jama.jamanetwork.com/ Retrieved 3 June 2012.

"Ongoing Influenza Defense Tactics." *Centers for Disease Control and Prevention/Pandemic Influenza*. 25 June 2001; http://www.cdc.gov/ Retrieved 14 October 2003.

Opie, E. L., et al. *Epidemic Respiratory Diseases: The Pneumonias and Other Infections of the Respiratory Tract Accompanying Influenza and Measles*. St. Louis: C. V. Mosby, 1921.

Orent, Wendy. "From a Bat, to a Pig, to You—Not Likely. *The Los Angeles Times/Op-Ed*. 25 September 2011; http://articles.latimes.com/ Retrieved 7 May 2013.

Osler, William. *The Principles and Practice of Medicine*. 4th ed. New York: D. Appleton, 1904; www.mcgovern.library.tmc.edu/ Retrieved 4 August 2012.

Osterholm, Michael T. "Preparing for the Next Epidemic." *The New England Journal of Medicine* 352, no. 18 (2005): 1839–1842.

_____, and John Schwartz. *Living Terrors: What America Needs to Know to Survive the Coming Bioterrorist Catastrophe*. New York: Delacorte Press, 2000.

O'Toole, Tara. "Smallpox: An Attack Scenario." *Centers for Disease Control and Prevention/Perspective* 5, no. 4 (August 1999); http://webcache,googleuser.com/ Retrieved 4 December 2011.

Outbreak. Perf. Dustin Hoffman, Rene Russo, Morgan Freeman. Dir. Wolfgang Petersen. Warner Brothers, 10 March 1995.

_____. *Internet Movie Database; http://www.imb.com/* Retrieved 10 June 2013.

Oxford, J. S. "The So-called Great Spanish Influenza Pandemic of 1918 May Have Originated in France in 1916." *Philosophical Transactions of the Royal Society: Biological Sciences* 356 (29 December 2001): 1857–1859; http://www.jstor.org/ Retrieved 9 December 2011.

_____, et al. "A Hypothesis: The Conjunction of Soldiers, Gas, Pigs, Ducks, Geese and Horses in Northern France during the Great War Provided the Conditions for the Emergence of the 'Spanish' Influenza Pandemic of 1918–1919." *Vaccine* 23, no. 7 (4 January 2005): 940–945; www.ncbi.nlm.nih.gov/ Retrieved 31 December 2012.

_____. "World War I May Have Allowed the Emergence of 'Spanish' Influenza." *The Lancet/Infectious Diseases. Origins of the Great Influenza Pandemic/ Historical Review* 2 (2002): 111–114; http://infection.thelancet.com/ Retrieved 9 December 2011.

The Oxford English Dictionary. 21 vols., supplement, and bibliography. Oxford: At the Clarendon Press, 1971.

Palese, Peter. "Don't Censor Life-saving Science." *Nature Magazine/Column: World View* 481, no. 115 (11 January 2012); http://www.nature.com/ Retrieved 4 April 2013.

_____, and Taia T. Wang. "Why Do Influenza Virus Subtypes Die Out? A Hypothesis." *mBio* 2, no. 5 (September/October 2011): 1–3; http://mbio.asm.org/ Retrieved 25 November 2013.

Palucka, Tim. "History of the Microscope:

Electron Microscopy." *History of Recent Science & Technology*. The Dibner Institute for the History of Science and Technology. 2001; www.authors.library.caltech.edu/ Retrieved 20 January 2013.

Pandemic Flu History; http://www.flu.gov/ Retrieved 11 January 2014.

"Pandemic Influenza/Ongoing Influenza Defense Tactics." *The Centers for Disease Control and Prevention*; www.cdc.gov/ Retrieved 14 October 2003.

"Pandemic Influenza/ Pandemics: How They Start, How They Spread, and Their Potential Impact." *The Centers for Disease Control and Prevention*; www.cdc.gov/ Retrieved 14 October 2003.

Pandemic Influenza Storybook; http://www.flu.gov/ Retrieved 11 January 2014.

"Pandemics and Pandemic Scares in the 20th Century/ Historical Overview." *The Centers for Disease Control and Prevention/Pandemic Influenza*. 25 June 2001; http://www.cdc.gov/ Retrieved 14 October 2003.

Park, David A. "Physics." *Encyclopedia of Time*. Edited by Samuel L. Macey. New York: Garland, 1994. 462–466.

Park, William H. "Bacteriology and Possibility of AntiInfluenza Vaccine as a Prophylactic." *New York Medical Journal* 108 (1918): 62.

_____. "Bacteriology of Recent Pandemic of Influenza and Complicating Infections." *The Journal of the American Medical Association* 73, no. 5 (2 August 1919): 318–321; www.google.com/ Retrieved 25 July 2012.

Parson, Robert P. *Trail to Light: A Biography of Joseph Goldberger*. Indianapolis: Bobbs-Merrill, 1943.

Paschall, Benjamin S. "Value of Vaccination Against Influenza." *The Journal of the American Medical Association* 71, no. 19 (9 November 1918): 1602; http://jama.ama-assn.org/ Retrieved 1 January 2012.

"Past Avian Influenza Outbreaks." *Centers for Disease Control and Prevention/ Avian* Influenza (Flu); www.cdc.gov/ Retrieved 21 June 2013.

Pasteur, Louis. "The Attenuation of the Causal Agent of Fowl Cholera" (1880). Translated by Thomas D. Brock. *Milestones in Microbiology*. 126–130.

_____. "On a Vaccine for Fowl Cholera and Anthrax" (1881). Translated by Thomas D. Brock. *Milestones in Microbiology*. 131.

_____. "Prevention of Rabies: A Method by Which the Development of Rabies after a Bite May Be Prevented (1885)." Translated by D. Berger. *Founders of Modern Medicine: Pasteur, Koch, Lister*. Edited by Elie Metschnikoff. New York: Walden, 1939. 379–387.

_____, and Louis Thuillier. *Correspondence of Pasteur & Thuillier, Concerning Anthrax and Swine Fever Vaccinations* [1881–1887]. Translated and edited by Robert M. Frank & Denise Wrotnowska. Preface by Louis Pasteur Vallery-Radot. University, AL: Univ. of Alabama Press, 1968.

"pathography." *The Compact Edition of the Oxford English Dictionary. Complete Text Reproduced Micrographically*. 2 vols. Oxford: At the Clarendon Press, 1971. I., 2049.

"pathography." *The Merriam-Webster Dictionary*. Edited by Frederick C. Mish. Springfield, MA: Merriam-Webster, 2004. 528.

Patterson, S. W. "The Pathology of Influenza in France." Introduction by Geoffrey Miller. *The Medical Journal of Australia* 1, no. 10 (6 March 1920): 201–210; www.authorsden.com/ Retrieved 19 February 2013.

"Pause on Avian Flu Transmission Research." *Sciencexpress/Letter*. 20 January 2012; www.sciencexpress.org/ Retrieved 28 March 2012.

Pavia, Andrew T. "Laboratory Creation of a Highly Transmissible H5N1 Influenza Virus: Balancing the Substantial Risks and Real Benefits." *Annals of Internal Medicine* 156 (2012): 463–465; www.annals.org/ Retrieved 2 April 2013.

Pettit, Dorothy A. *A Cruel Wind: Pandemic Flu in America, 1918–1920*. Edited by R. Neil Scott. Murfreesboro, TN: Timberlane Books, 2008.

Pfankuch, E., and G. A. Kausche. "Isolierung und ubermikroskopisiche Abbildung eines Bakteriophages." *Naturwissenschaften* 28 (1940): 46.

Pfeiffer, Richard. "The Influenza Bacillus: I.—Preliminary Communication on the Exciting Causes of Influenza. *The British Medical Journal* 1, no. 1620 (16 January 1892): 128; www.ncbi.nlm.nih.gov/ Retrieved 13 June 2012.

"A Piece of My Mind." *The Journal of the American Medical Association*. 1998- ; http://jama.jamanetwork.org.

Pocket Oxford Latin Dictionary. Edited and preface by James Morwood. 1994. New York: Oxford Univ. Press, 2005.

Population Reference Bureau; www.prb.gov/ Retrieved 4 July 2013.

Porter, Katherine Anne. *Pale Horse, Pale Rider: Three Short Novels*. 1936. New York: Harcourt Brace, 1990.

Potter, Polyxeni. "*This Time of Dying*, by Reina James" [Book Review]. *Emerging Infectious Diseases/Centers for Disease Control and Prevention* 14, no. 2 (February 2008): 358; http://www.ncbi.nlm.nih.gov/ Retrieved 18 April 2012.

"Preparing for the Next Pandemic." *The Centers for Disease Control and Prevention/National Vaccine Program; www.cdc.gov/* Retrieved 20 October 2003.

Preston, Richard. *The Cobra Event*. New York: Ballantine Books, 1997.

_____. *The Demon in the Freezer: A True Story*. New York: Random House, 2002.

_____. Foreword to *Smallpox: The Death of a Disease*. By D. A. Henderson. Amherst, NY: Prometheus Books, 2009. 11–18.

_____. *The Hot Zone: A Terrifying True Story*. New York: Anchor Books, 1994.

_____. *Panic in Level 4: Cannibals, Killer Viruses, and Other Journeys to the Edge of Science*. New York: Random House 2008.

_____. "The Reality behind *The Cobra Event*." In *The Cobra Event*. 419–422.

Program in Narrative Medicine. Columbia University, College of Physicians & Surgeons; www.narrativemedicine.org.

Program in Narrative Medicine. The University of California; www.ucmedicalhumanitiespress.com.

"Protocol for the Prohibition of the Use of Ashyxiating, Poisonous or Other Gases, and of Bacteriological Methods of Warfare. Geneva, 17 June 1925." *International Humanitarian Law—Treaties & Documents*; http://www.icrc.org/ Retrieved 18 August 2011.

"Public Health Threat of Highly Pathogenic Avian Influenza A (H5N1) Virus." *The Centers for Disease Control and Prevention;* www.cdc.gov/ Retrieved 4 May 2013.

"Quarantine & Inspection." *Public Health Service Act*. U.S. Department of Health & Human Services/U.S. Food & Drug Administration. Part G.: paragraphs 264–272; *http://www.fda.gov/* Retrieved 20 January 2014.

"Quarantine and Isolation in Influenza" [Editorial]." *The Journal of the American Medical Association* 71, no. 15 (12 October 1918): 1220; http://jamanetwork.com/ Retrieved 19 November 2013.

Rada, James, Jr. *October Mourning: A Novel of the 1918 Spanish Flu Pandemic*. Gettysberg, PA: Legacy, 2006.

Raup, David M. *Extinction: Bad Genes or Bad Luck?* Introduction by Stephen Jay Gould. New York: W. W. Norton, 1991.

"Recombinant DNA Research: Actions under the *NIH Guidelines for Research Involving Recombinant DNA Molecules (NIH Guidelines)*." *Department of Health and Human Services/National Institutes of Health*. Deputy Director, Lawrence A. Tabak. *Federal Register* 78, no. 35 (21 February 2013): 12074–12082; *pkisupport@gpo.gov/* Retrieved 11 April 2013.

Reed, Walter. "Yellow Fever." *Source Book of Medical History*. Compiled with notes by Logan Clendening. New York: Henry Schuman; New York: Dover, 1942. 479–484.

Reid, Ann H., T. G. Fanning, J. V. Hultin, and J. K. Taubenberger. "Origin and Evolution of the 1918 'Spanish' Influenza Virus Hemagglutinin." *Proceedings of the National Academy of the Sciences [of the United States of America]* 96 (1999): 1651–1656.

_____, and Jeffery K. Taubenberger. "The Origin of the 1918 Pandemic Influenza

Virus: A Continuing Enigma" [Abstract]. *Journal of General Virology* 84 (September 2003): 2285–2292; http://www.socgenmicrobial.org.uk/ Retrieved 5 December 2004.

Reid, Panthea. *Art and Affection: A Life of Virginia Woolf.* New York: Oxford Univ. Press, 1996.

Reimann, R. A. "An Acute Infection of the Respiratory Tract with Atypical Pneumonia: A Disease Probably Caused by a Filterable Virus." *The Journal of the American Medical Association* 3 (24 December 1938): 2377–2384.

"The Revelation to John." Introduction by Jean Pierre Ruiz. *The New Oxford Annotated Bible.* Edited by Michael D. Coogan et al. New York: Oxford Univ. Press, 2007. 420–449.

Richey, Mary B., Peter Palese, and Jerome L. Schulman. "Mapping of the Influenza Virus Genome, III. Identification of Genes Coding for Nucleoprotein, Membrane Protein, and Nonstructural Protein." *Journal of Virology* 20 (1976): 307–313.

Richter, Harvena. *Virginia Woolf: The Inward Journey.* Princeton, NJ: Princeton Univ. Press, 1970.

Rivers, Thomas M. "Recent Advances in the Study of Viruses and Viral Diseases." *The Journal of the American Medical Association* 18, no. 3 (18 July 1936): 206–210; http://jem.rupress.org/ Retrieved 23 February 2012.

_____. "Viruses and Koch's Postulates." *Journal of Bacteriology* 33, no. 1 (January 1937): 1–22; www.ncbi.nlm.nih.gov/ Retrieved 31 March 2013.

Roback, A. A. "P. J. Mobius [1853–1907]—The Originator of Pathography" [Abstract]. *History of Psychology and Psychiatry.* Secaucus, NJ: Citadel Press, 1961. xiii; APA PsycNET Direct; www.psychnet.apa.org/ Retrieved 12 January 2012.

Roberts, Edgar V., and Robert Zweig, eds. *Literature: An Introduction to Reading and Writing.* 10th ed. Boston: Longman/Pearson, 2012.

Robinson, C. R. "Koch's Postulates and the Modern Era in Virus Research." *Canadian Medical Association Journal* 79 (1 September 1958): 387–389; www.ncbi.nlm.nih.gov/ Retrieved 28 October 2012.

Robinson, Phyllis C. *Willa: The Life of Willa Cather.* Garden City, NY: Doubleday, 1983.

Robson, Stuart. *The First World War.* Seminar Series in History. Edited by Clive Emsley and George Martel. London: Longmans, 1998.

Roos, Robert. "Fouchier Study Reveals Changes Enabling Airborne Spread of H5N1." *Center for Infectious Disease Research & Policy.* 2012; http://www.cidrap.umn.edu/ Retrieved 7 December 2012.

Rosenau, Milton J. "Experiments to Determine Mode of Spread of Influenza." *The Journal of the American Medical Association* 73, no. 5 (2 August 1919): 311–313; www.Google.com/ Retrieved 25 July 2012.

_____, W. J. Keegan, and Joseph Goldberger. "Some Interesting Though Unsuccessful Attempts to Transmit Influenza Experimentally." *Hygienic Laboratory Bulletin. United States Public Health Reports* 34, no. 2 (10 January 1919): 33–36; http://www.jstor.org/ Retrieved 6 April 2012.

_____, W. J. Keegan, D. W. Richey, G. W. McCoy, J. Goldberger et al. "Experiments upon Volunteers to Determine the Cause and Mode of Spread of Influenza" [February and March 1919]. *Hygienic Laboratory Bulletin. United States Public Health Reports* 123 (1921): 54–99; http://www.ncbi.nlm.nih.gov/ Retrieved 25 June 2013.

Rosenow, E. C., and B. F. Sturdivant. "Studies in Influenza and Pneumonia: IV. Further Results of Prophylactic Inoculations." *The Journal of the American Medical Association* 73, no. 6 (9 August 1919): 396–401; www.Google.com/ Retrieved 25 July 2012.

Rosner, David. "Twentieth-Century Medicine." *The Columbia History of the Twentieth Century.* Edited by Richard W. Bulliet. New York: Columbia Univ. Press, 1998. 483–507.

Ross, Philip E. "Jurassic Virus?" *Scientific American* 269, no. 4 (October 1993): 28;

www.fulviofrisone.com/ Retrieved 9 September 2012.

Rous, Peyton. "A Sarcoma of the Fowl Transmissible by an Agent Separable from the Tumor Cells." *Journal of Experimental Medicine* 13, no. 4 (1 April 1911): 397–411; http://jem.rupress.org/ Retrieved 1 November 2013.

Rous, Peyton, and J. B. Murphy. "On the Causation of Filterable Agents of Three Distinct Chicken Tumors [Abstract]." *Journal of Experimental Medicine* 19, no. 1 (1 January 1914): 52–68; http://jem.rupress.org/ Retrieved 1 November 2013.

Royer, B. Franklin. "Precautions on the Part of Physicians to Avoid Influenza Infection" [Letter to the Editor]. *The Journal of the American Medical Association*71, no. 17 (26 October 1918):1431; http://jamanetwork.com/ Retrieved 19 November 2013.

Saey, Tina Hesman. "H5N1 influenza research moratorium ends." *ScienceNews: Magazine of the Society for Science & the Public* 183, no. 4 (23 January 2013): 17; http://www.sciencenews.org/ Retrieved 2 April 2013.

_____. "Second of Two Blocked Flu Papers Released." *ScienceNews: Magazine of the Society for Science & the Public* 182, no. 1 (14 July 2012); http://www.sciencenews.org/ Retrieved 7 December 2012.

Sagita, Dessy. "Health Warnings over New Strain of Avian Influenza." *The Jakarta Globe*. 28 December 2012; http://www.thejakartaglobe.com/ Retrieved 7 November 2013.

Schoch-Spana, Monica. "Bioterrorism: U.S. Public Health and a Secular Apocalypse." *Anthropology Today* 20, no. 5 (October 2004): 8–13.

_____. "Implications of Pandemic Influenza for Bioterrorism Response." *Clinical Infectious Diseases* 31, no. 6 (2000): 1409–1413; http://cid.oxfordjournals.org/ Retrieved 26 March 2012.

"Serums and Vaccines in Influenza" [Editorial]. *The Journal of the American Medical Association* 71, no. 17 (26 October 1918): 1408; http://jama.ama-assn.org/ Retrieved 1 January 2012.

Shane, Scott. "Panel of Psychiatrists Backs F.B.I.'s Finding That Scientist Sent Anthrax Letters." *The New York Times/National*. 24 March 2011, A19.

Shanks, G. Dennis, and John F. Brundage. "Deaths from Bacterial Pneumonia during the 1918–1919 Influenza Pandemic." *Emerging Infectious Diseases* 14, no. 8 (August 2008): 1193–1199; www.ncbi.nlm.nih.gov/ Retrieved 10 December 2012.

_____. "Pathogenic Responses among Young Adults during the 1918 Influenza Pandemic" [Abstract]. *Emerging Infectious Diseases* 18, no. 2 (February 2012): 201–207.

Shanks, G. Dennis, et al. "Determinants of Mortality in Naval Units during the 1918–1919 Influenza Pandemic." *The Lancet/Infectious Diseases* 11 (2011): 793–799.

_____. "Low but Highly Variable Mortality among Nurses and Physicians during the Influenza Pandemic of 1918–1919." *Influenza and Other Respiratory Viruses Journal* 5, no. 3 (2011): 213–219. *Medscape/Multispeciality*; http://www.medscape.com/ Retrieved 22 October2013.

"Shar'ia." *Glossary of Islamic Terms*. The Clarion Project; http://www.clarionproject.org/ Retrieved 13 December 2013.

Sheng, Zong-Mei, et al. "Autopsy Series of 68 Cases Dying before and during the 1918 Influenza Pandemic" [Abstract]. *Proceedings of the National Academy of Sciences* 108, no. 39 (27 September 2011): 16416–16421; http://www.pnas.org/ Retrieved 10 December 2011.

Sherestha, Sourya, et al. "Identifying the Interaction between Influenza and Pneumococcal Pneumonia Using Incidence Data." *Science Translational Medicine* 15, no. 191 (26 June 2013): 191ra84; http://stm.sciencemag.org/ Retrieved 7 October 2013.

Shooter, R. A., et al. *Report of the Investigation into the Cause of the 1978 Birmingham Smallpox Occurrence*. Ordered by the House of Commons to be Printed 22 July 1980. Foreword by Patrick Jenkin. The Secretary of State for Social Services. London: Her Majesty's Stationary Office, 1980; http://www.ncbi.nlm.nih.gov/ Retrieved 28 July 2013.

Shope, Richard E. "Immunization Experiments with Swine Influenza Virus" [Abstract] *The Journal of Experimental Medicine* 64, no. 1 (1 July 1936): 47–61; http://jem.rupress.org/ Retrieved 23 February 2012.

_____. "Immunological Relationship between the Swine and Human Influenza Viruses in Swine" *The Journal of Experimental Medicine* 66, no. 2 (26 April 1937): 151–168; http://jem.rupress.org/ Retrieved 18 February 2013.

_____. "The Incidence of Neutralizing Antibodies for Swine Influenza Virus in the Sera of Human Beings of Different Ages" [Abstract]. *The Journal of Experimental Medicine* 63, no. 5 (1 May 1936): 669–684; http://jem.rupress.org/ Retrieved 23 February 2013.

_____. "The Infection of Ferrets with Swine Influenza Virus." *The Journal of Experimental Medicine* 60, no. 1 (30 June 1934): 49–61; www.ncbi.nlm.nih.gov/ Retrieved 20 June 2013.

_____. "The Infection of Mice with Swine Influenza Virus." *The Journal of Experimental Medicine* 62, no. 4 (30 September 1935): 561–572; www.ncbi.nlm.nih.com/ Retrieved 20 June 2013.

_____. "Influenza: History, Epidemiology, and Speculation." *The R. E. Dyer Lecture. Public Health Reports* 73, no. 2 (February 1958): 165–179; www.ncbi.nlm.nih.org/ Retrieved 16 August 2012.

_____. "Porcine Contagious Pleuropneumonia: 1. Experimental Transmission, Etiology, and Pathology" [Abstract]. *The Journal of Experimental Medicine* 119, no. 3 (29 February 1964): 357–368; http://jem.rupress.org/ Retrieved 20 June 2013.

_____. "Serological Evidence for the Occurrence of Infection with Human Influenza Virus in Swine." *The Journal of Experimental Medicine* 67, no. 5 (1 May 1938): 739–748; http://jem.rupress.org/ Retrieved 20 June 2013.

_____. "Studies on Immunity to Swine Influenza" [Abstract]. *The Journal of Experimental Medicine* 56, no. 4 (30 September 1932): 575–585; http://jem.rupress.org/ Retrieved 23 February 2012.

_____."Swine Influenza: I. Experimental Transmission and Pathology" [Abstract]. *The Journal of Experimental Medicine* 54, no. 3 (1 September 1931): 349; http://jem.rupress.org/ Retrieved 23 February 2012.

_____. "Swine Influenza: III. Filtration Experiments and Etiology" [Abstract]. *The Journal of Experimental Medicine* 54, no. 3 (6 May 1931): 373–385; http://www.ncbi.nlm.nih.gov/ Retrieved 17 February 2012.

_____. "Swine Influenza: V. Studies on Contagion." *The Journal of Experimental Medicine* 59, no. 2 (31 January 1934): 201–211; www.ncbi.nlm.nih.gov/ Retrieved 20 June 2013.

Shope, Richard E., and Thomas Francis, Jr. "The Susceptibility of Swine to the Virus of Human Influenza." *The Journal of Experimental Medicine* 65, no. 5 (1 November 1936): 791–801; http://jem.rupress.org/ Retrieved 23 February 2012.

Shortridge, Kennedy F. "Severe Acute Respiratory Syndrome and Influenza: Virus Incursions from Southern China." *The American Journal of Respiratory Care Medicine* 168 (2003): 1416–1420; www.atsjournals.org/ Retrieved 3 December 2012.

Sipress, David. *The Fatal Strain: On the Trail of Avian Flu and the Coming Pandemic.* New York: Viking, 2009.

Smith, Wilson, C. H. Andrewes, and P. P. Laidlaw. "A Virus Obtained from Influenza Patients." *The Lancet* 222, no. 5732 (8 July 1933): 66–69; www.cnic.org.cn./ Retrieved 7 January 2012.

Snodgrass, May Ellen. *World Epidemics: A Cultural Chronology of Disease from Prehistory to the Era of SARS.* Jefferson, NC: McFarland, 2003.

Snow, C. P. *The Two Cultures.* Introduction by Stefan Collini. 1959 and 1964. Cambridge: Cambridge Univ. Press, 1998.

Söderblom, Jason D. "Risk Analysis in Suicide Bioterrorism." *Jane's Homeland Security & Resilience Monitor* 3, no. 1 (February 2004); www.rusi.org/rjhm.janes.com/ Retrieved 15 July 2013.

"Some Interesting Though Unsuccessful Attempts to Transmit Influenza Experimentally." *Public Health Reports* 34, no. 2 (10 January 1919): 33–36; http://www.jstor.org/ Retrieved 6 April 2012.

Sonne, Paul. "Anxiety in the Time of Influenza: A Flu Literary Review." *Wall Street Journal*. 14 August 2009; http://online.wsj.com/ Retrieved 19 December 2011.

Sontag, Susan. *Illness as Metaphor and AIDS and Its Metaphors*. New York: Farrar Straus Giroux, 1978.

Soper, George A. "The Influenza Pneumonia Pandemic in the American Army Camps during September and October, 1918." *Science Magazine* 48, no. 1245 (8 November 1918): 51–456; http://www.sciencemag.org/ Retrieved 13 January 2012.

Sorrell, Erin M., et al. "Minimal Molecular Constraints for Respiratory Droplet Transmission of an Avian-human H9N2 Influenza A Virus" [Abstract]. *Proceedings of the National Academy of Sciences of the United States of America* 106, no. 18 (5 May 2009): 7565–7570; www.pnas.org/ Retrieved 10 December 2012.

"Source List and Detailed Death Tolls for the Primary Megadeaths of the Twentieth Century." *Necrometrics. Twentieth Century Atlas*; http://www.necrometrics.com/ Retrieved 6 November 2013.

Spooner, Leslie H., Andrew Watson Sellards, and John H. Wyman. "Serum Treatment of Type I Pneumonia." *The Journal of the American Medical Association* 71, no. 16 (19 October 1918): 1310–1311; http://jama.ama-assn.org/ Retrieved 1 January 2012.

Starr, Isaac. "Influenza in 1918: Recollections of the Epidemic in Philadelphia." *Annals of Internal Medicine/History of Medicine* 145 (2006): 138–140; www.annals.org/ Retrieved 31 December 2012.

Stegner, Wallace. *The Big Rock Candy Mountain*. 1938. New York: Penguin Books, 1943.

_____. *On a Darkling Plain*. New York: Harcourt, Brace, 1940.

Stewart, George R. *Earth Abides*. 1949. New York: Ballantine Books, 2006.

Stokebury, James L. *A Short History of World War I*. New York: HarperCollins, 1981.

Stoll, Henry F. "Value of Convalescent Blood and Serum in Treatment of Influenza Pneumonia." *The Journal of the American Medical Association* 73, no. 7 (16 August 1919): 478–482; www.Google.com/ Retrieved 26 July 2012.

Stumpf, Richard. *War, Mutiny and Revolution in the German Navy: The World War I Diary of Seaman Richard Stumpf*. Edited and translated with an introducttion by David Horn. New Brunswick, NJ: Rutgers Univ. Press, 1967.

Sweeney, Frederick. "Unpublished Diary [27 September 1918 to 18 April 1918]." Archives & Special Collections. The University of Nebraska/Lincoln Libraries; www.libxml1a.unl.edu/ Retrieved 9 December 2013.

Symmers, Douglas. "Pathologic Similarity between Pneumonia of Bubonic Plague and of Pandemic Influenza." *The Journal of the American Medical Association* 71, no. 18 (1918): 1482–1485; http://jama.ama-assn.org/ Retrieved 1 January 2012.

Taubenberger, Jeffery K. "Genetic Characterization of the 1918 'Spanish' Influenza Virus." *The Spanish Influenza Pandemic of 1918–1919: New Perspectives*. 2003. 39–47.

_____. "The Origin and Virulence of the 1918 'Spanish' Influenza Virus" [Abstract]. *Proceedings of the American Philosophical Society* 150, no. 1 (March 2006): 86–112; www.ncbi.nlm.nih.gov/ Retrieved 12 September 2012.

_____. "Seeking the 1918 Spanish Influenza Virus: Gene Sequences of the Virus from the 1918 Influenza Pandemic are Yielding Insights into its Origin but Little about Virulence." *ASM News/American Society for Microbiology* 65, no. 7 (July 1999); http://www.aswmusa.org/ Retrieved 20 October 2003.

_____, Johan V. Hultin, and David M. Morens. "Discovery and Characterization of the 1918 Pandemic Influenza Virus in Historical Context/Review." *Antiviral Therapy* 12 (2007): 581–591; www.intermed.press.com/ Retrieved 18 March 2012.

_____, and David M. Morens. "1918 Influenza: The Mother of All Pandemics."

Emerging Infectious Diseases/Centers for Disease Control and Prevention/ Perspective 12, no. 1 (1 January 2006): 15–22; www.cdc.gov/ Retrieved 22 May 2011.

_____, and David M. Morens. "The Pathology of Influenza Virus Infections." *Annual Review of Pathology* 3 (11 August 2008): 499–522; http://www.ncbi.nlm.nih.gov/ Retrieved 15 March 2013.

_____, A. H. Reid, T. A. Janczewski, and T. G. Fanning. "Integrating Historical, Clinical and Molecular Genetic Data in Order to Explain the Origin and Virulence of the 1918 Spanish Influenza Virus" [Abstract]. *Philosophical Transactions of the Royal Society/ (London) Section B: Biological Science* 356, no. 1416 (29 December 2001): 1829–1839; http://www.ncbi.nlm.nih.gov/ Retrieved 5 December 2004.

_____, et al. "Characterization of the 1918 Influenza Virus Polymerase Genes." *Nature Magazine/Letters* 437 (6 October 2005): 889–893; www.nature.com/ Retrieved 21 June 2013.

_____, et al. "Initial Genetic Characterization of the 1918 'Spanish' Influenza Virus." *Science Magazine.* March 1997; 275 (5307): 1792–1796; http://www.sciencemag.org/ Retrieved 11 December 2011.

"Taubenberger, Jeffery: An Interview with." Conducted by Leonard Crane in May 1998; http://www.ninthday.com/ Retrieved 7 September 2012.

Taylor, David, and Shon Lewis. "Neurological Emergencies: Delirium." *Journal of Neurology, Neurosurgery, and Psychiatry* 56 (1993): 742–751.

Thomas, Louisa. *Conscience: Two Soldiers, Two Pacifists, One Family—A Test of Will and Faith in World War I.* New York: Penguin, 2011.

"Timeline of World War I"; http://en.wikipedia.org/ Retrieved 4 December 2013.

Todd, Charles. *An Unmarked Grave.* New York: HarperCollins, 2012.

Todkill, Anne Marie. "The Island of the Ill" [Review of "On Being Ill," by Virginia Woolf]. *Canadian Medical Association Journal* 169, no. 4 (19 October 2003): 320; http://www.cmaj.ca/ Retrieved 6 March 2012.

Tomkins, Sandra M. "The Failure of Expertise: Public Health Policy in Britain during the 1918–19 Influenza Pandemic" [Abstract]. *Social History of Medicine* 5, no. 3 (1992): 435–454; http://shm.oxfordjournals.org/ Retrieved 3 May 2012.

Tortora, Gerard J., and Bryan Derrickson. *Introduction to the Human Body: The Essentials of Anatomy and Physiology.* 8th ed. New York: John Wiley and Sons, 2010.

"Transmission of Avian Influenza A Viruses between Animals and People." *The Centers for Disease Control and Prevention/Seasonal Influenza (Flu)*; www.cdc.gov/ Retrieved 9 January 2012.

Tuchman, Barbara. *The Guns of August.* Foreword by Robert K. Massie. Preface by B. Tuchman. 1962. New York: Presidio/Random House, 2004.

Tucker, Jonathan B. "Historical Trends Related to Bioterrorism: An Empirical Anaysis." *Emerging Infectious Diseases/Centers for Disease Control and Prevention* 5, no. 4 (July-August 1999); http://www.cdc.gov/ Retrieved 29 August 2011.

_____. "National Health and Medical Services Response to Incidents of Chemical and Biological Terrorism." *The Journal of the American Medical Association/Policy Perspectives* 278, no. 5 (6 August 1997): 362–368; www.jama.ama-assn.org/ Retrieved 30 August 2011.

_____. *Scourge: The Once and Future Threat of Smallpox.* New York: Grove Press, 2001.

Tumpey, T. M., et al. "Characterization of the Reconstructed 1918 Spanish Influenza Pandemic Virus" [Abstract]. *Science Magazine* 310, no. 5745 (2005): 77–80.

Tuveson, Ernest. "Millenarianism." *Dictionary of the History of Ideas: Studies of Selected Pivotal Ideas.* Edited by Philip P. Wiener. 6 vols. New York: Scribner's, 1973. Volume III, 223–225.

Ungchusak, K., et al. "Probable Person-to-person Transmission of Avian Influenza A (H5N1)." *The New England Journal of Medicine* 352, no. 4 (27 January 2005): 333–340; www.ncbi.nlm.nih.gov/ Retrieved 10 December 2012.

United States Government Policy for Oversight of Life Sciences Dual Use Research of Concern [DURC]; www.oba.od.nih.gov/ Retrieved 4 April 2013.

"Unrest in Germany Naval Mutiny at Kiel." *The Mercury* (Hobart, Tasmania: 1860–1954) 11 November 1918, 4–5; http://nla.gov.au/nla.news-article/ Retrieved 5 December 2013.

Van Hartesveldt, Fred R. "The Doctors and the 'Flu': The British Medical Profession's Response to the Influenza Pandemic of 1918–1919." *International Social Science Review.* Spring-Summer 2010; http://findarticles.com/ Retrieved 1 May 2012.

_____. *The 1918–1919 Pandemic of Influenza: The Urban Experience in the Western World.* New York: The Edwin Mellen Press, 1993.

Van Helvoort, T. "A Bacteriological Paradigm in Influenza Research in the First Half of the Twentieth Century [Abstract]." *History and Philosophy of the Life Sciences* 15, no. 1 (1993): 3–21; http://www.ncbi.nlm.nih.gov/ Retrieved 6 November 2013.

Vaughan, Victor Clarence. *A Doctor's Memories: An Autobiography by Victor Clarence Vaughan.* Indianapolis: Bobbs-Merrill, 1962; www.vaughan.org/ Retrieved 1 January 2013.

Virus Taxonomy: Classification and Nomenclature of Viruses. Ninth Report of the International Committee on Taxonomy of Viruses. Edited by A. M. Q. King et al. San Diego: Elsevier Academic Press, 2012.

Voigt, Ellen Bryant. *Kyrie: Poems.* New York: W. W. Norton, 1995.

Von Magnus, Preben. "The Influenza Virus: Its Morphology, Immunology, and Kinetics of Multiplication." *Bulletin of the World Health Organization* 8, no. 5–6 (1953): 647–660; http://www.ncbi.nlm.nih.org/ Retrieved 23 November 2012.

Wald, Priscilla. *Contagious: Cultures, Carriers, and the Outbreak Narrative.* Durham: Duke Univ. Press, 2008.

Walker, O. J. "Pathology of Influenza-Pneumonia." *The Journal of Laboratory & Clinical Medicine* 5 (1919): 154.

Wang, H., et al. "Probable Limited Person-to-person Transmission of Highly Pathogenic Avian Influenza A (H5N1) Virus in China." *The Lancet* 371, no. 9622 (26 April 2008): 1427–1434; www.ncbi.nlm.nih.gov/ Retrieved 10 December 2012.

Waterson, A. P., and Elise Wilkinson. *An Introduction to the History of Virology.* New York: Cambridge Univ. Press, 1978.

Watson, John T., Michelle Gayer, Maire A. Connolly. "Epidemics after Natural Disasters." *Emerging Infectious Diseases* 13, no. 1 (January 2007): 1–5; http://www.ncbi.nlm.nih.gov/ Retrieved 26 January 2014.

Webster, R. G., et al. "Evolution and Ecology of Influenza A Viruses" [Abstract]. *Microbiology Review* 56, no. 1 (March 1992): 152–179; www.ncbi.nlm.nih.gov/ Retrieved 18 July 2012.

Webster, Robert G., and Elizabeth Jane Walker. "Influenza: The World is Teetering on the Edge of a Pandemic that Could Kill a Large Fraction of the Human Population." *American Scientist* 91 (March-April 2003): 122–129; http://www.voh.chem.ucla.edu/ Retrieved 9 July 2012.

Webster's Seventh New Collegiate Dictionary. Editor in chief, Philip B. Gove. Preface by Philip B. Gove. Springfield, MA: G & C. Merriam, 1971. 618.

Whitelaw, T. H. "The Practical Aspects of Quarantine for Influenza." *The Canadian Medical Journal* 9, no. 12 (1919): 1070–1074; www.ncbi.nlm.nih.gov/ Retrieved 27 May 2012.

Wilford, John Noble. "Quest for Frozen Pandemic Virus Yields Mixed Results." *The New York Times/Science.* 8 September 1998; http://www.nytimes.com/ Retrieved 11 December 2011.

Wilkinson, Lise. "The Development of the Virus Concept as Reflected in Corpora of Studies of Individual Pathogens: I. Beginnings at the Turn of the Century."

Medical History 18 (1974): 211–221; http://www.ncbi.nlm.nih.gov/ Retrieved 21 January 2012.

_____. "The Development of the Virus Concept as Reflected in Corpora of Studies on Individual Pathogens: 3. Lessons of the Plant Viruses—Tobacco Mosaic Virus." *Medical History* 20, no. 2 (April 1976): 111–134; http://www.ncbi.nlm.nih.gov/ Retrieved 21 January 2012.

Wilkinson, Lise, and A. P.Waterson. "The Development of the Virus Concept as Reflected in Corpora of Studies on Individual Pathogens: 2. The Agent of Fowl Plague—A Model Virus?" *Medical History* 19, no. 1 (January 1975): 52–72; www.ncbi.nlm.nih.gov/ Retrieved 1 August 2012.

Willman, David. *The Mirage Man: Bruce Ivins, the Anthrax Attacks, and America's Rush to War*. New York: Random House, 2011.

Willmott, W. P. *World War I*. New York: Darling Kindersley, 2003.

Wines, Michael. "China Reports a Second Bird Flu Death in Less Than a Month." *The New York Times/International*. 23 January 2012, A6.

Winter, J. M. *The Experience of World War I*. New York: Oxford Univ. Press, 1989.

Winternitz. Milton C., et al. *The Pathology of Influenza*. New Haven: Yale University Press, 1920.

Wolbach, S. Burt. "Comments on the Pathology and Bacteriology of Fatal Influenza Cases, as Observed at Camp Devens, Massachusetts." *The Johns Hopkins Hospital Bulletin* XXX, no. 338 (1919): 104–109.

_____. "The Filterable Viruses: A Summary." *The Journal of Medical Research*. New Series XII 38, no. 1 (September 1912): 1–25. http://www.ncbi.nlm.nih.org/ Retrieved 6 November 2013.

_____, and Channing Frothingham. "The Influenza Epidemic at Camp Devens in 1918: A Study of the Pathology of Fatal Cases." Chicago: The American Medical Association, 1923. 1–30.

Wolfe, Thomas. *Look Homeward, Angel: A Story of the Buried Life*. Introduction by Maxwell Perkins. 1929. New York: Simon & Schuster, 1957.

Woodress, James. *Willa Cather: A Literary Life*. Lincoln, NE, 1987.

Woodruff, A. M., and E. W. Goodpasture. "The Susceptibility of Chorioallantoic Membrane of Chicken Embryos to Infection with the Fowl-pox Virus." *American Journal of Pathology* 7 (1931): 209–222.

Woolf, Virginia. "On Being Ill" (1926). *The Collected Essays of Virginia Woolf*. 4 vols. 1925. New York: Harcourt, Brace & World, 1967. Vol. 4, 193–203.

_____. *The Voyage Out*. 1915. San Diego: a Harvest/HBJ Book, 1948.

Worldometers: Real Time World Statistics. "World Population (11 December 2013)"; http://www.worldometers.info/ Retrieved 11 December 2013.

Yamanouchi, T., S. Sakakami, and S. Iwashima. "The Infecting Agent in Influenza, an Experimental Research." *The Lancet* 1 (1919): 971.

Yen, Hui-Ling. "Inefficient Transmission of H5N1 Influenza Viruses in a Ferret Contact Model" [Abstract]. *Journal of Virology* 81, no. 13 (April 2007): 6890–6898; www.jui.asm.org/ Retrieved 9 December 2013.

Zimmer, Carl. "Amateurs Are New Fear In Creating Mutant Virus." *The New York Times/Science Times*. 6 March 2012, D6.

Zimmer, Shanta M., and Donald S. Burke. "Historical Perspective—Emergence of Influenza A (H1N1)." *The New England Journal of Medicine/Current Concepts* 361, no. 3 (16 July 2009): 279–284; www.nejm.org/ Retrieved 11 August 2011.

Index

www.ingramcontent.com/pod-product-compliance
Lightning Source LLC
Chambersburg PA
CBHW032050300426
44116CB00007B/672
* 9 7 8 0 7 8 6 4 9 5 8 9 4 *